Bayesian Design in Clinical Trials

Bayesian Design in Clinical Trials

Editors

Paola Berchialla
Ileana Baldi

MDPI • Basel • Beijing • Wuhan • Barcelona • Belgrade • Manchester • Tokyo • Cluj • Tianjin

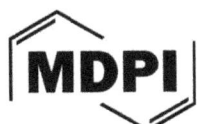

Editors
Paola Berchialla
University of Torino
Italy

Ileana Baldi
University of Padova
Italy

Editorial Office
MDPI
St. Alban-Anlage 66
4052 Basel, Switzerland

This is a reprint of articles from the Special Issue published online in the open access journal *International Journal of Environmental Research and Public Health* (ISSN 1660-4601) (available at: https://www.mdpi.com/journal/ijerph/special_issues/Bayesian_Design_Clinical_Trials?authAll=true).

For citation purposes, cite each article independently as indicated on the article page online and as indicated below:

LastName, A.A.; LastName, B.B.; LastName, C.C. Article Title. *Journal Name* **Year**, *Volume Number*, Page Range.

ISBN 978-3-0365-3333-9 (Hbk)
ISBN 978-3-0365-3334-6 (PDF)

© 2022 by the authors. Articles in this book are Open Access and distributed under the Creative Commons Attribution (CC BY) license, which allows users to download, copy and build upon published articles, as long as the author and publisher are properly credited, which ensures maximum dissemination and a wider impact of our publications.

The book as a whole is distributed by MDPI under the terms and conditions of the Creative Commons license CC BY-NC-ND.

Contents

About the Editors vii

Preface to "Bayesian Design in Clinical Trials" ix

Pavel Mozgunov, Rochelle Knight, Helen Barnett and Thomas Jaki
Using an Interaction Parameter in Model-Based Phase I Trials for Combination Treatments? A Simulation Study
Reprinted from: *Int. J. Environ. Res. Public Health* **2021**, *18*, 345, doi:10.3390/ijerph18010345 . . . **1**

Alessandra Giovagnoli
The Bayesian Design of Adaptive Clinical Trials
Reprinted from: *Int. J. Environ. Res. Public Health* **2021**, *18*, 530, doi:10.3390/ijerph18020530 . . . **21**

Fulvio De Santis, Stefania Gubbiotti
Sample Size Requirements for Calibrated Approximate Credible Intervals for Proportions in Clinical Trials
Reprinted from: *Int. J. Environ. Res. Public Health* **2021**, *18*, 595, doi:10.3390/ijerph18020595 . . . **37**

Miguel-Angel Negrín-Hernández, María Martel-Escobar and Francisco-José Vázquez-Polo
Bayesian Meta-Analysis for Binary Data and Prior Distribution on Models
Reprinted from: *Int. J. Environ. Res. Public Health* **2021**, *18*, 809, doi:10.3390/ijerph18020809 . . . **49**

Moreno Ursino and Nigel Stallard
Bayesian Approaches for Confirmatory Trials in Rare Diseases: Opportunities and Challenges
Reprinted from: *Int. J. Environ. Res. Public Health* **2021**, *18*, 1022, doi:10.3390/ijerph18031022 . . . **67**

Adrien Ollier, Sarah Zohar, Satoshi Morita and Moreno Ursino
Estimating Similarity of Dose–Response Relationships in Phase I Clinical Trials—Case Study in Bridging Data Package
Reprinted from: *Int. J. Environ. Res. Public Health* **2021**, *18*, 1639, doi:10.3390/ijerph18041639 . . . **77**

Danila Azzolina, Paola Berchialla, Dario Gregori and Ileana Baldi
Prior Elicitation for Use in Clinical Trial Design and Analysis: A Literature Review
Reprinted from: *Int. J. Environ. Res. Public Health* **2021**, *18*, 1833, doi:10.3390/ijerph18041833 . . . **93**

Danila Azzolina, Giulia Lorenzoni, Silvia Bressan, Liviana Da Dalt, Ileana Baldi and Dario Gregori
Handling Poor Accrual in Pediatric Trials: A Simulation Study Using a Bayesian Approach
Reprinted from: *Int. J. Environ. Res. Public Health* **2021**, *18*, 2095, doi:10.3390/ijerph18042095 . . . **115**

Manuela Robella, Paola Berchialla, Alice Borsano, Armando Cinquegrana, Alba Ilari Civit, Michele De Simone and Marco Vaira
Study Protocol: Phase I Dose Escalation Study of Oxaliplatin, Cisplatin and Doxorubicin Applied as PIPAC in Patients with Peritoneal Metastases
Reprinted from: *Int. J. Environ. Res. Public Health* **2021**, *18*, 5656, doi:10.3390/ijerph18115656 . . . **131**

Paola Berchialla, Veronica Sciannameo, Sara Urru, Corrado Lanera, Danila Azzolina, Dario Gregori and Ileana Baldi
Adjustment for Baseline Covariates to Increase Efficiency in RCTs with Binary Endpoint: A Comparison of Bayesian and Frequentist Approaches
Reprinted from: *Int. J. Environ. Res. Public Health* **2021**, *18*, 7758, doi:10.3390/ijerph18157758 . . . **141**

Valeria Sambucini
Bayesian Sequential Monitoring of Single-Arm Trials: A Comparison of Futility Rules Based on Binary Data
Reprinted from: *Int. J. Environ. Res. Public Health* **2021**, *18*, 8816, doi:10.3390/ijerph18168816 . . . **151**

Bethany Jablonski Horton, Nolan A. Wages and Ryan D. Gentzler
Bayesian Design for Identifying Cohort-Specific Optimal Dose Combinations Based on Multiple Endpoints: Application to a Phase I Trial in Non-Small Cell Lung Cancer
Reprinted from: *Int. J. Environ. Res. Public Health* **2021**, *18*, 11452, doi:10.3390/ijerph182111452 . **169**

About the Editors

Paola Berchialla is an Associate Professor of Biostatistics at the Department of Clinical and Biological Sciences of the University of Torino. She received a BS in Mathematics from the University of Torino and a PhD degree in Applied Statistics from the University of Firenze. During her PhD, she received a scholarship for the Department of Statistics at the Oxford University. Her expertise lies in statistical methodological development as well as general statistical applications. The methodological component of her research includes Bayesian networks and Bayesian design for clinical trials and machine learning. Her interdisciplinary research includes collaborations with physicians, geneticists, psychologists and nutritionists, among others.

Ileana Baldi is an Associate Professor of Medical Statistics at the Unit of Biostatistics Epidemiology and Public Health of the University of Padova, where she has been a faculty member since 2011. She holds a PhD in Statistics from the University of Milano-Bicocca and an MSc in Epidemiology from the University of Torino. During her previous research experience at the University of Torino (2002-2011), she developed skills in the design and analysis of early phase clinical trials. Her recent research interests encompass using machine learning techniques to address the analytical challenges posed by integrating real-world data into clinical drug development.

Preface to "Bayesian Design in Clinical Trials"

Bayesian designs have become increasingly popular in clinical trials, particularly in the early phase of drug and biologics development for evaluating their safety and efficacy [1], as well as medical device trials [2]. The Bayesian approach has been used to answer treatment questions and to foster novel designs [3]. The inability to estimate the probability of clinical benefit, a lack of mechanism for incorporating prior information and the difficulty in including multiple hypothesis testing are some inherent limitations to frequentist analysis that are overcome in the Bayesian framework [4].

In the last 10 years, the FDA has supported the development of Bayesian adaptive trials, and recently it has enhanced its capacity to review complex innovative designs [1]. The Bayesian approach leads to thinking about inference in terms of a probability distribution on the treatment effect, rather than a point estimate or confidence interval. Therefore, the Bayesian approach is oriented toward a progressive uncertainty reduction on a posterior distribution in treatment effect estimation. Prior information may contribute to the reduction of this uncertainty. The specification of the sample size in advance required by traditional clinical trials can be inefficient when limited information is available at the design stage, especially regarding the likely effect size. By incorporating knowledge from different resources, such as experts' opinions, the literature and historical data, a properly elicited prior distribution can improve the efficiency and reduce the sample size of a Bayesian trial, thus saving resources and minimizing the number of subjects exposed to an unpromising treatment [5].

In this regard, as uses of real world data become more familiar for trial design and regulatory submission, the increasing availability of open data holds immense potential, not only for expanding general scientific knowledge but also for strengthening Bayesian trials across the therapeutic continuum of medical product development, regulation and use. Even if Bayesian designs have many strengths, they do not provide solutions to all problems. It is acknowledged that implementing Bayesian methods in the regulated pharmaceutical industry does entail challenges. Prior elicitation, extensive simulations before launching the real trial, multidisciplinary collaboration during the design stage and less established reporting guidelines are just some of the challenges posed by Bayesian trials [6].

However, new methods and integrated software for study design, such as http://trialdesign.org, are available to overcome the traditional difficulty of implementing Bayesian methods.

It is important to find the right trade-off between innovation (i.e., software that can bring new methods but requires skilled programmers), and usability (i.e., software intended as a resource for the rapid construction of trial designs), which encourages exploration and experimentation as well.

This would be a key element to persuade clinical trialists and academics to better understand and exploit the benefit of Bayesian designs.

References

1. Fors, M.; González, P. Current status of Bayesian clinical trials for oncology, 2020. *Contemp. Clin. Trials Commun.* **2020**. [CrossRef]
2. Campbell, G. Bayesian methods in clinical trials with applications to medical devices. *Commun. Stat. Appl. Methods* **2017**, *24*, 561–581. [CrossRef]

3. Ryan, E.G.; Bruce, J.; Metcalfe, A.J.; Stallard, N.; Lamb, S.E.; Viele, K.; Young, D.; Gates, S. Using Bayesian adaptive designs to improve phase III trials: A respiratory care example. *BMC Med. Res. Methodol.* **2019**, *19*, 99. [CrossRef]

4. Greenland. S.; Senn, S.J.; Rothman, K.J.; Carlin, J.B.; Poole, C.; Goodman, S.N.; Altman, D.G. Statistical tests, P values, confidence intervals, and power: A guide to misinterpretations. *Eur. .J Epidemiol.* **2016**, *31*, 337–350. [CrossRef]

5. Medical Outreach Subteam of the Drug Information Association Bayesian Scientific Working Group. Why Are Not There More Bayesian Clinical Trials? Perceived Barriers and Educational Preferences Among Medical Researchers Involved in Drug Development. *Ther. Innov. Regul. Sci.* **2022**. [CrossRef]

6. Ferreira, D.; Vivot, A.; Diemunsch, P.; Meyer, N. Bayesian analysis from phase III trials was underused and poorly reported: A systematic review. *J. Clin. Epidemiol.* **2020**, *123*, 107–113. [CrossRef]

Paola Berchialla, Ileana Baldi
Editors

Article

Using an Interaction Parameter in Model-Based Phase I Trials for Combination Treatments? A Simulation Study

Pavel Mozgunov [1,*], Rochelle Knight [1], Helen Barnett [1] and Thomas Jaki [1,2]

1. Department of Mathematics and Statistics, Lancaster University, Lancaster LA1 4YF, UK; rochelleknight96@gmail.com (R.K.); h.barnett@lancaster.ac.uk (H.B.); thomas.jaki@mrc-bsu.cam.ac.uk (T.J.)
2. MRC Biostatistics Unit, University of Cambridge, Cambridge CB2 0SR, UK
* Correspondence: p.mozgunov@lancaster.ac.uk

Abstract: There is growing interest in Phase I dose-finding studies studying several doses of more than one agent simultaneously. A number of combination dose-finding designs were recently proposed to guide escalation/de-escalation decisions during the trials. The majority of these proposals are model-based: a parametric combination-toxicity relationship is fitted as data accumulates. Various parameter shapes were considered but the unifying theme for many of these is that typically between 4 and 6 parameters are to be estimated. While more parameters allow for more flexible modelling of the combination-toxicity relationship, this is a challenging estimation problem given the typically small sample size in Phase I trials of between 20 and 60 patients. These concerns gave raise to an ongoing debate whether including more parameters into combination-toxicity model leads to more accurate combination selection. In this work, we extensively study two variants of a 4-parameter logistic model with reduced number of parameters to investigate the effect of modelling assumptions. A framework to calibrate the prior distributions for a given parametric model is proposed to allow for fair comparisons. Via a comprehensive simulation study, we have found that the inclusion of the interaction parameter between two compounds does not provide any benefit in terms of the accuracy of selection, on average, but is found to result in fewer patients allocated to the target combination during the trial.

Keywords: dose-escalation; combination study; modelling assumption; interaction

1. Introduction

Traditionally, Phase I oncology trials predominantly investigated dose-finding for a single cytotoxic agent. In recent years, however, more complex dosing regimens are routinely considered. In particular combinations of drugs can have better therapeutic outcomes than a single anti-cancer drug treatment [1]. In a Phase I dual-agent combination trials, the aim is to determine the highest acceptable combination of doses known as the maximum tolerated combination (MTC) which is defined as the combination with probability of a dose-limiting toxicity (DLT) closest to the pre-specified target θ.

Single agent trials typically assume that toxicity increases monotonically with dose (also known as monotonicity assumption [2]) and hence there is only one target dose, the maximum tolerated dose (MTD). In combination trials, however, the monotonicity assumption typically does not hold for all combinations under study. This can be examplified where for the one level we have two drugs at two different doses, but the next level corresponds to an increase in one of the drugs but a decrease in the other. Here, the ordering of the toxicity probabilities is typically not known. The situation where the orderings between some dose combinations are known where others are not, is known as partial ordering [2]. A number of novel dose-finding design for combination trials were proposed [3,4]. The majority of novel designs are model-based and rely on a parametric model to fit the combination-toxicity relationship given the accumulating data. Typically, these models have between 4 and 6 parameteres [5–7] to be estimated given a small number of observations in the study.

There is, however, an ongoing discussion as to whether a model with more parameters can be adequately fit in the setting of small sample sizes (usually between 20 and 60 in total and as few as two when the model is fit for the first time).

Specifically, Cunanan et al. [8] found that early phase dose finding trials studying toxicity and efficacy together often relied on copula models to specify the joint distribution of toxicity and efficacy, which include an additional correlation parameter that can be difficult to estimate. This is because of the small sample size in early phase trials. It was also found that a simple model that assumes independence between toxicity and efficacy performs just as well due to difficulty in estimating the copula model correlation parameters from binary data.

Similar reasoning to that of modelling the interaction between toxicity and efficacy as independent is thought to be relevant for models used in combination trials. Specifically, the question translated into whether an interaction term between the two agents could be estimated on small samples. Mozgunov et al. [9] have recently proposed a model-free dose-finding design for combination studies that assumed no-interaction and was found to perform more accurately in the considered setting than a model-based partial ordering continual reassessment method (POCRM) [10] and an alternative model-free design, PIPE [11]. However, one potential drawback of not including an interaction term in the combination-toxicity model is that less flexible models can collapse in some situations. While it was not found to be the case for the model-free design [9] due its flexibility, the question of the trade-off between not capturing unexpected combination-toxicity relationships and the challenging estimation of additional parameters still stands for the model-based combination designs.

In this work, we investigate for one particular model, namely the 4-parameter logistic model by Riviere et al. [6], the effect of removing specific parameters from the dose combination-toxicity model. We propose two model modifications reducing the number of parameters to three. For a fair comparison in the presence of no prior information on the compounds, we also propose an extensive calibration procedure to find so-called operational prior parameters, parameters that results in high accuracy in a range of different scenarios. Using the operational prior for each model considered, we explore the trade-off between estimation and flexibility via a compherensive simulation study in a number of clinical plausible scenarios with various interaction mechanisms of the compounds.

2. Model-Based Dose-Finding Design

2.1. Setting

Consider a dual-agent Phase I clinical trial. Assume that there are J dose levels of agent 1 (indexed by j) and K dose levels of agent 2 (indexed by k). A combination of the jth dose of agent 1 and the kth dose of agent 2 is denoted by (j,k). Let Y_{ijk} be a Bernoulli random variable indicating whether a DLT occurs in patient i ($i = 1, \ldots, N$) given combination (j,k) where $Y_{ijk} = 0$ if no DLT is observed in patient i and $Y_{ijk} = 1$ if a DLT is observed. Let $\pi_{j,k}$ denote the toxicity probability given combination (j,k) and the logit function is defined as $logit(\pi_{j,k}) = \log\{\frac{\pi_{j,k}}{1-\pi_{j,k}}\}$. It is assumed that the dose-toxicity relationship increases monotonically with the dose-levels of each agent. The aim of the trial is to determine the MTC, the highest dose combination with a probability of toxicity closest to the corresponding target level of toxicity θ.

2.2. 4-Parameter Logistic Model

Riviere et al. [6] proposed the following logistic parametric form to model the combination-toxicity relationship:

$$Y_{ijk} \sim \text{Bernoulli}(\pi_{jk})$$

Model M0: $$logit(\pi_{j,k}) = \beta_0 + \beta_1 u_j + \beta_2 v_k + \beta_3 u_j v_k \qquad (1)$$

where β_0, β_1, β_2 and β_3 are unknown parameters that denote the intercept (β_0), the toxicity effect of agent 1 (β_1), agent 2 (β_2) and the interaction between the two agents (β_3), and $u_j = \log\left(\frac{p_j}{1-p_j}\right)$ and $v_k = \log\left(\frac{q_k}{1-q_k}\right)$ are the standardised doses of the two agents. The parameters $p_1, \ldots, p_J$, and $q_1, \ldots, q_K$, are the prior estimates of the toxicity probabilities for the dose levels of agent 1 and 2, respectively, when administered as monotherapy. The terms u_j and v_k are also known as the skeleton and are unchanged throughout the trial (with the estimation of the contribution of each agent to the combination toxicity being updated through the corresponding model parameters $\beta_1, \beta_2, \beta_3$).

Riviere et al. [6] defined the parameters β_0, β_1, β_2 and β_3 such that $\beta_1 > 0$ and $\beta_2 > 0$, ensuring that the toxicity probability is increasing with increasing dose levels of each agent alone; and $\forall k, \beta_1 + \beta_3 v_k > 0$ and $\forall j, \beta_2 + \beta_3 u_j > 0$, guaranteeing that the toxicity probability is increasing with increasing dose levels of both agents together; and the intercept $\beta_0 \in \mathcal{R}$. The model parameters are initialised by some prior distribution which describe beliefs about these parameters before any data are collected. We will refer to this original combination-toxicity model as "Model M0".

Assume that $n_{j,k}$ patients are assigned to combination (j,k) and a total of $t_{j,k} = \sum_{i=1}^{n_{j,k}} Y_{ijk}$ toxic responses are observed for this combination. We define $\mathbb{N} = (n_{1,1}, n_{1,2}, \ldots, n_{j,k}, \ldots, n_{J,K})$ and $\mathbb{T} = (t_{1,1}, t_{1,2}, \ldots, t_{j,k}, \ldots t_{J,K})$. Assuming some prior distribution of the model parameters $f(\beta_0, \beta_1, \beta_2, \beta_3)$ and applying Bayes Theorem, the posterior distribution of the model parameters is given by

$$f(\beta_0, \beta_1, \beta_2, \beta_3 | \mathbb{N}, \mathbb{T}) \propto \prod_{j=1}^{J} \prod_{k=1}^{K} \pi_{j,k}^{t_{j,k}} (1 - \pi_{j,k})^{n_{j,k} - t_{j,k}} f(\beta_0, \beta_1, \beta_2, \beta_3)$$

where $f(\beta_0, \beta_1, \beta_2, \beta_3)$ is the joint probability density function of the prior distribution of the parameters. In the original proposal, independent prior distributions for each parameters were considered. We investigate the case of dependent prior distributions for the model parameters in Section 5.1.

For the parametric model and set of prior distributions of the model parameters, MCMC was used to obtain posterior samples from each distribution, that were then used to approximate the posterior distribution as they do not, generally, have a closed form. Specifically, Gibbs Sampling as implemented in the R-package `rjags` [12] was used. To satisfy the constraints of $\beta_1 > 0$ and $\beta_2 > 0$, the prior distributions defined on the positive real line were chosen (see Section 3 for further details). To ensure that $\forall k, \beta_1 + \beta_3 v_k > 0$ and $\forall j, \beta_2 + \beta_3 u_j > 0$, only those posterior samples of the model parameters that satisfy these constraints are taken forwards. Once the posterior samples for each parameter were obtained, they were used to get the posterior distribution of toxicity probability at each combination. These toxicity probabilities are subsequently used to govern escalation/de-escalation decisions (see Section 2.3).

2.3. Original Dose Finding Design

Riviere et al. [6] proposed to use model (1) in a sequential dose-finding trial with cohorts of patients sequentially assigned to different combinations based on accumulating evidence gained throughout the trial. Dose escalation and de-escalation was restricted to one level at a time (i.e., dose escalation and de-escalation along the diagonal is not allowed). The decision about which combination to assign to the next cohort was made based on the escalation/de-escalation constraints that were defined as follows.

Let c_e be the probability threshold for dose escalation, c_d the probability threshold for dose de-escalation and θ be the target toxicity probability. It is required that $c_e + c_d > 1$. Let the current dose combination be (j,k) and $\{\mathbb{N}, \mathbb{T}\}$ be the current data available on the number of patients thus far assigned to dose combinations and the number of DLTs observed, then

- If $P\left(\pi_{j,k} < \theta | \mathbb{N}, \mathbb{T}\right) > c_e$, the combination dose level is escalated to an adjacent combination dose level $\{(j+1,k), (j,k+1), (j+1,k-1), (j-1,k+1)\}$ and the next allocated dose combination (j',k') is chosen such that it has a toxicity probability higher than the current value, $\tilde{\pi}_{j',k'} > \tilde{\pi}_{j,k}$, and a toxicity probability closest to θ

$$\min_{j',k'}\{\left|\tilde{\pi}_{j',k'} - \theta\right| : (j',k') \in (j+1,k), (j,k+1), (j+1,k-1), (j-1,k+1)\}$$

If the current combination is the highest of the combination space, (J,K), the next cohort of patients will receive the same combination.

- If $P\left(\pi_{j,k} > \theta | \mathbb{N}, \mathbb{T}\right) > c_d$, the combination dose level is de-escalated to an adjacent combination dose level $\{(j-1,k), (j,k-1), (j+1,k-1), (j-1,k+1)\}$ and the next allocated dose combination (j',k') is chosen such that it that has a toxicity probability lower than the current value, $\tilde{\pi}_{j',k'} < \tilde{\pi}_{j,k}$, and a toxicity probability closest to θ. If the current combination is the lowest of the combination space, $(1,1)$, the next cohort of patients will receive the same combination.
- If $P\left(\pi_{j,k} < \theta | \mathbb{N}, \mathbb{T}\right) \le c_e$ and $P\left(\pi_{j,k} > \theta | \mathbb{N}, \mathbb{T}\right) \le c_d$, the next cohort will be receive the current combination dose level.

Once the required sample size has been reached, the MTC is selected as the combination with the highest posterior probability of the risk of toxicity being within δ of the target probability, θ, $P(\pi_{j,k} \in [\theta - \delta; \theta + \delta])$, and which has been used to treat at least one cohort of patients. Here, the parameter δ reflects how close the toxicity risk of a combination should be to the target in order for this combination to be considered promising.

For the purposes of this manuscript, we will focus on this specification of the design without stopping rules to ensure that the model specification is responsible for differences in the results. Each model can, however, also be used with stopping rules. For example, the most common stopping rule is to stop for safety—none of the studied combinations are deemed safe given the current data and the trial is terminated [13]. Furthermore, a design could stop once a given number of patients has been assigned to the same combination [14].

2.4. Alternative Models for the Combination-Toxicity Relationship

To ease the estimation problem of the combination-toxicity relationship with small samples, we explore a similar type of combination-toxicity relationship but with a reduced number of parameters. We consider modelling the drug combination-toxicity relationship based on the model with no interaction term, β_3,

$$\text{Model M1:} \quad logit\left(\pi_{j,k}\right) = \beta_0 + \beta_1 u_j + \beta_2 v_k \qquad (2)$$

and the model with no intercept term, β_0

$$\text{Model M2:} \quad logit\left(\pi_{j,k}\right) = \beta_1 u_j + \beta_2 v_k + \beta_3 u_j v_k. \qquad (3)$$

The model in Equation (2) will be referred to as "Model M1" and the model in Equation (3) will be referred to "Model M2". Both models M1 and M2 use the same escalation and de-escalation criteria as outlined in Section 2.3 and all parameters within these models are as defined as before. Note that Model 2 resembles some of the features of the model by Thall et al. [5] but without the power parameters.

3. Choice of Prior Distribution

All combination-toxicity models described in the previous section employ a Bayesian paradigm for the sequential parameter estimation. Therefore, to initialise the model, prior distributions for each parameter should be defined before the trial commences. For each parameter, we use the same distributions as in the original work by [6]. In this section, using the example of the 4-parameter logistic design, we describe an algorithm for calibrating the hyper-parameters of the prior distributions of the model parameters β_0, β_1, β_2 and β_3. We will apply the same algorithm for all models considered in this manuscript.

The calibration of the hyper-parameters of the prior distributions for the model parameters will be performed through a grid search which consists of fitting a model for each of the possible combinations of hyper-parameters. The hyper-parameters of the models parameters—β_0, β_1, β_2 and β_3—will be calibrated using the following prior distributions:

$$\beta_0 \sim \mathcal{N}(0,a), \quad \beta_1 \sim Gamma(b,b), \quad \beta_2 \sim Gamma(c,c), \quad \beta_3 \sim \mathcal{N}(0,d) \tag{4}$$

for $a \in \mathcal{A}$, $b \in \mathcal{B}$, $c \in \mathcal{C}$, and $d \in \mathcal{D}$ where $\mathcal{A}$, $\mathcal{B}$, $\mathcal{C}$ and $\mathcal{D}$ are the grids of values of hyper-parameters for each of the prior distributions. Following the original proposal, we use the normal prior for β_0 and β_3 centred at 0 to allow for the parameters to take both positive and negative values with neither being favoured. The Gamma prior is used for β_2 and β_3, to ensure that the parameters are positive, and are centred at 1 [6]. The latter implies that the toxicity effect of both agents is considered to be similar and that neither agent is favoured to increase the toxicity effect with increasing dose level more than the other.

While a model can be calibrated under all scenarios that are considered clinically plausible, such a procedure can become computationally infeasible if there are many scenarios to be considered. Therefore, we propose to perform a grid search using a subset of scenarios such that these would represent noticeably different (but still clinically plausible) combination-toxicity relationships. For example, one scenario with many doses having toxicity probabilities far below the MTC, and another where most doses have toxicity probabilities far above the MTC would reflect different extreme settings [14,15]. Additionally, some of the scenarios selected for the calibration should reflect various interaction mechanism between the two compounds. We provide examples of such scenarios in Section 4.

For the purposes of this manuscript, the models will be calibrated in terms of their accurate, namely, the proportion of correct selections (PCS). Let $\eta_{a,b,c,d}^{(h)}$ be the PCS under scenario h using prior parameters a,b,c,d. Then, the parameters $a^\star, b^\star, c^\star, d^\star$ maximising the geometric mean of the PCS across H considered scenarios

$$\max_{a \in \mathcal{A}, b \in \mathcal{B}, c \in \mathcal{C}, d \in \mathcal{D}} \left(\prod_{h=1}^{H} \eta_{a,b,c,d}^{(h)} \right)^{\frac{1}{H}} \tag{5}$$

are selected for the model. The use of the geometric mean over the arithmetic mean is proposed as a model performing uniformly across the considered scenarios is desirable. The geometric mean penalises poor results which is advantageous when looking at the ability of a model to consistently find the MTC across a variety of scenarios.

We would like to stress that the calibration procedure in this work is solely based on one measure (5) for the purposes of the comparing the models in terms of the MTC selections. At the same time, when considering calibration of the design hyper-parameters for a particular dose-finding clinical trial, some of the choices of hyper-parameters might not be considered as favourable even if they imply the highest accuracy. If there are some additional constraints to be imposed on the prior, this can be embedded within the procedure. For example, one can target the hyper-parameters such that the PCS is maximised but the prior toxicity probability at the lowest combination is not above 15%.

4. Numerical Evaluation

4.1. Setting

In this section, we study how the different parametric models for the combination toxicity relationship defined in Section 2 perform in a variety of clinically plausible settings. To investigate the design under each model, we simulate independent replications of Phase I trials that evaluate dual-agent drug combinations. We focus on the setting originally considered by Riviere et al. [6]. Specifically we use five dose levels for agent 1 and three dose levels for agent 2, resulting in 15 dose combinations to be investigated. The target toxicity is fixed at $\theta = 0.3$ and for each trial, an overall sample size of $N = 60$ is used. A cohort size of 3 is used for all models and no stopping rules are used. For ethical reasons, each trial is started at the lowest dose combination (1,1). It was assumed in [6] that both agents were previously studied separately and intial guesses of toxicities for each dose of both agents administered as monotherapies can be provided by the clinical team. Specifically, for agent 1, the marginal initial guesses of toxicities, p_j, are specified as $p = (0.12, 0.2, 0.3, 0.4, 0.5)$ and for agent 2, q_k is specified as $q = (0.2, 0.3, 0.4)$. These prior guesses are used to construct the skeletons u_j and v_k in Equation (1). The probability thresholds used to guide dose escalation and de-escalation follow [6] and are set at $c_e = 0.85$ and $c_d = 0.45$. The length around the target interval, δ is set at $\delta = 0.1$.

The objective is to evaluate the models in terms of their accuracy and the ethical counterparts: how many patients are assigned to overly toxic combinations and often is the target combination assigned during the trial. Specifically, we study the properties of the designs in terms of

- the percentages of correct selections (PCS) reflecting how accurately the design selects the target combination;
- percentage of patients allocated to a true MTC during the trial, reflecting the potential benefit the patients could get from efficient combination assignment;
- the percentage of DLTs observed throughout the trial reflecting how many patients suffer from the adverse events under each design.

4.2. Scenarios

Twenty scenarios are used to represent a variety of clinically feasible true underlying combination-toxicity relationships (Table 1). We focus on finding one MTC at the end of the trial, regardless of if there are multiple possible correct combinations within the scenario.

In Scenarios 1–7, the MTC is located along each diagonal of the combination space, moving from the lower (1,1) corner of the combination space in scenario 1 to the upper (5,3) corner in Scenario 7. As it is unknown at the planning stage what the true combination-toxicity relationship is, it is important that all these scenarios are used to ensure good operating characteristics across all these scenarios. Scenarios 2 and 6 each have two possible MTC dose combinations. Two more variants of each of these scenarios were added.

Scenarios 2 and 6 were altered by replacing, in turn, one of the two MTCs with a dose combination with a toxicity probability different to 0.3 whilst ensuring that the monotonicity assumption still holds to form the Scenarios 2.1, 2.2, 6.1 and 6.2. The Scenarios 1, 2.1, 2.2, 6.1, 6.2 and 7 represent extreme examples of the dose-toxicity relationship. For Scenarios 1, 2.1 and 2.2, they represent a steep combination-toxicity relationship with many of the doses higher in the combination space having toxicity probabilities far above the MTC. Comparatively, for Scenarios 6.1, 6.2 and 7, they show a flat combination-toxicity relationship where many of the doses lower in the combination have toxicity probabilities space are far below the MTC. Note that Scenarios 2.1, 2.2, 6.1, 6.2 also correspond to cases when one compound increases the toxicity of the combination more than the other—when increasing the dose of one compound leads just to the target toxicity of 30% but increase in another corresponds to an overly toxic (40%) dose combination.

Scenarios 8–12 were proposed by Riviere et al. [6]. In Scenarios 8, 10, 11 and 12 there are multiple MTCs which are not located along the same diagonal but throughout the combination space and in Scenario 9 there is one MTC located in the centre of the combination space. Furthermore, under Scenarios 8, 10, and 12, it is assumed that one of the compounds is more toxic than the other (i.e., the combination toxicity relationship is steeper in one compound). Scenarios 13 and 14 represent the scenarios with only one MTC located for high doses of one of the agents.

Table 1. Toxicity scenarios for the dual-agent combinations. The true MTC combinations are in bold.

			Agent 1							
Agent 2	1	2	3	4	5	1	2	3	4	5
		Scenario 1					Scenario 2			
1	**0.30**	0.40	0.50	0.60	0.70	0.20	**0.30**	0.40	0.50	0.60
2	0.40	0.50	0.60	0.70	0.80	**0.30**	0.40	0.50	0.60	0.70
3	0.50	0.60	0.70	0.80	0.90	0.40	0.50	0.60	0.70	0.80
		Scenario 2.1					Scenario 2.2			
1	0.20	**0.30**	0.40	0.50	0.60	0.20	0.40	0.50	0.60	0.70
2	0.40	0.50	0.60	0.70	0.80	**0.30**	0.50	0.60	0.70	0.80
3	0.50	0.60	0.70	0.80	0.85	0.40	0.60	0.70	0.80	0.90
		Scenario 3					Scenario 4			
1	0.15	0.20	**0.30**	0.40	0.50	0.10	0.15	0.20	**0.30**	0.40
2	0.20	**0.30**	0.40	0.50	0.60	0.15	0.20	**0.30**	0.40	0.50
3	**0.30**	0.40	0.50	0.60	0.70	0.20	**0.30**	0.40	0.50	0.60
		Scenario 5					Scenario 6			
1	0.05	0.10	0.15	0.20	**0.30**	0.03	0.05	0.10	0.15	0.20
2	0.10	0.15	0.20	**0.30**	0.40	0.05	0.10	0.15	0.20	**0.30**
3	0.15	0.20	**0.30**	0.40	0.50	0.10	0.15	0.20	**0.30**	0.40
		Scenario 6.1					Scenario 6.2			
1	0.01	0.03	0.05	0.10	0.20	0.03	0.05	0.10	0.15	0.20
2	0.03	0.05	0.10	0.15	**0.30**	0.05	0.10	0.15	0.20	0.40
3	0.05	0.10	0.15	0.20	0.40	0.10	0.15	0.20	**0.30**	0.50
		Scenario 7					Scenario 8			
1	0.01	0.03	0.05	0.10	0.15	0.05	0.08	0.10	0.13	0.15
2	0.03	0.05	0.10	0.15	0.20	0.09	0.12	0.15	**0.30**	0.45
3	0.05	0.10	0.15	0.20	**0.30**	0.15	**0.30**	0.45	0.50	0.60
		Scenario 9					Scenario 10			
1	0.02	0.10	0.15	0.50	0.60	0.05	0.12	0.20	**0.30**	0.40
2	0.05	0.12	**0.30**	0.55	0.70	0.10	0.20	**0.30**	0.40	0.50
3	0.08	0.15	0.45	0.60	0.80	**0.30**	0.42	0.52	0.62	0.70
		Scenario 11					Scenario 12			
1	0.12	0.20	**0.30**	0.40	0.60	0.04	0.06	0.08	0.20	**0.30**
2	0.20	**0.30**	0.40	0.50	0.67	0.10	0.20	**0.30**	0.50	0.67
3	0.42	0.52	0.62	0.70	0.80	**0.30**	0.42	0.52	0.70	0.80
		Scenario 13					Scenario 14			
1	0.05	0.08	0.10	0.15	0.20	0.01	0.03	0.06	0.10	0.20
2	0.10	0.15	0.20	**0.30**	0.40	0.04	0.07	0.12	0.20	**0.30**
3	0.20	0.40	0.50	0.55	0.60	0.08	0.10	0.20	0.40	0.50
		Scenario 15					Scenario 16			
1	0.45	0.50	0.55	0.60	0.65	0.01	0.02	0.05	0.10	0.15
2	0.50	0.55	0.60	0.65	0.70	0.02	0.05	0.10	0.15	0.17
3	0.55	0.60	0.65	0.70	0.75	0.05	0.10	0.15	0.17	0.20

Under Scenario 15, all combinations are too toxic as the lowest combination already has the toxicity rate of 45%. In contrast, under scenario 16, all combinations are safe as the highest combination has a toxicity probability of 20%. Note that as the design does not include stopping rules, it is expected that a design with desirable properties would recommend the lowest and the highest dose in Scenarios 15 and 16, respectively.

Finally, Scenarios 11 and 14 were found to be well-approximated by the original 4-parameter logistic model but with the slope parameters for each agent being equal to $\beta_1 = \beta_2 = 0$. This implies that the underlying combination-toxicity relationships are fully determined by the interaction parameter β_3 and these are the scenarios where one could expect to see the most gain in benefit in including the interaction term. Therefore, we will be using these 2 scenarios to assess further potential losses of not including the interaction parameter.

4.3. Calibration

The sets of values for the grid search for the hyper-parameters have been selected as

$$\mathcal{A} = \{0.1, 1, 10, 100, 200, 400\},$$
$$\mathcal{B} = \{0.1, 1, 10\},$$
$$\mathcal{C} = \{0.1, 1, 10\},$$
$$\mathcal{D} = \{1, 10, 100, 200, 400\}$$

for each of the considered models. Note that the values of $a = 10$, $b = 1$, $c = 1$ and $d = 10$ correspond to the prior distributions specified by Riviere et al. [6]. Therefore, these grids were chosen to explore lower and higher variance around the mean of the parameters compared to the originally considered prior distribution. Due to the computational costs, the hyper-parameters to be tried were chosen to be noticeably different from each other, e.g., at least increasing the variance of the parameter twofold. This aims at locating an approximately optimal (in terms of PCS) values. We will use these values to compare whether the proposed calibration procedure can provide benefits in terms of the operating characteristics. For each set of hyper-parameters combinations, we simulate 500 trials to evaluate dual-agent drug combinations.

As discussed above, the choice of scenarios for the calibration is crucial. As the calibration over all 20 scenarios would have been to computationally demanding, we specify a subset of four scenarios to reduce the compuational costs while still adequately exploring the properties of the design specification under extreme scenarios. Specifically, Scenarios 2.1, 2.2, 6.1 and 6.2 from Table 1 are used for the calibration process. Scenarios 2.1 and 2.2 represent a steep combination-toxicity relationship with many of the doses higher in the combination space far above the MTC and Scenarios 6.1 and 6.2 show a flat combination-toxicity relationship where many of the doses lower in the combination space are far below the MTC. Importantly, we have selected scenarios with one MTC only as it was noted previously that model-based designs can strongly favour one of the MTC in scenarios with several of them. This undesirable favouring of particular combinations cannot be picked up via summary characteristics such as the PCS, and the inclusion of scenarios with one MTC only would mitigate this risk.

The results of the hyper-parameter calibration are given in Table 2.

Table 2. Calibrated prior parameters for each model and the corresponding PCS under 4 calibration scenarios. GM is the geometric mean of the PCS across the four scenarios. Results are based on 500 replications.

Model	β_0	β_1	β_2	β_3	Sc 2.1	Sc 2.2	Sc 6.1	Sc 6.2	GM
M0$^{(0)}$	$\mathcal{N}(0,10)$	G(1,1)	G(1,1)	$\mathcal{N}(0,10)$	-	-	-	-	-
M0	$\mathcal{N}(0,1)$	G(1,1)	G(1,1)	$\mathcal{N}(0,100)$	44.6	38.8	45.0	55.6	45.6
M1	$\mathcal{N}(0,400)$	G(1,1)	G(10,10)	-	41.3	40.8	43.3	40.5	41.4
M2	-	G(1,1)	G(1,1)	$\mathcal{N}(0,100)$	32.1	26.0	40.2	76.2	39.9

For completeness, we also include the prior distribution originally proposed for the 4-parameter model (to which we refer as M0$^{(0)}$) that will be further included in the simulation study. Note that the values of the hyper-parameters for M1 yielding the highest PCS were found to be on the bound of the selected grids of β_0 and β_2. We have further extended these grids to include $a = 400, 500, 600$ and $c = 10, 20, 40$ and it was found that indeed the hyper-parameters in Table 2 result in the highest PCS among the considered combinations of values (see Table 3).

Finally, the calibrated hyper-parameters choices imply various prior combination toxicity relationships, all of which could be plausible. For example, under Model M2, the prior point estimate is around 0.05% for the lowest combination (i.e., the starting combination is very safe) and the highest is nearly 40%. Such prior beliefs correspond to a sharp increase in toxicity on the 5th dose on one of the compounds. Then, for example, starting escalation at the lowest combination, if the earlier data would suggest that the highest dose is not as toxic as expected, the escalation to higher doses would be allowed.

Table 3. Further calibration of M1: the geometric mean of the PCS across scenario 2.1, 2.2, 6.1, 6.2 for various values of hyper-parameters $a = 400, 500, 600$, and $c = 10, 20, 40$. The highest PCS is in bold. Results are based on 500 replications.

	$c = 10$	$c = 20$	$c = 40$
$a = 400$	**41.4**	38.2	39.2
$a = 500$	40.7	38.9	37.1
$a = 600$	37.9	39.3	37.6

4.4. Comparator: Optimal Benchmark for Combination Studies

While the primary goal of this work is to compare the performance of different models to each other, the similarity of the parametric models defined (and the fact that all of the designs are model-based) could mean that all methods perform equally poorly on some scenarios. To provide a context for the comparison of operating characteristics, we include the performance of the non-parameteric benchmark for combination studies, a tool that provides an estimate for the upper bound on the PCS under the given combination-toxicity scenario [16]. The benchmark takes into account the "difficulty" of a scenario in terms of how close the toxicity risks for the combinations (under this scenario) to the target level of 30% are, and also accounts for the unknown monotonic ordering in the combination setting.

Specifically, at its first step, the benchmark utilises the concept of complete information [17], which assumes that the data for each patient given each dose is available (in contrast to the actual trials setting with this information for one dose only). Under complete information, the toxicity estimates at each combination are found. At the second step, the probabilities that these toxicity estimates come from various potential clinically feasible "orderings" of combination are found. These probabilities are assigned to the probability of each combination selection under the given ordering. We refer the reader to the recent work by Mozgunov et al. [16] for further technical details on the benchmark for combinations trials. We will refer to the benchmark design as "B".

4.5. Results

A summary of operating characteristics using 4000 replications for all 4 models under Scenarios 1–14 with at least one MTC is given in Table 4. As some designs are expected to outperform others in some scenarios and perform worse in others, we also provide the geometric mean (GM) of the PCS and its variance (Var) across scenarios.

Table 4. Percentage of correct selection in comparison of 5 dose-finding designs and the benchmark (B) under Scenarios 1–14. Percentage of patients allocated to a true MTC during the trial and percentage of observed DLTs throughout the trial. GM is the geometric mean and Var is the variance. In the top third of the table, the highest PCS and those within less than 3% across the dose-finding designs are shown in bold for each scenario. Results are based on 4000 simulations.

Sc	1	2	2.1	2.2	3	4	5	6	6.1	6.2	7	8	9	10	11	12	13	14	GM	Var
\multicolumn{21}{c}{Percentage of correct selection (PCS)}																			
$M0^{(0)}$	58	**59**	56	27	58	56	56	57	32	51	69	**64**	62	**62**	**61**	**61**	24	18	48.7	232.6
M0	59	53	48	35	54	**56**	**57**	64	**40**	54	68	61	53	57	57	58	28	22	49.6	152.0
M1	**75**	**60**	38	**42**	58	55	54	55	**41**	36	**76**	57	**68**	52	**59**	40	**46**	**31**	50.8	165.2
M2	47	37	30	26	35	41	47	**82**	39	**74**	57	28	33	39	43	36	11	23	37.0	296.6
B	82	61	49	46	57	54	57	61	46	42	83	65	58	53	50	56	32	41	53.8	166.1
\multicolumn{21}{c}{Percentage of patients allocated to a true MTC during the trial}																			
$M0^{(0)}$	45	45	38	17	42	36	34	36	23	24	38	36	24	44	38	40	14	16	30.9	105.6
M0	41	36	30	22	36	35	37	45	32	28	33	38	18	40	32	36	19	21	31.2	62.0
M1	56	40	21	32	38	34	31	36	25	21	48	35	37	33	34	26	19	22	31.4	91.8
M2	33	26	21	20	27	27	35	57	39	33	23	31	9	27	21	27	22	28	26.4	96.9
\multicolumn{21}{c}{Percentage of DLTs throughout the trial}																			
$M0^{(0)}$	37	33	35	36	30	28	26	24	23	25	20	28	33	30	32	30	28	26	28.6	21.1
M0	38	36	36	38	33	31	28	25	23	26	20	30	36	33	34	33	31	27	30.5	27.4
M1	36	33	34	34	31	29	28	25	25	27	21	29	31	31	32	32	30	27	29.4	13.2
M2	41	39	40	41	37	34	30	25	23	27	19	33	41	37	38	38	34	28	32.8	47.1

The calibrated model M2, the model with no intercept parameter, has a significantly lower average PCS of 37.0% compared to all other models. In 10 scenarios it has a PCS below 40% and has the lowest PCS amongst all models with a PCS of 11% in Scenario 13. The model M2 also has the lowest average percentage of patients allocated to a true MTC during the trial and the average percentage of DLTs throughout the trial is 32.8% which is the furthest from 30% compared to all other models. As this model is not performing comparably to all other models, it will not be considered further.

For model M0, which is the four-parameter model, two variations, with different set of prior parameters, are considered. The original model $M0^{(0)}$ and the calibrated M0 have the mean PCS of 48.7% and 49.6%, respectively. Therefore, the use of a calibrated prior allowed to increase the average PCS by nearly 1% on average under all considered scenarios. Comparing the average performance across scenarios that were not included in the calibration (i.e., excluding 2.1, 2.2, 6.1, 6.2), the models perform comparably—within 0.4% for the average PCS. At the same time, the calibrated model results in a noticeably more consistent performance in terms of the PCS across the scenarios—the variance of the PCS is 232.6 for the original prior and 152.0 for the calibrated one. Furthermore, the calibrated model results in nearly the same proportion of patients allocated to the true MTC (difference of 0.3%) but with noticeably lower variance across scenarios—62.0 for the calibrated model against 105.6 for the original prior. The costs for a better and more consistent performance for the calibrated model M0 is having an average percentage of observed DLTs slightly above the target rate, 30.5%, but still close to the target toxicity. Therefore, the model with the calibrated prior results in a more consistent performance of the design, and therefore the model under this prior is taken for further evaluation with the competing models.

Model M1, the model with no interaction parameter, had the highest average PCS of 50.8% compared to the other models 1.2% higher that for the calibrated model M0. At the same time, M0 has slightly lower variance in the PCS across the scenarios of 152.0 compared to 165.2 for M1. In eleven scenarios the model M1 has either higher PCS than the model M0 or is within 3% of it (for 9 scenarios the same can be said for M0). Additionally,

M1 allocated the highest average percentage of patients to a true MTC throughout the trial at 31.4% and has 1% lower average percentage of observed DLTs. We will now focus on comparing scenario-by-scenario performance as the two models M0 and M1 seem to perform somewhat comparably.

In scenarios with only one MTC, the two models show uneven performance depending on the location of the MTC. When the true MTC was located in either the lower (1,1) or higher (5,3) extremity or the centre (3,2) of the combination space, as in scenarios 1, 7 and 9 respectively, model M1 showed its best performances with PCS of 75%, 76% and 68% respectively. In all three of these scenarios the model M0 had a PCS at least 8% lower. Importantly, in scenario 1, the difference in PCS of 16% is observed between the two models in favour of the model M1. Scenario 1 shows a steep combination-toxicity relationship with all the doses higher in the combination space having a toxicity probability far above the MTC. Therefore, the significantly higher PCS for the model M1 is of particular preference in this scenario. The model M1 also allocates 56.1% of patients to the true MTC in scenario 1 which is the highest allocation across all scenarios compared to 41% for M0. The higher percentage of patients allocated to the true MTC for the model M1 suggests it is more conservative and less aggressive in its approach at allocating patients compared to the model M0. This is preferable, in particular in scenarios such as scenario 1 which shows such a steep combination-toxicity relationship. The most noticeable costs for this advantage of the model M1 is a loss of 18% PCS in scenario 12 with the target combination lying on various diagonals. The model M0 has a PCS of 58% compared to 40% for M1 that suggests that having a more flexible model (under the calibrated parameters) might be more beneficial under this scenario. Comparatively, in scenarios 2.1, 2.2, 6.1, 6.2, 13 and 14, both models show some of their poorest performances as these are the most challenging scenarios with a single MTC. It also confirmed by the benchmark that these scenarios are the most difficult—the benchmark results in its lowest PCS under these scenarios as well. In all these scenarios, both models have a PCS of 45% or lower.

Comparing the PCS in scenarios 11 and 14 which are approximately generated using the model with the intercept and interaction parameter model, $\beta_1 = \beta_2 = 0$, one can find that the calibrated 4-parameter and 3-parameter with no interaction models perform within 3% of each other under scenario 11, and M1 outperforms M0 by 9% under scenario 14. Therefore, in the scenarios determined by the interaction only, the 4-parameter model does not provide any tangible benefit and the 3-parameter model can approximate the combination-toxicity relationship well enough (or even better) to locate the true MTC.

Finally, comparing the performance of the models to the benchmark, as expected the benchmark results in the highest average PCS. Specifically, the ratio of the PCS compared to the benchmark, is 90% for $M0^{(0)}$ and are 92 and 94% for M0 and M1, respectively. Furthermore, the benchmark results in the highest PCS under the majority of scenarios, in 11 out of 18 scenarious, the benchmark results in either higher PCS or within the simulation error. The lowest ratio of the PCS compared to the benchmark is nearly 44% for $M0^{(0)}$ and around 71–72% for M0 and M1. In some of the scenarios, the models have shown to lead to super-efficiency [18], the phenomenon when the benchmark is outperformed. This can be explained by a design favouring particular combinations. The highest ratio of PCS compared to the benchmark is also achieved for M1 under Scenario 13–32% PCS for the benchmark versus 46% for M1 resulting in the ratio of 144%. This suggests that the design favours this combination under the calibrated hyper-parameters.

The model M1 assigned at least 30% of patients to a true MTC in more scenarios than M0. Of the two models, M0 was the only one in which for two scenarios—Scenario 9 and 13—the allocation was below 20%. For the model M0, the highest percentage of DLTs observed for all the scenarios was 38% in scenario 1 whereas for M1 this value is lower at 36%, also in scenario 1. This once again highlights that the model M0 is more aggressive in patients allocations. For the model M1, in six scenarios the percentage of observed DLTs lay in the interval [29%, 31%] compared to three scenarios for M0.

The results for scenarios 15 and 16 with no MTC are given in Table 5.

Table 5. Operating characteristics of the dose-finding designs under Scenarios 15 and 16. Results are based on 4000 simulations.

Sc	15	16
Selection Percentage of The Combination Closest to 30%		
$M0^{(0)}$	95.8	88.9
M0	96.1	88.3
M1	98.9	93.9
M2	92.7	79.8
Allocation Percentage To The Combination Closest to 30%		
$M0^{(0)}$	83.1	49.9
M0	78.1	45.4
M1	90.1	58.9
M2	61.7	31.3

Under the overly toxic scenario 15, all of the models select the lowest combination with at least 92% with the minimum value of 92.7% for M2 and the highest of 98.9% for M1 (nearly 3% higher than for the calibrated model M0). Similarly, M1 allocated nearly 90% of patients to the lowest combination, which is the highest proportion among all models. Concerning, the safe scenario 16, M2 correspond to the poorest performance and selects the highest combination in nearly 80% compared to nearly 88% for both M0 models and nearly 94% for M1. The proportion of allocation is again the lowest for M2 and the highest for M1. Therefore, under both scenarios, Model 1 selects the closest to the target level combination with the highest probability and allocated more patients to the right dose.

As it was noted above, under the scenarios with several target combinations, model-based designs can favour particular combinations that will be reflected in uneven selection proportion of the target combinations. To explore this aspect of the considered models, we study the variance of each MTC selection within the scenario. Table 6 shows the variance between the percentage of selections of each possible correct MTC within the scenario for the models $M0^{(0)}$, M0, and M1.

Table 6. Variance between correct selections of MTCs in different locations throughout the combination space. GM is geometric mean. Results are based on 4000 simulations.

Scenario	2	3	4	5	6	8	10	11	12	GM
$M0^{(0)}$	18	250.7	157.9	233.8	269.1	5.1	245.9	1223.9	348.8	141.9
M0	33.4	244.5	140.1	234.0	257.6	35.7	294.3	1336.4	449.2	196.4
M1	22.4	234.5	200.5	417.0	8.9	1365.0	313.0	116.7	428.1	163.5

All of the models show poor performance in evenly selecting between multiple MTC combinations across the scenarios. Comparing calibrated models, Model M1 has a lower average variance across these scenarios of 163.5 compared to 196.4 for M0. Despite having a lower average variance, the model M1 shows a greater range of values across the scenarios. In Scenario 8, M1 shows its highest variance of 1365.0. The model M0 has nearly the same range of variance across these scenarios, where its highest variance is 1336.4 in Scenario 11.

Overall, under the operational prior distributions calibrated to achieve the highest PCS under each parameter model, the model M1 without interaction parameter was found to have the best performance in the set of considered scenarios. The model M1 has the highest average PCS and has the greatest lowest ratio of the PCS compared to the benchmark across scenarios. The model M1 allocates the highest average percentage of patients to a true MTC throughout the trial. It has the closest average percentage of observed DLTs throughout the trial to the target value of 30%. The model M1 also has the highest proportion of MTC selections in the interval [0.2, 0.4] so is, on average, selecting combinations with toxicities around the target value of $\theta = 0.3$ more often. It has also demonstrated the most accurate performance in scenarios without the MTC. Furthermore, it contaions one fewer parameter that can reduce the computations complexity of the proposed calibration procedure noticeably. One of the main drawbacks of model M1 is that it shows high variability when selecting the MTC when there are multiple possible MTCs in the combination space (e.g., Scenario 8).

5. Sensitivity Analysis: Joint Prior Distribution

5.1. Joint Prior Distribution

In the previous sections, following the approach of Riviere et al. [6], we have considered the parameters of the drug combination-toxicity relationship models to be independent. This assumption may not necessarily hold true and so we are interested in investigating whether considering the parameters to be dependent in a Phase I setting can improve the model's performance. We therefore consider an alternative model that allows for dependence between the parameters in this section. Above, it was found that the calibrated three-parameter logistic model, M1, showed the best operating characteristics amongst the models considered and therefore we will use it her again but allow for a dependence structure between the three parameters β_0, β_1 and β_2 via a joint prior distribution with a given correlation structure.

We will model the joint distribution of the model parameters using a multivariate normal distribution. To ensure the conditions on parameters β_1 and β_2 to be positive, the following parameterisation will be used to

$$(\beta_0, \beta_1, \beta_2)^T = (\tau_1, \exp(\tau_2), \exp(\tau_3))^T$$

where the 3-dimensional random vector $\boldsymbol{\tau} = (\tau_1, \tau_2, \tau_3)^T$ follows a multivariate normal distribution $\boldsymbol{\tau} \sim \mathbb{N}_3(\boldsymbol{\mu}, \boldsymbol{\Sigma})$ with mean vector $\boldsymbol{\mu}$ and 3×3 covariance matrix $\boldsymbol{\Sigma}$.

5.2. Parameters Calibration

To calibrate the joint prior, we use the same algorithm as before. The main difference being that now one needs to calibrate with respect to the correlation parameters. Specifically, using previously found calibrated values of the variance for the parameter β_0, we parametrise the covariance matrix of vector $\boldsymbol{\tau}$ as

$$\boldsymbol{\Sigma} = \begin{bmatrix} 400 & 20\rho_0\sqrt{M} & 20\rho_0\sqrt{n} \\ 20\rho_0\sqrt{m} & m & \rho_1\sqrt{mn} \\ 20\rho_0\sqrt{n} & \rho_1\sqrt{mn} & n \end{bmatrix}, \tag{6}$$

with mean $\boldsymbol{\mu} = (0, -\frac{m}{2}, -\frac{n}{2})$ \hfill (7)

for $\rho_0 \in P_0$, $\rho_1 \in P_1$, $m \in \mathcal{M}$ and $n \in \mathcal{N}$ where P_0, P_1 are sets of correlation values between the parameters and $\mathcal{M}$, $\mathcal{N}$ are sets of hyper-parameters for the variance of the prior distributions of τ_2 and τ_3, respectively. To ease the computational burden, we have fixed the value of hyper-parameter corresponding to β_0 at the value found in Section 4.3, $a = 400$ as the marginal distribution of β_0 is unchanged under this parametrisation. We have also assumed that $\text{Corr}[\tau_1, \tau_2] = \text{Corr}[\tau_1, \tau_3] = \rho_0$. This is based on the assumption that it is reasonable to assume that $\text{Corr}[\beta_0, \beta_1] = \text{Corr}[\beta_0, \beta_2]$ as the assumption that the correlation between the parameter of interaction, β_0, and the toxicity effects of agent 1, β_1; and the correlation between the parameter of interaction, β_0, and the toxicity effects of agent 2, β_2 is the same. The correlation between the two parameters τ_2 and τ_3 will be $\text{Corr}[\tau_2, \tau_3] = \rho_1$. As before, we require β_0 to be centred at zero.

As in the model M1[1], we require the parameters β_1 and β_2 to be centred at 1 such that $E[\beta_1] = E[\beta_2] = 1$. The parameters β_1 and β_2 both follow a log-normal distribution, hence, we take $\mu_2 = E[\tau_2] = -\frac{m}{2}$ and $\mu_3 = E[\tau_3] = -\frac{n}{2}$ to guarantee it.

To calibrate the covariance matrix, the following values of the hyperparameters were tried.

$$\mathcal{M} = \{0.5, 1, 1.3, 1.4, 1.5, 1.6, 2, 2.5, 5\}$$
$$\mathcal{N} = \{0.05, 0.1, 0.2, 0.4, 0.5, 0.6, 0.7, 0.8, 1\}$$
$$P_0 = \{-0.25, 0, 0.1, 0.25, 0.3, 0.4, 0.5, 0.6, 0.8\}$$
$$P_1 = \{-0.25, 0, 0.1, 0.2, 0.25, 0.3, 0.4\}$$

Under the prior distributions in model M1, its hyper-parameter values correspond to $m = 1$ and $n = 0.1$ relating to the variance of β_1 and β_2; and $\rho_0 = \rho_1 = 0$ as all the parameters in the model are independent. Higher values of m and n relate to higher variance which indicates a greater level of uncertainty for the parameters β_1 and β_2, respectively. Higher positive values of ρ_0 and ρ_1 reflect a stronger positive correlation between the two parameters in question, whilst lower negative values of ρ_0 and ρ_1 reflect a stronger negative correlation. The values of $\mathcal{M}$ and $\mathcal{N}$ on the grid were selected so that the variance of the model parameters could be both increased and decreased compared to the values in the model M1. The values of ρ_0 and ρ_1 were selected so that the parameters could be both positively and negatively correlated.

The final calibrated model M3 uses the hyper-parameter values $m = 1.6$, $n = 0.5$ and $\rho_0 = \rho_1 = 0.3$ which corresponds to a weak positive prior correlation in the parameters. This combination of hyper-parameters provided the highest average PCS across the four calibration scenarios. This model will be referred to as M3.

5.3. Results

The model M3 was used in a large scale simulation study to assess its ability to determine the MTC under the scenarios in Table 1. The simulation study setting used was the same as described in Section 4.1. Again, we use 4000 replication to provide the results. We compare the model M3 to model M1. A summary of operating characteristics are given in Table 7.

Table 7. Percentage of correct selection in comparison of 2 dose-finding designs and under the benchmark (B). Percentage of patients allocated to a true MTC during the trial and percentage of observed DLTs throughout the trial. GM is the geometric mean and Var is the variance. In the top third of the table, the highest PCS and those within less than 3% among the dose-finding designs are shown in bold for each scenario. Results are based on 4000 simulations.

Sc	1	2	2.1	2.2	3	4	5	6	6.1	6.2	7	8	9	10	11	12	13	14	GM	Var
							Percentage of correct selection (PCS)													
M1	75	60	38	42	58	55	54	55	41	36	76	57	68	52	59	40	46	31	50.8	165.2
M3	73	60	46	36	57	54	52	55	31	38	76	56	70	51	60	57	44	32	51.1	172.4
B	82	61	49	46	57	54	57	61	46	42	83	65	58	53	50	56	32	41	53.8	166.1
						Percentage of patients allocated to a true MTC during the trial														
M1	56	40	21	32	38	34	31	36	25	21	48	35	37	33	34	26	19	22	31.4	91.8
M3	56	38	24	26	36	32	30	35	20	20	48	28	36	31	33	31	21	21	30.2	90.9
							Percentage of DLTs throughout the trial													
M1	36	33	34	34	31	29	28	25	25	27	21	29	31	31	32	32	30	27	29.4	13.2
M3	36	33	35	34	31	30	28	25	25	27	21	29	31	31	32	32	30	27	29.6	14.2

The model M3 has the higher average PCS of the two models of 51.1% compared to 50.8% for model M1. Both models show a similar variance in PCS across the eighteen scenarios, however the variance is higher for the model M3 at 172.4 compared to 165.2 for M1. For 14 scenarios, the PCS for each model is within 3% of the other. In scenarios 2.1, 2.2,

6.1 and 12, the two models have PCS results that have a difference of greater than 3%. The model M1 has the higher PCS in scenarios 2.2 and 6.1. Both represent extreme examples of the dose-toxicity relationship where for scenario 2.2, many of the doses higher in the combination space are far above the MTC and for scenario 6.1, many of the doses lower in the combination space are far below the MTC. The largest difference in PCS between the two is in scenario 12 where it is possible to gain an additional 17% in PCS by selecting the model M3. At the same time, in scenario 6.1, model M3 has a PCS that is 10% lower than that of model M1. Comparing the performances to the benchmark, both model results in the ratio of average PCS of around 94%. Although, the lowest ratio of the PCS compared to the benchmark is nearly 71% for M1 under scenario 12 and 67% under scenario 6.1 for M3. Similarly to the findings for M1 above, super-efficiency can still be observed for M3, the ratio of the PCS is 138% under scenario 13 versus around 144% under the same scenario.

The model M1 on average allocates 31.4% of patients to a true MTC throughout the trial which is higher than for the model M3 which allocates 30.2%. In 14 scenarios the model M1 allocates a higher percentage of patients to a true MTC compared to only three scenarios for the model M3. In one scenario the allocation is the same. The average percentage of DLTs observed throughout the trial is highly similar for the two models at 29.6% for the model M3 compared to 29.4% for the model M1. In sixteen scenarios, the percentage of observed DLTs for each model was within 0.5% of the other and of these sixteen scenarios, the percentage of observed DLTs was the same for the two models in six scenarios.

Overall, for the operating characteristics we have studied, neither of the two models, M1 and M3, uniformly outperforms the other. The model M3 has a slightly higher average PCS so is able to locate a true MTC correctly more often under the scenarios investigated than the model M1. However, the model M1 allocates a higher average percentage of patients to a MTC throughout the trial, and allocates a higher percentage of patients to combinations with toxicity around the target value. The percentage of DLTs observed throughout the trial is similar for both models where the average values for each model is close to the targeted value of 30%. For both models, compromises in performance in one area needs to be made to achieve better performance in another.

6. Sensitivity Analysis: Different Sample Sizes

The results above concerned the setting with a sample size of up to $N = 60$ patients enrolled in the trial. One can argue that the interaction parameter could be fitted more accurately with such a sample size but not with smaller sample sizes. Therefore, in this section, we study the behaviour of various models under different sample sizes under all considered scenarios.

Specifically, we will focus on the calibrated 4-parameter model M0, calibrated 3-parameter model M1, and calibrated 3-parameter model M3 with joint prior distribution on model parameters. These were found to result in similar operating characteristics and provide the most benefit in terms of the PCS while delivering safe designs. We consider 3 sample sizes, $N = 60$ as before, and lower sample sizes $N = 48$ and $N = 30$ and fix the cohort size to be $c = 3$ in each setting. Note that the values of prior parameters for each sample size will be the same for the given model, and these parameters were calibrated for $N = 60$ and are given in Sections 4 and 5.

The results for the three model and various sample sizes based on 4000 replications are given in Figure 1.

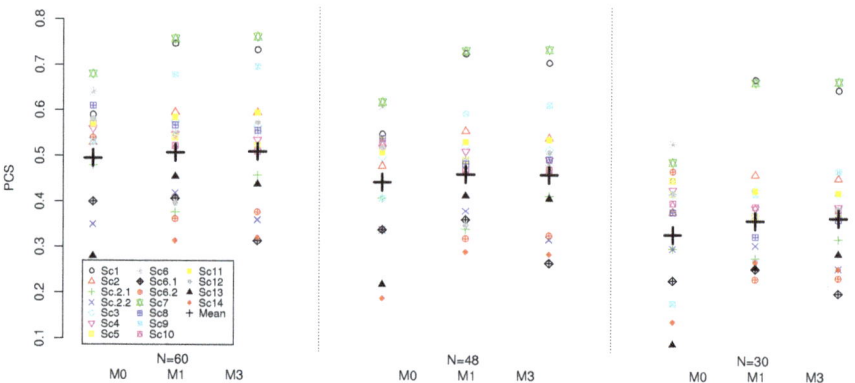

Figure 1. PCS for M0, M1 and M3 models under 18 scenarios and the sample sizes of $N = 60, 48, 30$. Results are based on 4000 replications.

Considering the PCS for each model individually, the lower sample size results in lower mean PCS for all models. The reduction in the sample size from $N = 60$ to $N = 48$ results in 5% mean PCS reduction for all three models. Further reduction from $N = 48$ to $N = 30$ results in additional nearly 9–11% for all models. Therefore, as expected, the sample size does have a major impact on accuracy of all model and larger sample sizes should be advocated for (regardless of the model used) in Phase I combination trials in order to achieve reliable recommendation of the MTC.

Comparing the models amongst themselves for a given sample size, a similar pattern as for $N = 60$ discussed in previous section can be found. The 3-parameter models perform within 0.5%, on average, for all considered sample sizes and result in higher mean PCS compared to the M0 model: nearly 1% for $N = 60$, nearly 2% for $N = 48$, and approximately 3–4% for $N = 30$. As a result, for lower sample sizes, the benefit provided by the models with fewer model parameters increases. Therefore, the interaction parameter does not seem to provide benefit in the mean PCS under the considered scenarios and, on the contrary, was found to result in lower average PCS as sample size decreases. The variance of PCS for all considered models under three considered sample sizes is similar across all three methods.

Considering other operating characteristics, the proportion of patients allocated to the MTC and the average proportion of the DLTs, all of the design performed similarly and the conclusion for $N = 60$ stand. We refer the reader to the Supplementary Materials for the complete set of results for the lower sample sizes.

Overall, under the calibrated prior distribution targeting the highest PCS, the model with interaction resulted in 1–3% lower PCS across various sample sizes compared to the model with fewer parameters while resulting in nearly the same performance on other characteristics.

7. Discussion

In this work, we have conducted an extensive simulation study of various model-based dose-finding design for combination trials. Firstly, we have proposed a formal calibration procedure for the hyper-parameters under a given parametric curve to obtain an operation prior—the prior leads that leads to high PCS across many various scenarios. Applying the same procedure to each of the models allowed for a fairer comparison between models with various parameters. This is crucial as by definition, for the same hyper-parameters, a model with fewer model parameter would bare less uncertainty. We have shown that the proposed procedure allows for the improvement of the performance of the original 4-parameter model under the considered scenarios—it resulted in slightly higher average

PCS yet noticeably more consistent performance across scenarios (reflected in the lower variance of the PCS).

Secondly, it was found that under the considered logistic-type models and the operational prior distributions calibrated to achieve the highest PCS for each model, the interaction parameters provided no benefit in terms of the PCS but resulted in lower ratio of the PCS compared to the benchmark than a model with the interaction term. The reduced number of parameters in the model has also had no negative effect on the performance under scenarios generated by the model with an interaction parameter only. Given a lower computations costs needed to calibrate fewer parameters, a logistic model with 3 parameters, the intercept, and a slope corresponding to each compound, is recommended for the consideration. We have also found that this recommendtion is consistent for various sample sizes, $N = 30, N = 48, N = 60$. Importantly, this conclusion is obtained under the assumption when no reliable prior information on the interaction between the compounds (i.e., on β_3) is available. If, however, such information is available and is indeed correct, one can expect that the model with interaction parameter can have certain benefits.

Finally, comparing the 3-parameter models, specifying the joint prior distribution for the model parameters has not provided any tangible benefit in terms of the PCS. However, it did result in lower computational costs and, therefore, could be considered in practice to speed up the calibration process proposed. Again, the conclusion is consistent across the various sample sizes.

Building on the computation aspect of the proposed calibration, it should be noted that the procedure is indeed quite computational costly given that it involves a grid search over each of the parameters. At the same time, the resulting hyper-parameters lead to good operating characteristics across many scenarios that enabled a more consistent aproach to the prior choice under the assumption of no prior knowledge about the compounds that is desired to be incorporated. If the calibration under various scenarios are parallised, it has found to result in feasible computation time. Moreover, the reader might use the parameters calibrated as the starting point in the the settings with similar numbers of doses of the compounds. At the same time, a less computationally demanding (yet reliable) procedure could be of interest and will be explored in the future.

In this work, we have focused on the comparison of designs that employ various parametric models for the combination-toxicity relationships but do not have any early stopping contraints. Constraints for stopping for safety (if all of the combinations are deemed unsafe) and stopping early for reaching a particular number of patients on one combination can easily be added.

Importantly, in this work, we have focused on a single form of the parametric curves for the combination-toxicity relationship—the logistic curve. While one could reasonably expect similar patterns under alternative parameter forms, this could be checked for a desirable model when taking a particular design forward in an actual trial. This could be done in a similar scheme to the simulation study as proposed in this manuscript. At the same time, the findings of this manuscript would warrant such an exploration.

Finally, the dual-agent setting is considered in this manuscript. However, combination studies looking at 3 and more agents could also be of interest. The extension of the proposed parametric model to more than 2 agents can be achieved via including the variables reflecting each compound. Then, the question will again be whether inclusion of the interaction terms can provide any benefits in terms of the operating characteristics and how these interaction should be included (e.g., only pairwise or should be interaction of 3 compounds be considered too). Given the findings of this work, the benefits of including interaction terms (that would complicate the estimation problem even further) should be scrutinised. It is also important to mention that the calibration procedure proposed for the setting more than 2 agents can be even more computational costly and might not be always feasible. For such cases, alternative (yet robust) approaches to the specification of the operational prior distribution should be studied.

8. Conclusions

Our study finds that carefully calibrated prior distributions can result in improved performance of the 4-parameter logistic model used for combination dose-finding. Moreover we show that only marginal benefits (if any) are seen when using an interaction term in the combination-toxicity model that are outweight by the additional complexity of the model.

Supplementary Materials: The following are available online at https://www.mdpi.com/1660-4601/18/1/345/s1. Complete set of results for the lower sample sizes.

Author Contributions: P.M. and T.J. conceptualized the research; R.K. and P.M. undertook the simulations and wrote the initial draft. H.B. undertook the calibrations and simulations for the revision of the manuscript. T.J. and H.B. reviewed and edited the manuscript. All authors have read and agreed to the published version of the manuscript.

Funding: This report is independent research supported by the National Institute for Health Research (NIHR Advanced Fellowship, Pavel Mozgunov, NIHR300576; and Jaki's Senior Research Fellowship, NIHR-SRF-2015-08-001). The views expressed in this publication are those of the authors and not necessarily those of the NHS, the National Institute for Health Research or the Department of Health and Social Care (DHCS). T Jaki received funding from UK Medical Research Council (MC_UU_0002/14).

Informed Consent Statement: Not applicable.

Data Availability Statement: R codes implementing the considered designs are available on request from the corresponding author.

Conflicts of Interest: The authors declare no conflict of interest.

Abbreviations

The following abbreviations are used in this manuscript:

MDPI	Multidisciplinary Digital Publishing Institute
DOAJ	Directory of open access journals
TLA	Three letter acronym
LD	Linear dichroism

References

1. Lu, D.Y.; Lu, T.R.; Wu, H.Y. Personalized cancer therapy, a perspective. *Clin. Exp. Pharmacol.* **2014**, *4*, 153. [CrossRef]
2. Wages, N.A.; Conaway, M.R.; O'Quigley, J. Dose-finding design for multi-drug combinations. *Clin. Trials* **2011**, *8*, 380–389. [CrossRef] [PubMed]
3. Hirakawa, A.; Wages, N.A.; Sato, H.; Matsui, S. A comparative study of adaptive dose-finding designs for phase i oncology trials of combination therapies. *Stat. Med.* **2015**, *34*, 3194–3213. [CrossRef] [PubMed]
4. Riviere, M.K.; Dubois, F.; Zohar, S. Competing designs for drug combination in phase I dose-finding clinical trials. *Stat. Med.* **2015**, *34*, 1–12. [CrossRef] [PubMed]
5. Thall, P.F.; Millikan, R.E.; Mueller, P.; Lee, S.J. Dose-finding with two agents in phase I oncology trials. *Biometrics* **2003**, *59*, 487–496. [CrossRef] [PubMed]
6. Riviere, M.K.; Yuan, Y.; Dubois, F.; Zohar, S. A Bayesian dose-finding design for drug combination clinical trials based on the logistic model. *Pharm. Stat.* **2014**, *13*, 247–257. [CrossRef] [PubMed]
7. Neuenschwander, B.; Matano, A.; Tang, Z.; Roychoudhury, S.; Wandel, S.; Bailey, S. A Bayesian industry approach to phase I combination trials in oncology. In *Statistical Methods in Drug Combination Studies*; Zhao, W., Yang, H., Eds.; Chapman & Hall/CRC Press: Boca Raton, FL, USA, 2015; Chapter 6, pp. 95–135.
8. Cunanan, K.; Koopmeiners, J.S. Evaluating the performance of copula models in phase I-II clinical trials under model misspecification. *BMC Med. Res. Methodol.* **2014**, *14*, 51. [CrossRef] [PubMed]
9. Mozgunov, P.; Gasparini, M.; Jaki, T. A Surface-Free Design for Phase I Dual-Agent Combination Trials. *Stat. Methods Med. Res.* **2020**, *29*, 3093–3109. [CrossRef] [PubMed]
10. Wages, N.A.; Conaway, M.R.; O'Quigley, J. Continual reassessment method for partial ordering. *Biometrics* **2011**, *67*, 1555–1563. [CrossRef] [PubMed]
11. Mander, A.P.; Sweeting, M.J. A product of independent beta probabilities dose escalation design for dual-agent phase i trials. *Stat. Med.* **2015**, *34*, 1261–1276. [CrossRef] [PubMed]

12. Plummer, M. *rjags: Bayesian Graphical Models Using MCMC*; R package version 4-10; 2019. Available online: https://CRAN.R-project.org/package=rjags (accessed on 4 January 2020).
13. Zohar, S.; Chevret, S. The continual reassessment method: Comparison of bayesian stopping rules for dose-ranging studies. *Stat. Med.* **2001**, *20*, 2827–2843. [CrossRef] [PubMed]
14. Wheeler, G.M.; Mander, A.P.; Bedding, A.; Brock, K.; Cornelius, V.; Grieve, A.P.; Jaki, T.; Love, S.B.; Weir, C.J.; Yap, C.; et al. How to design a dose-finding study using the continual reassessment method. *BMC Med. Res. Methodol.* **2019**, *19*, 1–15. [CrossRef] [PubMed]
15. Brock, K.; Billingham, L.; Copl, ; M.; Siddique, S.; Sirovica, M.; Yap, C. Implementing the EffTox dose-finding design in the Matchpoint trial. *BMC Med. Res. Methodol.* **2017**, *17*, 112. [CrossRef] [PubMed]
16. Mozgunov, P.; Paoletti, X.; Jaki, T. A benchmark for dose finding studies with unknown ordering. *Biostatistics* **2020**. [CrossRef]
17. O'Quigley, J.; Paoletti, X.; Maccario, J. Non-parametric optimal design in dose finding studies. *Biostatistics* **2002**, *3*, 51–56. [CrossRef] [PubMed]
18. Paoletti, X.; O'Quigley, J.; Maccario, J. Design efficiency in dose finding studies. *Comput. Stat. Data Anal.* **2004**, *45*, 197–214. [CrossRef]

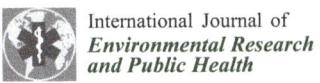

Review

The Bayesian Design of Adaptive Clinical Trials

Alessandra Giovagnoli †

Department of Statistical Sciences, University of Bologna, 40126 Bologna, Italy; alessandra.giovagnoli@unibo.it
† Retired.

Abstract: This paper presents a brief overview of the recent literature on adaptive design of clinical trials from a Bayesian perspective for statistically not so sophisticated readers. Adaptive designs are attracting a keen interest in several disciplines, from a theoretical viewpoint and also—potentially—from a practical one, and Bayesian adaptive designs, in particular, have raised high expectations in clinical trials. The main conceptual tools are highlighted here, with a mention of several trial designs proposed in the literature that use these methods, including some of the registered Bayesian adaptive trials to this date. This review aims at complementing the existing ones on this topic, pointing at further interesting reading material.

Keywords: adaptive designs; adaptive randomization; Bayesian designs; clinical trials; predictive power; target allocation

Citation: Giovagnoli, A. The Bayesian Design of Adaptive Clinical Trials. *Int. J. Environ. Res. Public Health* **2021**, *18*, 530. https://doi.org/10.3390/ijerph18020530

Received: 25 November 2020
Accepted: 6 January 2021
Published: 10 January 2021

Publisher's Note: MDPI stays neutral with regard to jurisdictional clai-ms in published maps and institutio-nal affiliations.

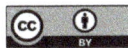

Copyright: © 2021 by the author. Licensee MDPI, Basel, Switzerland. This article is an open access article distributed under the terms and conditions of the Creative Commons Attribution (CC BY) license (https://creativecommons.org/licenses/by/4.0/).

1. Introduction

This paper is a bird's eye view of the recent literature on adaptive designs of clinical trials from a Bayesian perspective. Statistics plays a prominent role in the design as well as the analysis of the results of a clinical study and Bayesian ideas are well received by clinicians. In their book, Spiegelhalter and his coauthors [1] make a strong case in favour of Bayesian methods in health care, and in the last two decades Bayesian statistics has had a large impact in the medical field (see the superb review by Ashby [2]), the more so as its implementation gets easier thanks to better computational facilities. "Bayesian clinical trials: no more excuses" is the title of an editorial in Vol 6(3) of *Clinical Trials* [3]. The Bayesian approach has a good reputation at producing scientific openness and honesty.

The Bayesian paradigm is especially appropriate at the planning stage of a clinical trial, when external information, such as historical data, findings from previous studies, and expert opinions, is often available and awaiting to be made the most of. As Donald Berry and his colleagues state in [4], we are all Bayesian at the design stage! Health authorities have issued important statements on the statistical, clinical and regulatory aspects of Bayesian clinical trials ([5,6]), recently allowing and even advocating the use of innovative methods, in particular adaptive design; as the editors of this Special Issue point out, most statistical and biomedical journals have recently hosted proposals of trial designs with a Bayesian slant, in some cases virtual re-executions of published trials. A search carried out in PubMed in August 2020 has returned nearly 300 publications (half of them published in the last decade) which either propose or use Bayesian adaptive methods in the design of a clinical trial. This may be also thanks to the popularization by Donald Berry [7–11] and the efforts made by statisticians working in the pharmaceutical industry, one of the main players in the design of clinical trials, to incorporate Bayesian methods. This is shown in leading journals in clinical trial methodology, like *Pharmaceutical Statistics*, *The Journal of Biopharmaceutical Statistics* or *Biometrical Journal*.

Some confusion occasionally arises between the concepts of "Bayesian" and of "adaptive" design, because of similarities in the outlook: in the Bayesian paradigm, accrued data are used to update the prior distribution on the parameters, via Bayes' Theorem, and in response-adaptive experiments the accrued data are used at each step, namely after each observation or predefined group of observations, to update the next planning decision. Either approach (Bayesian or adaptive) can stand on its own, and has developed independently of the other: we clarify this point later.

We are interested in trial designs that are both Bayesian and adaptive. The data are recursively evaluated during the experiment: the posterior parameter distribution is recursively updated and used to modify the execution of the trial according to *a previously established rule*. The textbook by Berry, Carlin, Lee, and Muller [12] successfully illustrates Bayesian adaptive methods in clinical research and deals with design issues too. It goes almost without saying that randomization is a must in a clinical trial (for Bayesians too), to counteract several types of bias, for instance selection bias.

The subject is advancing fast in many directions and it is impossible to keep up with all the different threads. Dealing with this topic properly would require several books. In this paper it has been chosen to focus on the methodology, followed by several examples of instances in which the methods are applied. The subject matter is organized as follows: Section 2 is a general discussion of Bayesian designs. In Section 3 we summarize the theory of response-adaptive designs from the *frequentist* viewpoint, with emphasis on their importance in clinical studies. Moving on to Bayesian adaptive trial designs, Section 4 deals with the different methodological approaches (utility-based, probability-only, predictive) and their use for randomization, sample size determination and early stopping. Section 5 reports examples from the literature. Section 6 lists some well-known real life trials performed according to a Bayesian adaptive design. In Section 7 we mention the on-going debate on the relevance of response-adaptive randomization designs in clinical trials, although at present the controversy is not directly addressed to Bayesian methods. Conclusions are drawn in Section 8.

2. Bayesian Designs

To start with, the very meaning of the term "Bayesian design" has to be contextualized. It is important to specify whether the Bayesian approach relates just to the pre-experimental plan, or to the analysis of the data as well. Because "Bayesian" is sometimes taken to mean "subjective", for clinical trials an "objective" data analysis is often preferred. In clinical trials in particular the operating characteristics of the design often include the power of some statistical test, strictly speaking a non-Bayesian feature. So some studies are hybrid: the inference is frequentist, but a prior probability on the parameters is used at the design stage. Several authors, for example Ventz et al. [13] have presented ways of combining Bayesian models and frequentist analyses in clinical trials. At the start, design issues were neglected by Bayesian statisticians, but Bayesian design has latterly become a well-established subdiscipline, as shown by the outstanding number of quotations of Chaloner and Verdinelli's [14] paper throughout the years. Unfortunately, that review has never been updated, and does not mention the topic of adaptive design, which at the time was only beginning to appear in the literature.

As is well known, in the Bayesian model-based paradigm, the parameters of the model are treated as random quantities and the a priori knowledge about unknown effects of the interventions is expressed by means of a prior probability distribution on the model parameters. In the non-adaptive case, the experiment is designed entirely before the new data are acquired, and its performance may depend on the data still to be observed The fully Bayesian way to designing the trial would be a utility-based one, in accordance with Lindley [15]. In the model-based approach, the utility $\mathcal{U}$ will be a function of the experimental plan, the data y, and the model parameter values θ. A design action (deterministic or randomized) is chosen so as to maximize the expectation of the utility function with respect to the joint distribution of the parameters *and* the future data.

In the eighties Smith and Verdinelli [16], Giovagnoli and Verdinelli [17] and Chaloner [18] proposed Bayesian designs that maximize the precision of the posterior distribution of the treatment effects under a linear statistical model. For non-linear models, Chaloner and Larntz [19] suggested choosing the design that optimizes the expectation, with respect to the parameters' prior, of one of the well-known design criteria: the best known ones—the so-called D-optimality and trace-optimality for instance ("Optimal design" [20])—have also Bayesian interpretations. Since optimality criteria are functions of the Fisher information matrix, which is already an average over the possible responses, this approach too is not conditional on the data. This suggestion has become very popular and keeps being used in the literature, with many variants, not all of which are entirely convincing.

It should be stressed that the choice of a suitable utility function is related to the objectives of the trial. The specification of the function $\mathcal{U}$ is certainly demanding, as various aspects of the decision context have to be formally quantified. The main purpose of any experiment is obviously inference. Even if the subjects are patients, the main goal of a trial is knowledge, not healthcare, so the expected gain in information is a relevant component of $\mathcal{U}$. In the past, designs for Bayesian analysis of the data would mostly choose utility functions based on Shannon information or on a quadratic loss. Nowadays, it is not uncommon to find Bayesian designs motivated by the precision of the estimates and power of the tests, in view of the fact that the experimental data will be analysed by frequentist tools. On the other hand, in a clinical trial the utility function may also need to reflect care for the subjects involved in the experiment. An opposite, rather extreme, example in the binary response case is the 0–1 utility: the gain is 1 for success, 0 for failure, which takes no account of inference. Since a clinical trial is a multi-objective experiment, the utility will more likely be a trade-off between several purposes: ethical, inferential and possibly economic. Verdinelli and Kadane [21] suggested a utility function which is a linear combination of the total expected value of future observations and the Shannon's information of the experiment. Clyde and Chaloner [22] too have proposed weighted combinations of utility functions, which are still mathematically valid utilities. In this way optimal designs for multiple objectives can be handled in the decision-theoretic framework, so long as the utilities are standardized to a comparable scale. For instance with binary outcomes one of the usual optimality criteria—determinant or trace, standardized—can be combined with the percentage of expected successes. Clyde and Chaloner [22] show that this approach is equivalent to finding the optimal experiment under one (primary) criterion subject to constraints on the minimal efficiency of the experiment under criteria for other objectives. The weights will be chosen by the experimenter to reflect the relative importance given to each utility component: it is advisable that the ethical and/or economic impact should not completely outweigh the inferential goal.

Bayesian non-adaptive design has had numerous applications in clinical trials up to the end of the nineties and beyond, as shown in the paper by Ashby [2].

3. Adaptive Designs: The Frequentist Approach

Response-adaptive—or simply adaptive—experiments are those in which the accrued data and the past allocations are used at each step to choose how to perform the next observations, according to pre-established rules. In statistics, "response-adaptive" (sometimes also "flexible") is a technical term. It means a predefined step-wise sequential algorithm which prescribes the modalities of the next step as a (deterministic or probabilistic) function of the accrued data. The choice of the pre-established rule is an essential part of the design—as indicated by the FDA [6]— and must be taken into account to draw correct inferences. Response-adaptive design does not mean simply that at any stage you may want to change your plans. It should be stressed that the updating process of an experiment cannot take place in a haphazard manner, which could undermine the ensuing statistical analysis of the data. Typically it could lead to miscalculating the variance of the estimates or to drawing wrong conclusions. Burman and Sonesson [23] give a very clear-minded discussion. Thus the correct design of adaptive experiments poses challenging statistical problems: because of the dependence on the past data, the design itself will be a stochastic process, whose realization is the sequence of actual assignments of the experiment.

A good introduction to adaptive designs is Chapter 1 of the collective volume edited by Pong and Chow [24]. It is useful to distinguish among the different types of adaptation useable in clinical trials:

(1) Adaptive allocation rule—change in the randomization procedure to modify the allocation proportion.
(2) Adaptive sampling rule—change in the number of study subjects (sample size) or change in study population: entry criteria for the patients change.
(3) Adaptive stopping rule—during the course of the trial, a data-dependent rule dictates whether and when to stop for harm/futility/efficacy.
(4) Adaptive enrichment: during the trial, treatments are added or dropped.

A more detailed classification is the one by Huskins et al. [25]. All types of adaptation may also take into account covariates, i.e., the patient's prognostic factors/biomarkers. Adaptation may aim to ensure approximate balance of categorical covariates between the treatment arms in randomization (minimization and stratified randomization methods) or to best suit the characteristics of the subjects in the trial, when the covariates are of the "predictive" type, namely they interact with the treatments.

Despite the intricacies of the theory, including whether inference should be conditional on the design or unconditional as Baldi-Antognini and Giovagnoli point out [26], adaptive methods are attractive to experimenters: they look and sometimes are more flexible, efficient, ethical and/or economical, and proceeding sequentially seems to reflect real life practice. Among the possible applications, at present the clinical ones are playing a prominent role, to the point that response-adaptive designs are almost identified with clinical trials, notwithstanding their relevance in other disciplines: experimental economics, computer science, aerodynamics, combustion engineering, psychology, social sciences, and many others, as a simple search in Google Scholar easily shows. Altogether, adaptive design seems to be a more congenial perspective for practicing clinicians. Adaptive procedures are often feasible in clinical trials, in which typically the recruitment of subjects takes place sequentially, especially when they are healthy volunteers. In particular, they are fairly frequent in early phase studies, because of the inherently adaptive nature of such trials. The "steps" may consist of just one observation at-a-time, or more than one, as explained earlier. They may also represent natural stages of the experiment. Even a two-stage trial may be regarded as adaptive, if it is ruled in advance what decisions will be made conditional on the first stage data. Clearly such step-by-step procedures must be described and justified in the study protocol. A review of the literature unfortunately shows that some trials described as adaptive report not-so-rigorous ad-hoc adjustments of the experimental design along the way.

A quick overview of non-Bayesian adaptive designs methods may be helpful, to present the main ideas. An authoritative starting point is Rosenberger's 1996 review [27] but important methodological advances have been made since.

3.1. Dose Finding

Trials for new drug development involve dose-finding. In Phase I we are usually interested in finding which value of the dosage x will produce a prescribed mean response, typically a small tolerated amount of toxicity. The experimental problem is essentially adaptive by its very nature: after each observation a decision has to be taken as to whether to leave the dosage unaltered for the next cohort or change it. There are the so-called rule-based designs without assumptions on the dose-toxicity response curve, like the notorious 3 + 3 rule. I have chosen not to dwell on these non-Bayesian methods, since a description can be easily found in several books about statistical methods in clinical trials. Another non parametric method is the Up-and-Down design, in which the assignment rule of the next patient involves a random component: see for instance Baldi-Antognini and Giovagnoli [26] for the theoretical properties. Surprisingly, only few developments of the Up-and-Down incorporating Bayesian ideas have taken place.

In the parametric set-up, the mean response is modelled as a smooth increasing function Q(x, θ) of the dose, depending on an unknown vector parameter θ. Frequent choices for Q(x, θ) are the logistic quantile function and the probit function. The parameter θ can be recursively estimated through Maximum Likelihood. The design problem is how to modify the doses efficiently each time.

Adaptive ideas show their potential also in "seamless" designs for Phase I and Phase II simultaneously ([28]), or Phase II together with Phase III ([29]).

3.2. Response-Adaptive Randomization

When equal allocation to the treatment arms was regarded as optimum, the only accepted randomization rule with two treatments was "tossing a fair coin". Since Efron ([30]), randomization schemes that move away from the traditional equal allocation have gained consent. Efron's *Biased Coin* is a randomization rule skewed in favour of the under-represented treatment(s), regardless of the data; response-adaptive randomization, on the other hand, is a "biased coin" that skews the allocations using the accrued data, usually to favour the best performing treatment. An important introduction to the mathematics of response adaptive randomization in clinical trials is the book by Hu and Rosenberger [31].

For two treatments A and B with binary responses and p_A and p_B success probabilities, basic methods are the well-known Play-the-Winner and Randomized Play-the-Winner: see the book by Rosenberger and Lachin [32] for details and also for recent theoretical developments in adaptive randomization. The modern approach consist in first choosing an ideal allocation proportion of the treatments—a "target"—obtained by a trade-off between several purposes: ethical, inferential and possibly economic, as suggested by Baldi-Antognini and Giovagnoli [33]: see also [34]. Then an adaptive, possibly randomized, procedure is devised with the property of converging to this target allocation for all values of the unknown model parameters. Suggested adaptive rules that achieve this purpose are the Sequential Maximum Likelihood design, the Doubly-adaptive Biased Coin Design and the Efficient Randomized Adaptive Design (ERADE), which is a response-adaptive version of Efron's Biased Coin rule. These are explained, for instance, in Chapter 1 of the collective book edited by Sverdlov [35] that contains a description of the state-of-the art in adaptive randomization in clinical trials. The other contributions in the same volume dwell on further developments.

3.3. Sequential Monitoring

Selecting the sample size is the number one design concern in almost all experiments. In frequentist statistics the sample size is usually calculated so as to achieve a prescribed power for the statistical test of interest, under reasonable assumptions for the true state of nature. An adaptive approach to this problem is typically applied in clinical trials, when the trial design is in two or more stages. At the end of each stage the appropriate sample size for the next stage gets re-estimated, making use of the accrued data.

The sample size issue is also related to early stopping, since as is well-known in clinical trials another approach is to fix a (maximum) number for the sample and include the possibility to stop earlier, if certain conditions are met. Interim analyses of the data at predetermined time periods are conducted before the data collection has been completed, in order to stop the trial early if some of the treatments tested show to be clearly harmful or clearly useless, or obviously superior. This is the oldest practice in adaptive design, usually referred to as *group-sequential*. Decision rules for stopping consist in setting boundaries for a predetermined test statistic so that some error probability requirements are satisfied. There is a rich literature on this topic [36–39]. Adaptive early termination has been applied, for instance, in the recent 2020 World Health Organization Solidarity Trial for COVID-19 [40].

In bio-pharmaceutical experiments the attention has focussed in particular on stochastic curtailment ([41]). The stochastic curtailment rule computes the conditional power, i.e., the conditional probability that the summary statistics at the end of the trial is in the rejection region, given the current data available, under the null hypothesis of no effect or the alternative hypothesis (a clinically significant difference). This approach is based on a "prediction", thus it leans towards the Bayesian philosophy.

Group-sequential designs in general do not consider treatment allocations other than equal size randomization. For some models, however, Jennison and Turnbull [42] have shown that response-adaptive randomization can be incorporated into a general family of group sequential tests without affecting the error probabilities. Zhu and Hu [43] have studied both theoretical and finite sample properties of designs which combine sequential monitoring with response-adaptive randomization.

4. The Bayesian Viewpoint in Response-Adaptive Designs

Adaptive designs are (deterministic or randomized) rules that at each stage of the trial, conditionally on the accrued data, prescribe how to choose the treatment assignments and/or include new or drop old treatments and/or choose the sample size for the next experimental stage and/or choose the next patients, and/or decide whether to stop the trial. In the Bayesian set-up, in order to choose the next step's or stage's settings in an optimal way the design rule makes use of the posterior distribution of the parameters, updated each time. If the approach is decision-based, the design rule recursively optimizes the posterior expected utility. Posterior distributions may also be used in more direct ways in the design of the experiment, without the decision theoretic framework, as we shall see in Section 4.1 about adaptive randomization. In the binary case, posterior probabilities correspond to the choice of the simplistic utility, where the gain is 1 for success, 0 for failure. An essential Bayesian tool is also the predictive probability of yet unobserved events, conditional on past data. Predictive distributions are useful in many adaptive design contexts, like trial monitoring and also deciding whether to conduct a future trial. Their use is shown in many clinical contexts in the book by Berry et al. [12].

Recently, Bayesian methods are more and more to be found naturally embedded in most of the emergent adaptive design ideas: the Continuous Reassessment Method for dose-finding in Phase I (see Section 5) is a typical example. Important review articles are by Chevret [44], who searched adaptive Bayesian design in the medical literature up to 2010, and by Rosner [45], who deals with Bayesian adaptive design in drug development.

Bayesian adaptive designs are sometimes called BAD, not a very exciting acronym! When the randomization rule is adaptive, they are called Bayesian Adaptive Randomization (BAR), Bayesian RAR or Bayesian Response-Adaptive Randomization (BRAR); we prefer Bayesian Adaptively Randomized Designs (BARDs), a much more inspiring acronym. In the literature there is occasionally a temptation to describe as Bayesian some adaptive designs that make no use of priors or posteriors, like the Bayesian Biased Coin Design by Atkinson and Biswas [46].

4.1. Bayesian Adaptive Randomization

The need to randomize treatments to patients is mandatory in all clinical trials, and is used in each Phase whenever possible, although it tends to be studied with particular reference to Phase III: these are multicenter case-control studies on large patient groups (300–3000 or more), aimed at assessing how effective the proposed new intervention(s) is in comparison with the current "gold standard".

In spite of the popularity of Bayesian adaptive methods, Bayesian adaptive randomization for clinical trials does not seem to have been investigated extensively, as pointed out in the book by Atkinson and Biswas [47]. There is no straightforward Bayesian equivalent of Play-the-Winner for the case of binary data and two treatments, which is not surprising since Play-the-Winner is a myopic strategy, based on the most recent result, whereas the Bayesian paradigm is characterized by its use of all the past data.

The very early paper by Thompson [48] is worth a special mention, because its Bayesian way to randomization in the binary model—reminiscent of the Randomized Play-the-Winner, and called "probability only"—is still very popular to this day.

"If P is the probability estimate (meaning the posterior probability) that one treatment is better than a second, as judged by data at present available, then we might take some monotone increasing function of P, say f(P), to fix the fraction of such individuals to be treated in the first manner until more evidence may be utilised, where $0 \leq f(P) \leq 1$; the remaining fraction of such individuals $(1 - f(P))$ to be treated in the second manner; or we may establish a probability of treatment by the two methods of f(P) and $1 - f(P)$, respectively". (Thompson, [48])

When $f(P) = P$ this method is referred to as *randomized probability matching*: it is ethical from the patients' viewpoint but pays no attention to inference. However the function f may be chosen so as to act as a stabilizing transformation, to avoid excess variability which has a negative effect on the inferential efficiency. It has become customary to take $f(P)$ and $1 - f(P)$ proportional to $[\Pr(p_A > p_B \mid y)]^v$ and $[\Pr(p_B > p_A \mid y)]^v$, respectively, where v is a positive quantity that modulates the tradeoff between the exploration (gaining information) and the exploitation (benefit for the patients) aims of the experiment. The value of v recommended by Thall and Wathen [49], based on empirical experience, is $v = \frac{1}{2}$, or $v = n/2N$, where n is the present sample size and N the total proposed one. Extensions of the theory allow the progressive reassessment of v based on interim analysis data.

In principle, the idea of adaptive randomized designs converging to a prescribed target can be used in a Bayesian context as well. A utility function is chosen and at each step, a "temporary" target is found by optimizing the posterior expected utility. This pseudo-target—which is conditional on the data and gets updated each time—will be used, possibly after a suitable transformation, as the allocation probability of the randomization scheme. The intuitive meaning is to try to allocate the treatments—at each step—in the way that is optimal according to the present information. It may be looked at as a Bayesian equivalent of the frequentist Sequential Maximum Likelihood design mentioned in Section 3.2.

4.2. Sample Size Determination and Early Stopping

Although for a Bayesian analysis of the data in principle there is no need for pre-planned sample sizes, nevertheless Bayesian design does consider sample size selection, both for practical reasons and for a potential classical inferential analysis. The prior distribution of the unknown quantities may be incorporated into finding the appropriate sample size in more ways than one (utility-based, pre-posterior, ecc.); see for instance [50]. Instead of the conditional power, the predictive power is often used, namely the predictive probability of rejecting the null hypothesis of no effect, or of no difference among effects: this approach indicates how the sample size of a clinical trial is to be adjusted so as to claim a success at the conclusion of the trial with an expected probability. The same ideas can be used when the trial is planned to be performed adaptively; at the end of each step the sample size of the next step will be selected.

As to sequential monitoring, Donald Berry [51] and Spiegelhalter and Freedman [52] were perhaps the very first to suggest the application of Bayesian tools for the decision to stop the trial before the planned sample size is reached. Monitoring can be based on the posterior probabilities of the hypotheses of interest, like the posterior probability that the treatment benefit lies above or below some boundary, or based on the predictive probabilities of the consequences of continuing the study; the predictive power, namely the expectation of the power function with respect to the distribution of the true underlying effect size, is often relevant when deciding on whether to stop a clinical trial for futility. Useful references are [53,54]. Alternatively, the decision of whether to interrupt the trial may derive from a proper utility function that quantifies the gain associated with the consequences of stopping or continuing. A good discussion of the appropriateness of the different Bayesian decision rules is found in the books by Spiegelhalter et al. [1] and Berry et al. [12], and in [55].

5. Suggestions of Bayesian Adaptive Design from the Literature

The best known Bayesian adaptive rule is the Continual Reassessment Method (CRM) by O'Quigley et al. [56,57] for Phase I: Cheung [58] devotes an entire book to it. It is aimed at finding a given quantile of the dose-response function $Q(x, \theta)$, with θ the unknown vector parameter. Often the response is toxicity and we are looking for the dose x_p^* corresponding to a given maximum probability p^* of toxicity, called Maximum Tolerated Dose (MTD). Given a prior on θ, the expected value of x_p^* is calculated and the next set of observations is taken at the dose level nearest to it. The process is then iterated recusively and it can be proved to converge to the MTD. The main advantage of this design is that the majority of observations are centered around the dosage of interest.

Many variants of the CRM have appeared over the years to handle different clinical scenarios, such as separate groups or late-onset toxicity. In particular:

- The TITE-CRM by Cheung and Chappell [59] incorporates the time-to-event of each patient allowing patients to be entered in a staggered fashion.
- Escalation with Overdose Control (EWOC) by Babb and Rogatko [60]: it is the same as CRM, except for the use of the αth-quantile of the MTD's posterior, instead of its mean, when selecting the next dose. This allows rapid dose escalation while controlling the probability of exceeding MDT. The extension of EWOC to covariate utilization permits personalization of the dose level for each specific patient.
- The STARPAC design [61] uses a traditional rule-based design until the first patient has a dose limiting toxicity and then switches to a modified CRM.
- Yin and Yuan [62] use the rather controversial idea of averaging the statistical model with respect to the parameter prior in conjunction with the Continuous Reassessment Method.

Still about dose-finding trials of Phase I with a binary toxicity endpoint, examples of Bayes design rules obtained in a decision theoretic framework are:

- The modified Toxicity Probability Interval (mTPI) design [63]. The decision to escalate or de-escalate the dose is made by partitioning the probability interval into three subintervals. The posterior probability that p^* is in each subinterval is calculated, divided by the width of the subinterval. The interval with the highest posterior probability mass dictates the dose decision for the next patient. The mTPI possesses desirable large- and small-sample properties. These designs are compared in a numerical study in [64].
- The Adaptive Bayesian Compound Design by McGree et al. [65]: the authors use a compound utility functions to account for the dual experimental goals of estimating the MTD and addressing the safety of subjects.

Bayesian optimal design theory is used adaptively in a two-stage Phase I design by Haines et al. [66].

There has been a widespread use of Bayesian response-adaptive randomization methods.

- Thompson's idea for adaptive randomization, extended from the case of two treatment arms to several arms, has been applied by Thall, Inoue and Martin [67] to the design of a lymphocyte infusion trial.
- Under a beta-binomial model, Yuan, Huang and Liu [68] design a trial for leukemia. The randomization assigns an incoming patient to the treatment arm such that the imbalance of a prognostic score across the treatments is minimized. This score depends on an unknown parameter whose posterior mean is continuously updated during the ongoing trial.
- Still for the Beta Binomial model, in Giovagnoli [69] the trace criterion is used as the utility function and a recursive "biased coin" is found that maximizes the posterior utility. The sequential randomized treatment allocation is shown to converge to Neyman's classical target, namely the optimal one according to the trace criterion.
- Under the same model, Xiao et al. [70] have defined a Bayesian Doubly-adaptive Biased Coin Design, using the posterior probabilities of $p_A > p_B$ and of $p_B > p_A$, for the target and an assignment rule similar to the ERADE mentioned in Section 3.2. They

derive some asymptotic properties of their Bayesian design, namely convergence and asymptotic normality of the allocation proportion.

➢ Giovagnoli and Verdinelli [71] choose a recursive target that optimizes the posterior expectation of a compound utility function and the ERADE algorithm for convergence.

Turning to sample size determination and early stopping, sequential stopping is mainly associated with Phase II trials, but as early as 1994, Thall and Simon [72] developed a design with continuous monitoring until a high posterior probability is achieved that a drug is promising or that it is not promising, or until reaching the maximum sample size. This idea has been further refined and modified by a multitude of authors.

- Wang [73] predicts how the sample size of a clinical trial needs to be adjusted so as to claim a success at the conclusion of the trial with an expected probability.
- An interesting evaluation paper is by Uemura et al. [74].
- Continuous monitoring by means of predictive probabilities is given by Lee and Liu [75]: for the binary case, under a beta-binomial model, and a given maximum sample size, they recursively calculate the predictive probability of concluding the study rejecting the hypothesis of no efficacy of the new treatment. They search for the design parameters within the given constraints such that both the size and power of the test can be guaranteed.
- Yin, Chen and Lee [76] have coupled Thompson's adaptive randomization design with predictive probability approaches for Phase II.
- Zhong et al. [77] introduce a two-stage design with sample size re-estimation at the interim stage which uses a fully Bayesian predictive approach to reduce an overly large initial sample size when necessary.

Decision-theoretic methods have been applied in this context too, for example by Cheng and Shen [78] for a comparative two-armed clinical trial. They specify a loss function, based on the cost for each patient and the costs of making incorrect decisions at the end of the trial. At each interim analysis, the decision to terminate or to continue the trial is based on the expected loss function while concurrently incorporating efficacy, futility and cost. The maximum number of interim analyses is determined adaptively by the observed data.

6. Bayesian Adaptive Designs in Registered Trials

Adaptive designs are mathematically sophisticated instruments. Their development is fairly recent, and the split that can be observed between theory and practice is not at all surprising. There are several obstacles—both technical and practical—to launching an adaptive trial, beyond the significant time and effort required by any clinical trial. Among other things, adaptive design requires updating information on accrued data, the speed of acquisition may be highly variable so there is the need to identify short-term endpoints that can be used to accurately predict treatment responses such as long-term mortality in terms of a gold-standard endpoint. The steps required to establish this type of design in a novel context are indeed fairly complex, as some case studies show (see for instance Mason et al. [79]. As to the Bayesian approach, this may include specialized software programs to run the study design, only made possible by recent advancements in computational algorithms and computer hardware ([80]).

Nevertheless, it is worth remarking that the philosophy of Bayesian adaptive designs has already made its way into the clinic. They are now fairly well established in cancer research ([10]), and to a lesser extent, in other clinical areas. As well as single study designs, Bayesian adaptive methods are being employed to build "platform" designs (Adaptive Platform Trials). These are trials for simultaneous testing of multiple treatment strategies in separate groups, with plans to discontinue any group that is definitively inferior at planned interim analyses. Trial patients are enrolled in a continuous manner via a common master protocol, with interventions entering and leaving the platform on the basis of a predefined decision algorithm. Several Adaptive Platform Trials are now funded in various disease areas (see Angus et al. [81], Brown et al. [82] and Talisa et al. [83] for a discussion).

The following is a non-exhaustive list of recent or still on-going clinical trials that incorporate Bayesian adaptive design features:

- The Randomized Embedded Multifactorial Adaptive Platform Trial in Community Acquired Pneumonia (REMAP-CAP): see [84]. It has set-up a sub-platform called "REMAP–COVID" on which the evaluation of specific treatments for COVID-19 is run.
- Anti-Thrombotic Therapy to Ameliorate Complications of COVID-19 (ATTACC) (see [85]), similar in purpose to RECAP-COVID.
- GBM AGILE, an adaptive clinical trial to deliver improved treatments for glioblastoma, now open and enrolling patients ([86]).
- STURDY, a randomized clinical trial of Vitamin D supplement doses for the prevention of falls in older adults ([87]).
- The SPRINT trial on safety and efficacy of neublastin in painful lumbosacral radiculopathy ([88]).
- SARC009: A Phase II study in patients with previously treated, high-grade, advanced sarcoma ([89]).
- The SHINE clinical trial for hyperglycaemia in stroke patients ([90,91]).
- The EPAD project in neurology ([92]).
- The BATTLE and BATTLE-2 trials for lung cancer ([93,94]).
- The I-SPY 2 platform for breast cancer chemotherapy ([95]; see also [96–98]).
- A study on Lemborexant, for the treatment of insomnia disorder ([99]).
- A Phase I non-randomized trial of a combination therapy in patients with pancreatic adenocarcinoma ([100]).
- A first-in-human study of RG7342 for the treatment of schizophrenia in healthy male subjects ([101]).
- A newly started Phase II trial in Japan for sarcoma ([102]) also shows the utility of a Bayesian adaptive design.
- A Bayesian response-adaptive trial in tuberculosis is the endTB trial ([103]).
- Acute Stroke Therapy by Inhibition of Neutrophils (ASTIN) was a Bayesian adaptive phase 2 dose-response study to establish whether UK-279,276 improves recovery in acute ischemic stroke. The adaptive design facilitated early termination for futility ([104]).

7. Controversies

There is an on-going debate on adaptive designs in clinical trials. The criticisms are not addressed specifically to Bayesian methods, nor to the general class of adaptive designs, but circle around the value of response-adaptive randomization in clinical trials. The much criticized Michigan ECMO trial (see [105,106]), which took place 35 years ago, is often advocated to discourage the use of response-adaptive randomization in practice. It is not an aim of this paper to get involved in these controversies: among the rest, there are still too many open methodological questions surrounding the use of adaptive designs and their inference, whether Bayesian or not. On the other hand, it would be unfair not to mention the existence of this debate.

First of all the usefulness of adaptive randomized design is questioned: Korn and Freidlin [107] and Yuan and Yin [108] suggest that in the binary case outcome-adaptive randomization might not have substantial advantages over fixed-ratio when the response rate of the experimental treatment is not substantially higher than that of the standard treatment. Berry [109], however, disproves their conclusion. Korn and Freidlin [110] examine further the negative effects of response-adaptive randomization in some well-known trials. Lee, Chen and Yin [111] give a balanced view, as the result of extended simulations.

Another issue is whether adaptive randomization designs are ethical: Hey and Kimmelman [112] and Wathen and Thall [113] argue that the chance that adaptive random allocation will assign more patients to an inferior arm is too high. Other authors

(Wason et al. [114]) worry that these designs may be too complex for use and that standard analysis methods of analyzing results from adaptive trials are valid only asymptotically. Another main concern is bias from temporal trends ([115]).

In conclusion, Thall, Fox and Wathen [116] state that adaptive randomization produces inferential problems that decrease potential benefit to future patients, and may decrease benefit to patients enrolled in the trial. These problems should be weighed against its putative ethical benefit. For randomized comparative trials to obtain confirmatory comparisons, designs with fixed randomization probabilities and group sequential decision rules appear to be preferable to adaptive randomization, scientifically and ethically.

Whereas this controversy has been useful to learn how response-adaptive randomization might be used appropriately, for instance by introducing a burn-in period of equal randomization in some adaptive trials, the class of adaptive designs is really vast, so any discussion should focus around the value of a specific type of adaptive design in the specific context for which it is being proposed. Unfortunately, the arguments are often generic and not applied to the special features of adaptive procedures, as also Villar et al. [117] underline. In particular, as mentioned in Section 2 about the choice of the utility function, priorities about the very purpose or purposes of the experiment should be made clear in advance.

8. Conclusions

"Bayesian adaptive clinical trials: a dream for statisticians only?" asks Chevret [44]. Clearly, Bayesian adaptive experiments are not easy to design, let alone to implement. For a start, elicitation of a prior is not a simple matter. In clinical trials it is generally assumed to be based on historical data. In their book ([1]) Spiegelhalter, Abrams and Myles recommend attempting both an "enthusiastic" and a "skeptical" prior. On the other hand, Bayesian statistics exercises greater appeal than frequentist on most applied researchers, and the same can be said of adaptive design rules. This explains why the presence of Bayesian and adaptive design methods combined together has become massive in the biostatistical literature, notwithstanding the fact that adaptive algorithms are more complex than non-adaptive.

It is this author's opinion that although there is a widespread consensus that the Bayesian and the adaptive approaches to design go very well together, the field is still rather fragmented. The development has taken place in a relatively short time and Bayesian adaptive designs are still awaiting in-depth investigation. It is a sad state of affairs that in general there is no sounder way to evaluate the performance of Bayesian (and non-Bayesian) designs other than by computer simulations. Often the simulation scenarios are chosen on the basis of the researchers' personal preferences, so the conclusions may be debatable.

The book by Yin [118] is a thorough presentation of both Bayesian and frequentist adaptive methods in clinical trial design, but the two approaches are based on fundamentally different paradigms and a comparison of Bayesian and non-Bayesian designs is possible only in restricted cases. As an example, when several experimental treatments are available for testing, Wason and Trippa [119] compare Bayesian adaptive randomization, which allocates a greater proportion of future patients to treatments that have performed well, to multi-arm multi-stage designs, which use pre-specified stopping boundaries to determine whether experimental treatments should be dropped. The authors show that in this case both are efficient, but neither is superior: it depends on the true state of nature.

In conclusion, it is worth quoting the words of Stallard et al. [120]: *"Bayesian adaptive methods are often more bespoke than frequentist approaches . . . They require more design work than the use of a more standard frequentist method but can be advantageous in that design choices and their consequences are considered carefully"*.

Funding: This research received no funding.

Institutional Review Board Statement: Not applicable.

Informed Consent Statement: Not applicable.

Acknowledgments: The author wishes to express her deep gratitude and affection to Isabella Verdinelli for numberless conversations on the topic of Bayesian designs, for her help and criticisms which led to a substantial improvement of the paper, and for her continuous encouragement.

Conflicts of Interest: The author declares no conflict of interest.

References

1. Spiegelhalter, D.J.; Abrams, K.R.; Myles, J.P. *Bayesian Approaches to Clinical Trials and Health-Care Evaluation*; John Wiley & Sons: Hoboken, NJ, USA, 2004.
2. Ashby, D. Bayesian statistics in medicine: A 25 year review. *Stat. Med.* **2006**, *25*, 3589–3631. [CrossRef]
3. EDITORIAL Bayesian clinical trials: No more excuses. *Clin. Trials* **2009**, *6*, 203–204. [CrossRef]
4. Biswas, S.; Liu, D.D.; Lee, J.J.; Berry, D.A. Bayesian clinical trials at the University of Texas M. D. Anderson Cancer Center. *Clin. Trials* **2009**, *6*, 205–216. [CrossRef]
5. European Medicines Agency. *Reflection Paper on Methodological Issues in Confirmatory Clinical Trials Planned with an Adaptive Design*; European Medicines Agency: Amsterdam, The Netherlands, 2007; CHMP/EWP/2459/02.
6. Food and Drug Administration, USA. *Adaptive Designs for Clinical Trials of Drugs and Biologics Guidance for Industry*; Docket Number: FDA-2018-D-3124; U.S. Food and Drug Administration: Silver Spring, MD, USA, 2019.
7. Berry, D.A.; Müller, P.; Grieve, A.; Smith, M.; Parke, T.; Blazek, R.; Mitchard, N.; Krams, M. Adaptive Bayesian designs for dose-ranging drug trials. In *Case Studies in Bayesian Statistics*; Gatsonis, C., Kass, R.E., Carlin, B., Carriquiry, A., Gelman, A., Verdinelli, I., West, M., Eds.; Springer: New York, NY, USA, 2002; Volume 162, pp. 99–181.
8. Berry, D.A. Statistical innovations in cancer research. In *Cancer Medicine*, 6th ed.; Holland, J., Frei, T., Eds.; BC Decker: London, UK, 2003; pp. 465–478.
9. Berry, D.A. Bayesian clinical trials. *Nat. Rev. Drug Discov.* **2006**, *5*, 27–36. [CrossRef] [PubMed]
10. Berry, D.A. Adaptive clinical trials in oncology. *Nat. Rev. Clin. Oncol.* **2012**, *9*, 199–207. [CrossRef] [PubMed]
11. Stangl, D.; Lurdes, Y.T.I.; Telba, Z.I. Celebrating 70: An interview with Don Berry. *Stat. Sci.* **2012**, *27*, 144–159. [CrossRef]
12. Berry, S.M.; Carlin, B.P.; Lee, J.J.; Muller, P. *Bayesian Adaptive Methods for Clinical Trials*; Chapman & Hall/CRC Biostatistics Series; Chapman and Hall/CRC: Boca Raton, FL, USA, 2011.
13. Ventz, S.; Parmigiani, G.; Trippa, L. Combining Bayesian experimental designs and frequentist data analyses: Motivations and examples. *Appl. Stoch. Model Bus.* **2017**, *33*, 302–313. [CrossRef]
14. Chaloner, K.; Verdinelli, I. Bayesian experimental design: A review. *Stat. Sci.* **1995**, *10*, 273–304. [CrossRef]
15. Lindley, D.V. *Bayesian Statistics: A Review*; SIAM: Philadelphia, PA, USA, 1972.
16. Smith, A.F.M.; Verdinelli, I. A note on Bayes designs for inference using a hierarchical linear model. *Biometrika* **1980**, *67*, 613–619. [CrossRef]
17. Giovagnoli, A.; Verdinelli, I. Bayes D-optimal and E-optimal block designs. *Biometrika* **1983**, *70*, 695–706. [CrossRef]
18. Chaloner, K. Optimal Bayesian experimental design for linear models. *Ann. Stat.* **1984**, *12*, 283–300. [CrossRef]
19. Chaloner, K.; Larntz, K. Optimal Bayesian design applied to logistic regression experiments. *J. Stat. Plan. Inference* **1989**, *21*, 191–208. [CrossRef]
20. Wikipedia. Optimal Design. 2020. Available online: https://en.wikipedia.org/wiki/Optimal_design (accessed on 27 December 2020).
21. Verdinelli, I.; Kadane, J.B. Bayesian designs for maximizing information and outcome. *J. Am. Stat. Assoc.* **1992**, *87*, 510–515. [CrossRef]
22. Clyde, M.; Chaloner, K. The equivalence of constrained and weighted designs in multiple objective design problems. *J. Am. Stat. Assoc.* **1996**, *91*, 1236–1244. [CrossRef]
23. Burman, C.-F.; Sonesson, C. Are flexible designs sound? *Biometrics* **2006**, *62*, 664–669. [CrossRef]
24. Pong, A.; Chow, S.-C. (Eds.) *Handbook of Adaptive Designs in Pharmaceutical and Clinical Development*; Chapman & Hall: Boca Raton, FL, USA, 2011; pp. 3:1–3:19.
25. Huskins, W.C.; Fowler, V.G., Jr.; Evans, S. Adaptive designs for clinical trials: Application to healthcare epidemiology research. *Clin. Infect. Dis.* **2018**, *66*, 1140–1146. [CrossRef]
26. Baldi-Antognini, A.; Giovagnoli, A. *Adaptive Designs for Sequential Treatment Allocation*; Chapman and Hall/CRC Biostatistics Series; Chapman and Hall/CRC: Boca Raton, FL, USA, 2015; 216p, ISBN 9781466505759.
27. Rosenberger, W.F. New directions in adaptive designs. *Stat. Sci.* **1996**, *11*, 137–149. [CrossRef]
28. Dragalin, V. Seamless Phase I/II Designs. In *Handbook of Adaptive Designs in Pharmaceutical and Clinical Development*; Pong, A., Chow, S.-C., Eds.; Chapman & Hall: Boca Raton, FL, USA, 2011; pp. 12:1–12:22.
29. Maca, J. Phase II/III Seamless Designs. In *Handbook of Adaptive Designs in Pharmaceutical and Clinical Development*; Pong, A., Chow, S.-C., Eds.; Chapman & Hall: Boca Raton, FL, USA, 2011; pp. 13:1–13:8.
30. Efron, B. Forcing sequential experiments to be balanced. *Biometrika* **1971**, *58*, 403–417. [CrossRef]
31. Hu, F.; Rosenberger, W.F. *The Theory of Response-Adaptive Randomization in Clinical Trials*; John Wiley & Sons: Hoboken, NJ, USA, 2006.
32. Rosenberger, W.F.; Lachin, J.M. Randomization in Clinical Trials. In *Wiley Series in Probability and Statistics*, 2nd ed.; John Wiley & Sons: Hoboken, NJ, USA, 2016.
33. Baldi-Antognini, A.; Giovagnoli, A. Compound optimal allocation for individual and collective ethics in binary clinical trials. *Biometrika* **2010**, *97*, 935–946. [CrossRef]

34. Sverdlov, O.; Rosenberger, W.F. On recent advances in optimal allocation designs in clinical trials. *J. Stat. Theory Pract.* **2013**, *7*, 753–773. [CrossRef]
35. Sverdlov, O. (Ed.) *Modern Adaptive Randomized Clinical Trials: Statistical and Practical Aspects*; Chapman & Hall/CRC Press: Boca Raton, FL, USA, 2016.
36. Pocock, S.J. Group sequential methods in the design and analysis of clinical trials. *Biometrika* **1977**, *64*, 191–199. [CrossRef]
37. O'Brien, P.C.; Fleming, T.R. A multiple testing procedure for clinical trials. *Biometrics* **1979**, *35*, 549–556. [CrossRef] [PubMed]
38. Whitehead, J. *The Design and Analysis of Sequential Clinical Trials*; John Wiley & Sons: Hoboken, NJ, USA, 1997.
39. Jennison, C.; Turnbull, B.W. *Group Sequential Methods with Applications to Clinical Trials*; Chapman & Hall: New York, NY, USA, 2000.
40. World Health Organization. "Solidarity" Clinical Trial for COVID-19 Treatments. Available online: https://www.who.int/emergencies/diseases/novel-coronavirus-2019/global-research-on-novel-coronavirus-2019-ncov/solidarity-clinical-trial-for-covid-19-treatments (accessed on 7 January 2021).
41. Lachin, J.M. A review of methods for futility stopping based on conditional power. *Stat. Med.* **2005**, *24*, 2747–2764. [CrossRef] [PubMed]
42. Jennison, C.; Turnbull, B.W. Group sequential tests with outcome-dependent treatment assignment. *Seq. Anal.* **2001**, *20*, 209–234. [CrossRef]
43. Zhu, H.; Hu, F. Sequential monitoring of response-adaptive randomized clinical trials. *Ann. Stat.* **2010**, *38*, 2218–2241. [CrossRef]
44. Chevret, S. Bayesian adaptive clinical trials: A dream for statisticians only? *Stat. Med.* **2012**, *31*, 1002–1013. [CrossRef]
45. Rosner, G.L. Bayesian adaptive design in drug development Chap 8. In *Bayesian Methods in Pharmaceutical Research*; Lesaffre, E., Baio, G., Boulanger, B., Eds.; Chapman & Hall/CRC Press: Boca Raton, FL, USA, 2020.
46. Atkinson, A.C.; Biswas, A. Bayesian adaptive biased-coin designs for clinical trials with normal responses. *Biometrics* **2005**, *61*, 118–125. [CrossRef]
47. Atkinson, A.C.; Biswas, A. *Randomised Response-Adaptive Designs in Clinical Trials*; Chapman & Hall/CRC Press: Boca Raton, FL, USA, 2014.
48. Thompson, W.R. On the likelihood that one unknown probability exceeds another in view of the evidence of two samples. *Biometrika* **1933**, *25*, 285–294. [CrossRef]
49. Thall, P.F.; Wathen, J.K. Practical Bayesian adaptive randomization in clinical trials. *Eur. J. Cancer* **2007**, *43*, 859–866. [CrossRef]
50. Gubbiotti, S.; De Santis, F. A Bayesian method for the choice of the sample size in equivalence trials. *Aust. Nz. J. Stat.* **2011**, *53*, 443–460. [CrossRef]
51. Berry, D.A. Interim analyses in clinical trials: Classical vs. Bayesian approaches. *Stat. Med.* **1985**, *4*, 521–526. [CrossRef] [PubMed]
52. Spiegelhalter, D.J.; Freedman, L.S. A predictive approach to selecting the size of a clinical trial, based on subjective clinical opinion. *Stat. Med.* **1986**, *5*, 1–13. [CrossRef] [PubMed]
53. Rufibach, K.; Burger, H.U.; Abt, M. Bayesian predictive power: Choice of prior and some recommendations for its use as probability of success in drug development. *Pharm. Stat.* **2016**, *15*, 438–446. [CrossRef] [PubMed]
54. Harari, O.; Hsu, G.; Dron, L.; Park, J.J.H.; Thorlund, K.; Mills, E.J. Utilizing Bayesian predictive power in clinical trial design. *Pharm. Stat.* **2020**, 1–16. [CrossRef]
55. Gsponer, T.; Gerber, F.; Bornkamp, B.; Ohlssen, D.; Vandemeulebroecke, M.; Schmidli, H. A practical guide to Bayesian group sequential designs. *Pharm. Stat.* **2014**, *13*, 71–80. [CrossRef]
56. O'Quigley, J.; Pepe, M.; Fisher, L. Continual Reassessment Method: A practical design for Phase 1 clinical trials in cancer. *Biometrics* **1990**, *46*, 33–48. [CrossRef]
57. O'Quigley, J.; Conaway, M. Continual Reassessment and related dose-finding designs. *Stat. Sci.* **2010**, *25*, 202–216. [CrossRef]
58. Cheung, Y.K. *Dose Finding by the Continual Reassessment Method*; Chapman & Hall/CRC Press: New York, NY, USA, 2011.
59. Cheung, Y.K.; Chappell, R. Sequential Designs for Phase I Clinical Trials with Late-Onset Toxicities. *Biometrics* **2000**, *56*, 1177–1182. [CrossRef]
60. Babb, J.S.; Rogatko, A. Patient specific dosing in a cancer Phase I clinical trial. *Stat. Med.* **2001**, *20*, 2079–2090. [CrossRef]
61. North, B.; Kocher, H.M.; Sasieni, P. A new pragmatic design for dose escalation in phase 1 clinical trials using an adaptive continual reassessment method. *BMC Cancer* **2019**, *19*, 632. [CrossRef]
62. Yin, G.; Yuan, Y. Bayesian approach for adaptive design. In *Handbook of Adaptive Designs in Pharmaceutical and Clinical Development*; Pong, A., Chow, S.-C., Eds.; Chapman & Hall: Boca Raton, FL, USA, 2011; pp. 3:1–3:19.
63. Ji, Y.; Liu, P.; Li, Y.; Bekele, B.N. A modified toxicity probability interval method for dose-finding trials. *Clin. Trials* **2010**, *7*, 653–663. [CrossRef] [PubMed]
64. Zhou, H.; Yuan, Y.; Nie, L. Accuracy, safety, and reliability of novel Phase I trial designs. *Clin. Cancer Res.* **2018**, *24*, 4357–4364. [CrossRef] [PubMed]
65. McGree, J.M.; Drovandi, C.C.; Thompson, M.H.; Eccleston, J.A.; Duffull, S.B.; Mengersen, K.; Pettitt, A.N.; Goggin, T. Adaptive Bayesian compound designs for dose finding studies. *J. Stat. Plan. Inference* **2012**, *142*, 1480–1492. [CrossRef]
66. Haines, L.M.; Perevozskaya, I.; Rosenberger, W.F. Bayesian optimal design for Phase I clinical trials. *Biometrics* **2003**, *59*, 591–600. [CrossRef] [PubMed]
67. Thall, P.F.; Inoue, L.Y.T.; Martin, T.G. Adaptive decision making in a lymphocyte infusion trial. *Biometrics* **2002**, *58*, 560–568. [CrossRef]

68. Yuan, Y.; Huang, X.; Liu, S. A Bayesian response-adaptive covariate-balanced randomization design with application to a leukemia clinical trial. *Stat. Med.* **2011**, *30*, 1218–1229. [CrossRef]
69. Giovagnoli, A. Bayesian optimal experimental designs for binary responses in an adaptive framework. *Appl. Stoch. Model Bus.* **2017**, *33*, 260–268. [CrossRef]
70. Xiao, Y.; Liu, Z.; Hu, F. Bayesian doubly adaptive randomization in clinical trials. *Sci. China Math.* **2017**, *60*, 2503–2514. [CrossRef]
71. Giovagnoli, A.; Verdinelli, I. Bayesian randomized adaptive designs with compound utility functions. 2020; Manuscript submitted.
72. Thall, P.F.; Simon, R. A Bayesian approach to establishing sample size and monitoring criteria for phase II clinical trials. *Cont. Clin. Trials* **1994**, *15*, 463–481. [CrossRef]
73. Wang, M.-D. Sample Size Re-estimation by Bayesian Prediction. *Biom. J.* **2007**, *49*, 365–377. [CrossRef]
74. Uemura, K.; Ando, Y.; Matsuyama, Y. Utility of adaptive sample size designs and a review example. *J. Stat. Sci. Appl.* **2017**, *5*, 1–15. [CrossRef]
75. Lee, L.L.; Liu, D.D. A predictive probability design for Phase II cancer clinical trials. *Clin. Trials* **2008**, *5*, 93–106. [CrossRef] [PubMed]
76. Yin, G.; Chen, N.; Lee, J.J. Phase II trial design with Bayesian adaptive randomization and predictive probability. *Appl. Stat.* **2012**, *61*, 219–235. [CrossRef] [PubMed]
77. Zhong, W.; Koopmeiners, J.S.; Carlin, B.P. A two-stage Bayesian design with sample size re-estimation and subgroup analysis for phase II binary response trials. *Cont. Clin. Trials* **2013**, *36*, 587–596. [CrossRef]
78. Cheng, Y.; Shen, Y. Bayesian adaptive designs for clinical trials. *Biometrika* **2005**, *92*, 633–646. [CrossRef]
79. Mason, A.J.; Gonzalez-Maffe, J.; Quinn, K.; Doyle, N.; Legg, K.; Norsworthy, P.; Trevelion, R.; Winston, A.; Ashby, D. Developing a Bayesian adaptive design for a Phase I clinical trial: A case study for a novel HIV treatment. *Stat. Med.* **2017**, *36*, 754–771. [CrossRef]
80. Lee, J.J.; Chu, C.T. Bayesian clinical trials in action. *Stat. Med.* **2012**, *31*, 2955–2972. [CrossRef]
81. Angus, D.C.; Alexander, B.M.; Berry, S.; Buxton, M.; Lewis, R.; Paoloni, M. Adaptive platform trials, definition, design, conduct and reporting considerations. *Nat. Rev. Drug Discov.* **2019**, *18*, 797–807.
82. Brown, A.R.; Gajewski, B.J.; Aaronson, L.S.; Mudaranthakam, D.P.; Hunt, S.L.; Berry, S.M.; Quintana, M.; Pasnoor, M.; Dimachkie, M.M.; Jawdat, O.; et al. A Bayesian comparative effectiveness trial in action: Developing a platform for multi-site study adaptive randomization. *Trials* **2016**, *17*, 428. [CrossRef]
83. Talisa, V.B.; Yende, S.; Seymour, C.W.; Angus, D.C. Arguing for adaptive clinical trials in sepsis. *Front. Immunol.* **2018**, *9*, 1502. [CrossRef]
84. Angus, D.C.; Berry, S.; Lewis, R.J.; Al-Beidh, F.; Arabi, Y.; van Bentum-Puijk, W.; Bhimani, Z.; Bonten, M.; Broglio, K.; Brunkhorst, F.; et al. The Randomized Embedded Multifactorial Adaptive Platform for Community-Acquired Pneumonia (REMAP-CAP) study: Rationale and design. *Ann. Am. Thorac. Soc.* **2020**. [CrossRef]
85. Houston, B.L.; Lawler, P.R.; Goligher, E.C.; Farkouh, M.E.; Bradbury, C.; Carrier, M.; Zarychanski, R. Anti-Thrombotic Therapy to Ameliorate Complications of COVID-19 (ATTACC): Study design and methodology for an international, adaptive Bayesian randomized controlled trial. *Clin. Trials* **2020**, *17*, 491–500. [CrossRef] [PubMed]
86. Alexander, B.M.; Ba, S.; Berger, M.S.; Berry, D.A.; Cavenee, W.K.; Chang, S.M.; Cloughesy, T.F.; Jiang, T.; Khasraw, M.; Li, W.; et al. Adaptive global innovative learning environment for glioblastoma. *Clin. Cancer Res.* **2018**, *24*, 737–743. [CrossRef] [PubMed]
87. Michos, E.D.; Mitchell, C.M.; Miller, E.R., 3rd; Sternberg, A.L.; Juraschek, S.P.; Schrack, J.A.; Szanton, S.L.; Walston, J.D.; Kalyani, R.R.; Plante, T.B.; et al. Rationale and design of the Study to Understand Fall Reduction and Vitamin D in You (STURDY): A randomized clinical trial of Vitamin D supplement doses for the prevention of falls in older adults. *Contemp. Clin. Trials* **2018**, *73*, 111–122. [CrossRef] [PubMed]
88. Backonja, M.; Williams, L.; Miao, X.; Katz, N.; Chen, C. Safety and efficacy of neublastin in painful lumbosacral radiculopathy: A randomized, double-blinded, placebo-controlled phase 2 trial using Bayesian adaptive design (the SPRINT trial). *Pain* **2017**, *158*, 1802–1812. [CrossRef] [PubMed]
89. Schuetze, S.M.; Wathen, J.K.; Lucas, D.R.; Choy, E.; Samuels, B.L.; Staddon, A.P.; Ganjoo, K.N.; von Mehren, M.; Chow, W.A.; Loeb, D.M.; et al. SARC009: Phase 2 study of Dasatinib in patients with previously treated, high-grade, advanced sarcoma. *Cancer* **2016**, *122*, 868–874. [CrossRef] [PubMed]
90. Connor, J.T.; Broglio, K.R.; Durkalski, V.; Meurer, W.J.; Johnston, K.C. The Stroke Hyperglycemia Insulin Network Effort (SHINE) trial: An adaptive trial design case study. *Trials* **2015**, *16*, 72. [CrossRef]
91. Johnston, K.; Bruno, A.; Pauls, Q.; Hall, C.E.; Barrett, K.M.; Barsan, W.; Fansler, A.; Van de Bruinhorst, K.; Janis, S.; Durkalski-Mauldin, V.L. for the Neurological Emergencies Treatment Trials Network and the SHINE Trial Investigators. Intensive vs standard treatment of hyperglycemia and functional outcome in patients with acute ischemic stroke: The SHINE randomized clinical trial. *J. Am. Med. Assoc.* **2019**, *322*, 326–335. [CrossRef]
92. Ritchie, C.W.; Molinuevo, J.L.; Truyen, L.; Satlin, A.; van der Geyten, S.; Lovestone, S. Development of interventions for the secondary prevention of Alzheimer's dementia: The European Prevention of Alzheimer's Dementia. *Lancet Psych.* **2015**, *3*, 179–186. [CrossRef]
93. Kim, E.S.; Herbst, R.S.; Wistuba, I.I.; Lee, J.J.; Blumenschein, G.R.; Tsao, A.; Stewart, D.J.; Hicks, M.E.; Erasmus, J., Jr.; Gupta, S.; et al. The BATTLE trial: Personalizing therapy for lung cancer. *Cancer Discov.* **2011**, *1*, 44–53. [CrossRef]

94. Papadimitrakopoulou, V.; Lee, J.J.; Wistuba, I.; Tsao, A.; Fossella, F.; Kalhor, N.; Gupta, S.; Byers, L.A.; Izzo, J.; Gettinger, S.; et al. The BATTLE-2 Study: A biomarker-integrated targeted therapy study in previously treated patients with advanced non-small-cell lung cancer. *J. Clin. Oncol.* **2016**, *34*, 3638–3647. [CrossRef] [PubMed]
95. Barker, A.D.; Sigman, C.C.; Kelloff, G.J.; Hylton, N.M.; Berry, D.A.; Esserman, L.J. I-SPY 2: An adaptive breast cancer trial design in the setting of neoadjuvant chemotherapy. *Clin. Pharmacol. Ther.* **2009**, *86*, 97–100. [CrossRef] [PubMed]
96. Carey, L.A.; Winer, E.P. I-SPY 2: Toward more rapid progress in breast cancer treatment. *N. Eng. J. Med.* **2016**, *375*, 83–84. [CrossRef] [PubMed]
97. Park, J.W.; Liu, M.C.; Yee, D.; Yau, C.; van't Veer, L.J.; Symmans, W.F.; Paoloni, M.; Perlmutter, J.; Hylton, N.M.; Hogarth, M.; et al. for the I-SPY 2 Investigators. Adaptive randomization of Neratinib in early breast cancer. *N. Eng. J. Med.* **2016**, *375*, 11–22. [CrossRef] [PubMed]
98. Rugo, H.S.; Olopade, O.I.; DeMichele, A.; Yau, C.; van't Veer, L.J.; Buxton, M.B.; Hogarth, M.; Hylton, N.M.; Paoloni, M.; Perlmutter, J.; et al. Adaptive randomization of Veliparib-Carboplatin treatment in breast cancer. *N. Engl. J. Med.* **2016**, *375*, 23–34. [CrossRef] [PubMed]
99. Murphy, P.; Moline, M.; Mayleben, D.; Rosenberg, R.; Zammit, G.; Pinner, K.; Dhadda, S.; Hong, Q.; Giorgi, L.; Satlin, A.; et al. Dual Orexin Receptor Antagonist (DORA) for the treatment of insomnia disorder: Results from a Bayesian, adaptive, randomized, double-blind, placebo-controlled study. *J. Clin. Sleep Med.* **2017**, *13*, 1289–1299. [CrossRef]
100. Cook, N.; Basu, B.; Smith, D.M.; Gopinathan, A.; Evans, J.; Steward, W.P.; Palmer, D.; Propper, D.; Venugopal, B.; Hategan, M.; et al. A Phase I trial of the γ-secretase inhibitor MK-0752 in combination with Gemcitabine in patients with pancreatic ductal adenocarcinoma. *Br. J. Cancer* **2018**, *118*, 793–801. [CrossRef]
101. Sturm, S.; Delporte, M.L.; Hadi, S.; Schobel, S.; Lindemann, L.; Weikert, R.; Jaeschke, G.; Derks, M.; Palermo, G. Results and evaluation of a first-in-human study of RG7342, an mGlu5 positive allosteric modulator, utilizing Bayesian adaptive methods. *Br. J. Clin. Pharmacol.* **2018**, *84*, 445–455. [CrossRef]
102. Hirakawa, A.; Nishikawa, T.; Yonemori, K.; Shibata, T.; Nakamura, K.; Ando, M.; Ueda, T.; Ozaki, T.; Tamura, K.; Kawai, A.; et al. Utility of Bayesian single-arm design in new drug application for rare cancers in Japan: A case study of Phase 2 trial for sarcoma. *Ther. Innov. Regul. Sci.* **2018**, *52*, 334–338. [CrossRef]
103. Cellamare, M.; Ventz, S.; Baudin, E.; Mitnick, C.D.; Trippa, L. A Bayesian response-adaptive trial in tuberculosis: The end TB trial. *Clin. Trials* **2017**, *14*, 17–28. [CrossRef]
104. Krams, M.; Lees, K.R.; Hacke, W.; Grieve, A.P.; Orgogozo, J.M.; Ford, G.A. Acute Stroke Therapy by Inhibition of Neutrophils (ASTIN). An adaptive dose-response study of UK-279,276 in acute ischemic stroke. *Stroke* **2003**, *34*, 2543–2548. [CrossRef] [PubMed]
105. Ware, J.H. Investigating therapies of potentially great benefit: ECMO. *Stat. Sci.* **1989**, *4*, 298–306. [CrossRef]
106. Burton, P.R.; Gurrina, L.C.; Hussey, M.H. Interpreting the clinical trials of extracorporeal membrane oxygenation in the treatment of persistent pulmonary hypertension of the newborn. *Semin. Neonatol.* **1997**, *2*, 69–79. [CrossRef]
107. Korn, E.L.; Freidlin, B. Outcome-adaptive randomization: Is it useful? *J. Clin. Oncol.* **2011**, *29*, 771–776. [CrossRef]
108. Yuan, Y.; Yin, G. On the usefulness of outcome-adaptive randomization. *J. Clin. Oncol.* **2010**, *29*, e390–e392. [CrossRef]
109. Berry, D.A. Adaptive Clinical Trials: The Promise and the Caution. *J. Clin. Oncol.* **2011**, *29*, 606–609. [CrossRef]
110. Korn, E.L.; Freidlin, B. Commentary. Adaptive clinical trials: Advantages and disadvantages of various adaptive design elements. *J. Natl. Cancer Inst.* **2017**, *109*. [CrossRef]
111. Lee, J.J.; Chen, N.; Yin, G. Worth adapting? Revisiting the usefulness of outcome-adaptive randomization. *Clin. Cancer Res.* **2012**, *18*, 4498–4507. [CrossRef]
112. Hey, S.P.; Kimmelman, J. Are outcome adaptive allocation trials ethical? *Clin. Trials* **2015**, *12*, 102–106. [CrossRef]
113. Wathen, J.K.; Thall, P.F. A simulation study of outcome adaptive randomization in multi-arm clinical trials. *Clin. Trials* **2017**, *14*, 432–440. [CrossRef]
114. Wason, J.M.S.; Brocklehurst, P.; Yap, C. When to keep it simple—Adaptive designs are not always useful. *BMC Med.* **2019**, *17*, 1–7. [CrossRef] [PubMed]
115. Proschan, M.; Evans, S. The temptation of response-adaptive randomization. *Clin. Infect. Dis.* **2020**, *71*, 3002–3004. [CrossRef] [PubMed]
116. Thall, P.F.; Fox, P.S.; Wathen, J.K. Statistical controversies in clinical research: Scientific and ethical problems with adaptive randomization in comparative clinical trials. *Ann. Oncol.* **2015**, *26*, 1621–1628. [CrossRef] [PubMed]
117. Villar, S.S.; Robertson, D.S.; Rosenberger, W.F. The Temptation of Overgeneralizing Response-Adaptive Randomization. *Clin. Infect. Dis.* **2020**, in press. [CrossRef]
118. Yin, G. *Clinical Trial Design: Bayesian and Frequentist Adaptive Methods*; Wiley & Sons: Hoboken, NJ, USA, 2012; 368p.
119. Wason, J.M.S.; Trippa, L. A comparison of Bayesian adaptive randomization and multi-stage designs for multi-arm clinical trials. *Stat. Med.* **2014**, *33*, 2206–2221. [CrossRef]
120. Stallard, N.; Todd, S.; Ryan, E.G.; Gates, S. Comparison of Bayesian and frequentist group-sequential clinical trial designs. *BMC Med. Res. Methodol.* **2020**, *20*, 4. [CrossRef]

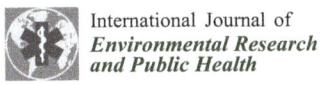

Article

Sample Size Requirements for Calibrated Approximate Credible Intervals for Proportions in Clinical Trials

Fulvio De Santis [†] and Stefania Gubbiotti *,[†]

Dipartimento di Scienze Statistiche, Sapienza University of Rome, Piazzale Aldo Moro n. 5, 00185 Rome, Italy; fulvio.desantis@uniroma1.it
* Correspondence: stefania.gubbiotti@uniroma1.it
† These authors contributed equally to this work.

Abstract: In Bayesian analysis of clinical trials data, credible intervals are widely used for inference on unknown parameters of interest, such as treatment effects or differences in treatments effects. Highest Posterior Density (HPD) sets are often used because they guarantee the shortest length. In most of standard problems, closed-form expressions for exact HPD intervals do not exist, but they are available for intervals based on the normal approximation of the posterior distribution. For small sample sizes, approximate intervals may be not calibrated in terms of posterior probability, but for increasing sample sizes their posterior probability tends to the correct credible level and they become closer and closer to exact sets. The article proposes a predictive analysis to select appropriate sample sizes needed to have approximate intervals calibrated at a pre-specified level. Examples are given for interval estimation of proportions and log-odds.

Keywords: bayesian inference; highest posterior density intervals; normal approximation; predictive analysis; sample size determination

---

Citation: De Santis, F.; Gubbiotti, S. Sample Size Requirements for Calibrated Approximate Credible Intervals for Proportions in Clinical Trials. *Int. J. Environ. Res. Public Health* **2021**, *18*, 595. https://doi.org/10.3390/ijerph18020595

Received: 1 November 2020
Accepted: 8 January 2021
Published: 12 January 2021

Publisher's Note: MDPI stays neutral with regard to jurisdictional clai-ms in published maps and institutio-nal affiliations.

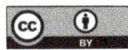

Copyright: © 2021 by the authors. Licensee MDPI, Basel, Switzerland. This article is an open access article distributed under the terms and conditions of the Creative Commons Attribution (CC BY) license (https://creativecommons.org/licenses/by/4.0/).

1. Introduction

The use of Bayesian methods for design, analysis and monitoring of clinical trials is becoming more and more popular. For instance, in some recent contributions [1,2] the Authors note that "compared with its frequentist counterpart, the Bayesian framework has several unique advantages, and its incorporation into clinical trial design is occurring more frequently." Acknowledgements have been arriving also from official institutions. In 2010 FDA, recognizing the merits of Bayesian inference, authorized and encouraged its use in medical device clinical trials. Similarly Bittle and He observe that "[...] in a major shift, the American College of Cardiology and American Heart Association have recently proposed using Bayesian analysis to create clinical trials guidelines" [3].

There are at least two main motivations for using Bayesian methods. The first is that, unlike frequentist analysis, the Bayesian approach allows the integration of information from a current experiment with pre-trial knowledge. The second advantage is that Bayesian inferential methods are derived from probability distributions that are directly defined on the quantity of interest in the trial (i.e., the parameter). This makes communication between statisticians and experts in the field much more effective than it is when frequentist methods are employed.

With no significant loss of generality, suppose we are concerned with inference on the unknown effect of a new treatment, that we assume to be our parameter of interest. Bayesian methodology is based on elaborations of the posterior distribution of the parameter, which merges pre-experimental knowledge (i.e., the prior distribution) and trial information (i.e., the likelihood function) on this parameter via Bayes theorem. Inferential tools—such as point estimates, set estimates or test statistics—are simply special functionals of the posterior distributions. Nowadays analytic and computational methods for handling complex Bayesian problems are available, even in high dimensional settings.

Nevertheless, the availability of closed-form expressions makes the use of Bayesian analysis more accessible also to non-statisticians. For this reason a relevant part of the available Bayesian literature in clinical trials resorts heavily to normal approximations [4].

Interval estimation is one of the most common techniques used to summarize information on an unknown parameter. Bayesian inference usually relies on exact Highest Posterior Density intervals (HPD). The $(1-\gamma)$-HPD interval is the subset of the parameter space of probability $(1-\gamma)$ whose points have density higher than the density of any value of the parameter outside the interval. When the posterior distribution is symmetric, HPDs are also equal-tails (ET) intervals, i.e., they are limited respectively by the $\gamma/2$ and the $1-\gamma/2$ quantiles of the posterior density of the parameter. HPDs are, typically, not easy to compute, but of minimal length among intervals of given credibility. For a predictive comparison between HPDs and ETs see [5]. Explicit closed-form expressions for the bounds of common exact credible intervals are in most of the cases, not available even in very common models. However, their computation can be simplified by approximating the exact posterior distribution with a normal density and finding the equal-tails intervals, i.e., the $\gamma/2$ and the $1-\gamma/2$ quantiles of the approximated (symmetric) normal density.

In many standard models the posterior density has a unique mode internal to its support. The degree of skewness of the posterior distribution with respect to its mode depends on the shapes of the likelihood function and of the prior distribution [6]. As shown in Figure 1 asymmetry affects the quality of approximate credible intervals that in general may differ substantially from exact HPDs. This means that, in general, for approximate intervals: (a) their actual posterior probability is not equal to the nominal credibility of the exact interval; (b) they are not the shortest intervals among those of given posterior probability.

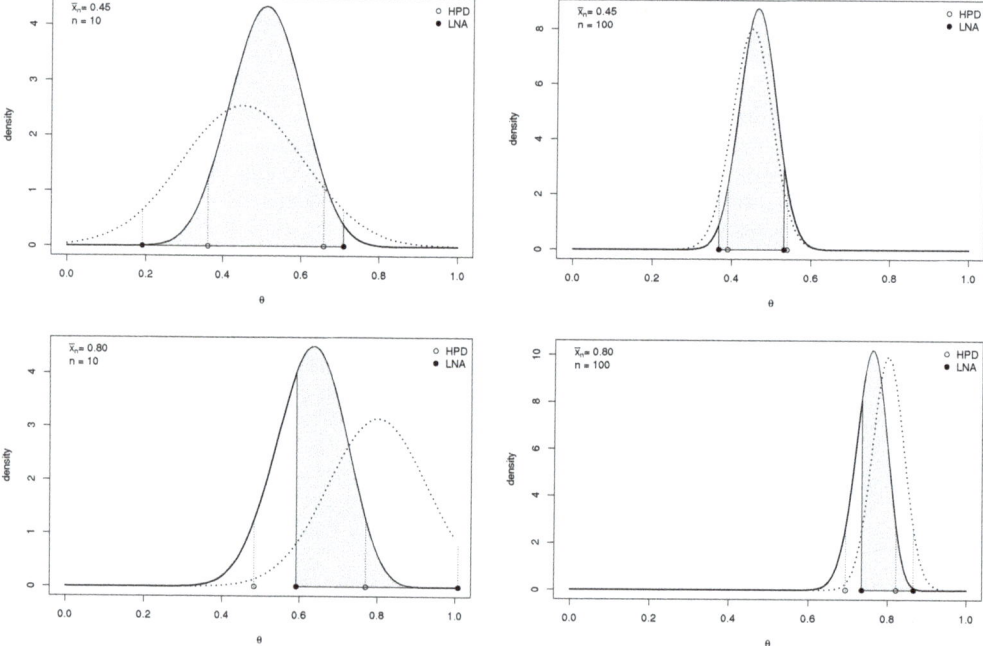

Figure 1. Posterior density, given a prior density of hyperparameters $(\alpha, \beta) = (10.8, 9.2)$, and likelihood approximation, given $\bar{x}_n = 0.45$ (*top row*) and $\bar{x}_n = 0.8$ (*bottom row*) for $n = 10$ (*left column*) and $n = 100$ (*right column*). Exact credible intervals (HPD: Highest Posterior Density) are denoted by empty circles, likelihood approximated credible intervals (LNA: Likelihood Normal Approximation) are denoted by black circles. The probability that θ belongs to the approximate interval under the exact posterior distribution is highlighted in grey.

Under standard and fairly general conditions [7], the degree of asymmetry of the likelihood function is strictly related to the sample size: as the number of experimental units increases, the shape of the likelihood becomes closer and closer to a Gaussian function whose mode is the maximum likelihood estimate and whose precision is measured by the square root of the observed Fisher Information [8]. Likelihood normalization carries along the same tendency of the posterior distribution and, for sufficiently large sample sizes, the posterior density can be approximated by a normal density with data-dependent parameters. This is the so-called Bayesian Central Limit Theorem. As a consequence, as the sample size increases, exact and approximate intervals become closer and closer and the accuracy of approximate intervals improves.

Example 1 (*Single arm phase II trial*). Let us consider an example for binary data, where θ is the probability of response to a treatment. The setup, the choice of the prior hyperparameters and a sensitivity analysis will be fully described in Section 4. A Beta prior of mean 0.54 is considered. Figure 1 shows the Beta posterior distributions of θ (solid line) and their normal approximations based on the likelihood (dotted line) for four different data sets. It also reports bounds of approximate intervals (black circle) and of exact HPD intervals (empty circles). Gray areas highlight the probability of the approximate intervals w.r.t. the exact posterior probability distributions. More specifically, when comparing right panels ($n = 100$) and left panels ($n = 10$) better approximations of the posteriors are observed, due to the larger sample size. Furthermore, the comparison between the two rows of panels (sample mean $\bar{x}_n = 0.45$ and $\bar{x}_n = 0.80$, respectively) shows that the distance between the posterior mode and the likelihood mode (i.e., the maximum likelihood estimate) affects the quality of the approximation: in this example, the larger the difference, the greater the discrepancy between exact and approximate intervals.

The problem we discuss in this paper is the selection of the minimal number of observations to obtain approximate sets that are sufficiently accurate. This sample size determination (SSD) problem is addressed from a pre-posterior perspective, i.e., by taking into account the randomness of the posterior density and of credible intervals.

In the existing literature besides a very general introduction to credible intervals [6,7,9,10] one can find reviews on Bayesian SSD in [11–13], articles specifically dedicated to Bayesian SSD using credible intervals in [14–17] and some contributions focused on binomial proportions, such as [18–20]. Recently, methods that take into account the variability of prior opinion have been developed: for instance, some contributions [15,21,22] deal with robustness with respect to the prior distribution, whereas a more recent proposal is about a consensus-based SSD criterion in the presence of a community of priors [23]. The idea of controlling the conflict between alternative procedures is also used for point estimation [24,25].

In the framework of Bayesian SSD based on credible intervals, our innovative purpose is to look for a sample size sufficiently large so that the approximate likelihood interval provides an accurate approximation to the HPD interval determined from the exact posterior distribution of the parameter of interest. It is worth recalling that whereas the HPD interval is obtained from the prior-to-posterior analysis, the likelihood normal approximation is independent on the prior distribution. In this sense our proposed criterion yields the smallest sample size such that the role of the prior in the posterior distribution is made negligible by the information provided by the data. This provides an additional motivation for our proposal, i.e., to find the study dimension that guarantees a substantial equivalence between closed-form formulas based on the normal approximation and exact Bayesian intervals, or, conversely, to evaluate the expected discrepancy between approximate intervals and exact Bayesian intervals.

The paper is organized as follows. In Section 2, after introducing notation, we propose a measure of discrepancy between exact and approximate intervals to be analyzed from a preposterior perspective: we select the minimal sample size so that the expected discrepancy is sufficiently small. Section 3 specifically refers to the Beta-Binomial model when the paramer of interest is the proportion (Section 3.1) and the logodds (Section 3.2) respectively. Section 4 illustrates some numerical examples related to the setup of the phase II clinical trial of Example 1 and makes comparison with other SSD methods. Finally, Section 5 contains some concluding remarks.

2. Methodology

Assume that $X_1, X_2, \ldots, X_n$ is a sample from $f_n(\cdot|\theta)$ (either a density or a probability mass function), where $\theta \in \Theta$ is an unknown scalar parameter and Θ is the parameter space. The quantity of interest may be either θ or a relevant function $\psi = g(\theta)$. Following the Bayesian inferential approach, we assume that prior information on θ is available (from experts or from historical data) and converted in a prior probability density function, denoted as $\pi(\cdot)$. Given an observed sample $x_n = (x_1, x_2, \ldots, x_n)$, let

$$\pi(\theta|x_n) = \frac{f_n(x_n|\theta)\pi(\theta)}{m(x_n)}$$

be the posterior distribution of θ, where $m(x_n) = \int_\Theta f_n(x_n|\theta)\pi(\theta)d\theta$ denotes the marginal distribution of the the data, computed at the observed x_n. In the following we assume that $\pi(\theta|x_n)$ has a unique mode.

2.1. Exact and Approximate Intervals

Let $C(x_n) = [\ell(x_n), u(x_n)]$ be an exact credible interval of level $1 - \gamma$, that is a subset of the parameter space such that

$$\mathbb{P}[\theta \in C(x_n)|x_n] = 1 - \gamma. \tag{1}$$

In the following, we will focus on HPD intervals. C is HPD if

$$\pi(\theta|x_n) \geq \pi(\theta'|x_n), \qquad \forall \theta \in C(x_n) \quad \text{and} \quad \forall \theta' \notin C(x_n),$$

or, equivalently, if

$$C(x_n) = \{\theta \in \Theta : \pi(\theta|x_n) \geq k_\gamma\},$$

where k_γ is such that (1) holds. The values of ℓ and u are the roots of the two equations

$$\pi(\ell|x_n) = \pi(u|x_n) \quad \text{and} \quad \int_\ell^u \pi(\theta|x_n)d\theta = 1 - \gamma,$$

and they typically do not have a closed-form expression.

In general, $\pi(\theta|x_n)$ is not symmetric with respect to its unique mode. Its level of skewness depends on the constitutive elements of Bayesian analysis—the likelihood (i.e., model and observed data) and the prior distribution— and it determines the level of discrepancy between approximate and exact credible intervals. However, as the sample size increases, the shape of both the likelihood function and the posterior density tend to become more and more Gaussian. This happens under standard regularity conditions: (a) the support of the X_i's does not depend on θ; (b) the derivatives with respect to θ of likelihood and posterior density at least up to the second order exist; (c) the maximum likelihood estimate of θ, $\hat{\theta}$, is in the interior of the parameter space [6–8]. More specifically, for sufficiently large n we have that

$$\theta|x_n \approx N[\hat{\theta}, I_n(\hat{\theta})^{-1}], \tag{2}$$

where $I_n(\theta) = -\frac{d^2}{d\theta^2} \ln L(\theta; x_n)$ is the expected Fisher Information and $L(\theta; x_n)$ is the likelihood function. Note that this approximation of the posterior distribution does not take into account the prior. From Equation (2) the $(1 - \gamma)$-likelihood approximate interval for θ is defined as $\tilde{C}(x_n) = [\tilde{\ell}(x_n), \tilde{u}(x_n)]$ where

$$\tilde{\ell} = \hat{\theta} - z_{1-\frac{\gamma}{2}} I_n(\hat{\theta})^{-1/2} \quad \text{and} \quad \tilde{u} = \hat{\theta} + z_{1-\frac{\gamma}{2}} I_n(\hat{\theta})^{-1/2}, \tag{3}$$

with z_ϵ denoting the ϵ-quantile of the standard normal distribution. As a consequence, as n increases, any measure of discrepancy between a chosen feature of exact and approximate intervals tends to become more and more negligible.

When the quantity of interest is $\psi = g(\theta)$, under the same regularity conditions stated above and assuming that the first derivative of g exists and is not equal to 0, the delta method provides the following normal approximation [26]

$$\psi | x_n \approx N[g(\hat{\theta}), g'(\hat{\theta})^2 \, I_n(\hat{\theta})^{-1}], \tag{4}$$

and the bounds of the $(1-\gamma)$ *likelihood approximate* credible interval for ψ are respectively

$$\tilde{\ell} = g(\hat{\theta}) - z_{1-\frac{\gamma}{2}} \cdot |g'(\hat{\theta})| \cdot I_n(\hat{\theta})^{-1/2} \quad \text{and} \quad \tilde{u} = g(\hat{\theta}) + z_{1-\frac{\gamma}{2}} \cdot |g'(\hat{\theta})| \cdot I_n(\hat{\theta})^{-1/2}. \tag{5}$$

2.2. A Measure of Discrepancy and Predictive Analysis

The set $\tilde{C} = [\tilde{\ell}, \tilde{u}]$ is calibrated if its exact posterior probability is equal to $1 - \gamma$:

$$\mathbb{P}(\theta \in \tilde{C} | x_n) = F(\tilde{u} | x_n) - F(\tilde{\ell} | x_n) = (1-\gamma), \tag{6}$$

where $F(\cdot | x_n)$ is the exact posterior cumulative distribution function of the parameter of interest. The departure from this situation can be measured by

$$|\mathbb{P}(\theta \in \tilde{C} | x_n) - (1-\gamma)| \tag{7}$$

which quantifies the discrepancy between the actual posterior *probability* of $\tilde{C}$ (the gray area of each panel of Figure 1 in Example 1) and its nominal value $1 - \gamma$. Notice that, under the typical assumption $0 < \gamma \ll \frac{1}{2}$, this discrepancy takes values in $(0, 1-\gamma)$. More specifically, it is equal to 0 when $\tilde{C}$ is perfectly calibrated and it is equal to $1 - \gamma$ when $\mathbb{P}(\theta \in \tilde{C} | x_n) = 0$. Hence, a relative measure based on (7) is

$$P(x_n) = \frac{|\mathbb{P}(\theta \in \tilde{C} | x_n) - (1-\gamma)|}{1-\gamma} \tag{8}$$

Before observing the data, $P(X_n)$ is a random object. Therefore the progressive calibration of $\tilde{C}(X_n)$ can be studied by looking at its expected value

$$e_n^P = \mathbb{E}_d[P(X_n)],$$

that is computed with respect to the sampling distribution of the data $f_n(\cdot | \theta_d)$ for a design value θ_d. In the following we assume that all the required regularity conditions hold such that the numerical sequence $\{e_n^P, n \in \mathbb{N}\}$ converges to zero.

In order to obtain a calibrated approximate interval, we must select the smallest sample size such that e_n^P is sufficiently small. More formally, for a suitable threshold $\epsilon_P > 0$,

$$n_P^\star = \min\{n \in \mathbb{N} : e_n^P < \epsilon_P\}. \tag{9}$$

In some cases the values of e_n^P can be obtained with exact calculations. More often they are obtained via Monte Carlo (MC) simulation. In the latter case, for each sample size n and design value θ_d, we proceed according to the following steps:

(i) draw N samples $x_n^{(1)}, \ldots, x_n^{(N)}$ from $f_n(\cdot; \theta_d)$;
(ii) compute $\tilde{\ell}(x_n^{(j)})$ and $\tilde{u}(x_n^{(j)})$, for $j = 1, \ldots, N$;
(iii) compute $P(x_n^{(j)})$, for $j = 1, \ldots, N$;
(iv) set $e_n^P \simeq \frac{\sum_{j=1}^N P(x_n^{(j)})}{N}$;
with a large number of draws, e.g., $N = 10000$.

In the following example, in order to assess the discrepancy between $\tilde{C}$ and C we also consider the absolute distance between their *bounds*

$$B(x_n) = |\tilde{\ell}(x_n) - \ell(x_n)| + |\tilde{u}(x_n) - u(x_n)|$$

and we compare $n_P^\star$ with

$$n_B^\star = \min\{n \in \mathbb{N} : e_n^B < \epsilon_B\}, \tag{10}$$

where

$$e_n^B = \mathbb{E}_d[B(X_n)],$$

and $\epsilon_B > 0$ is a chosen threshold. Note that, unlike $P(x_n)$ (and e_n^P), the discrepancy $B(x_n)$ (and e_n^B) depends on the unit of measurement of the data and its range is case-specific. Therefore the choice of ϵ_B is a critical issue, unless the parameter space is bounded (as in Example 1 where the parameter space is $(0,1)$). Similar measures of discrepancy based on the bounds of credible intervals have been recently proposed [23].

3. Examples: The Beta-Binomial Model

In order to illustrate the ideas sketched above we now consider an example within the Beta-Binomial model. Let $X_i|\theta \sim \text{Ber}(\theta)$, $i = 1, \ldots, n$ (i.i.d.), $\theta \in (0,1)$ and $\theta \sim \text{Be}(\alpha, \beta)$, $\alpha, \beta > 0$. Then, from standard results [6], $\theta|x_n \sim \text{Be}(\tilde{\alpha}, \tilde{\beta})$, where $\tilde{\alpha} = \alpha + s_n$, $\tilde{\beta} = \beta + n - s_n$ and $s_n = \sum_{i=1}^n x_i$. In the following we first analyze credible intervals for θ and then for the log-odds $\psi = g(\theta) = \ln \frac{\theta}{1-\theta}$.

3.1. Credible Intervals for a Proportion

In this model exact HPD credible intervals for θ do not have closed-form expressions. However, HPD bounds are easily obtained using the hdi() function of the HDInterval package of R, [27], which simply requires the R function qbeta() in input. Conversely, closed-form expressions for approximate intervals are easily obtained as follows. Recalling that $\hat{\theta} = \bar{x}_n$ and $I_n(\theta) = \frac{n}{\theta(1-\theta)}$, from Equation (3) the bounds of the *likelihood approximate interval* are

$$\tilde{\ell} = \bar{x}_n - z_{1-\frac{\gamma}{2}}\sqrt{\frac{\bar{x}_n(1-\bar{x}_n)}{n}} \quad \text{and} \quad \tilde{u} = \bar{x}_n + z_{1-\frac{\gamma}{2}}\sqrt{\frac{\bar{x}_n(1-\bar{x}_n)}{n}}.$$

3.2. Credible Intervals for the Log-odds

As before, exact credible intervals for ψ do not have a closed-form expression. HPD bounds can be otained via MC simulation as follows:

(i) draw $\theta^{(1)}, \ldots, \theta^{(M)}$ from the posterior Beta density, where M is a large number;
(ii) compute $\psi^{(j)} = g(\theta^{(j)})$, for $j = 1, \ldots, M$;
(iii) use the R function HDInterval::hdi with the MC draws $\psi^{(1)}, \ldots, \psi^{(M)}$ in input.

Closed-form expression of approximate credible intervals for ψ are obtained from Equation (5) noting that

$$g(\hat{\theta}) = \ln \frac{\bar{x}_n}{1-\bar{x}_n} \quad \text{and} \quad g'(\hat{\theta}) = \frac{1}{\bar{x}_n(1-\bar{x}_n)}.$$

Specifically, we have

$$\tilde{\ell} = \ln \frac{\bar{x}_n}{1-\bar{x}_n} - z_{1-\frac{\gamma}{2}} \cdot \sqrt{\frac{1}{n\bar{x}_n(1-\bar{x}_n)}} \quad \text{and} \quad \tilde{u} = \ln \frac{\bar{x}_n}{1-\bar{x}_n} + z_{1-\frac{\gamma}{2}} \cdot \sqrt{\frac{1}{n\bar{x}_n(1-\bar{x}_n)}}.$$

Note that in the Beta-Binomial model the values of e_n^P can be obtained using either exact calculations or MC simulations as described in Section 2.2.

4. Application to Clinical Trials

Let us assume that in an early phase trial we are interested in estimating the rate of response, θ, to an experimental treatment using a credible interval. As in Example 1 we consider the setup of a single-arm phase II trial. Specifically, the goal of the study is to test the combination of lenalidomideandrituximab in patients with recurrent indolent non-follicular lymphoma [28–30]. The endpoint is the overall response rate $\hat{\theta}$, that is the proportion of eligible patients who achieved complete, unconfirmed or partial response.

In the trial conducted between 2009 and 2011, 21 responses were observed out of 39 eligible patients. These hystorical data are used to elicit a Beta prior density for θ. More specifically, we set the prior mean equal to $\alpha/(\alpha+\beta) = 0.54$ and we consider several values for the prior sample size (i.e., the amount of information contained in the prior) that for the Beta model is $\alpha + \beta$ [31]. For illustrative purposes in the following example we set $\alpha + \beta$ equal to 5, 10 and 20. Moreover, for comparison, we also consider a uniform density as non-informative prior (e.g., $\alpha = \beta = 1$). The design value θ_d is set equal to 0.45, that is the lowest acceptable value for the overall response rate [28]. In order to evaluate the impact of the design parameter we also consider $\theta_d = 0.8$ that represents a much more optimistic design scenario.

Figure 2 shows the behaviour of e_n^P for increasing values of the sample size n under different prior assumptions. Table 1 reports the optimal sample sizes $n_P^\star$ and $n_B^\star$ obtained using criteria (9) and (10) for several choices of the prior hyperameters, when $\theta_d = 0.45$ and $\theta_d = 0.8$, given $\epsilon_P = \epsilon_B = 0.01$ (i.e., 1% of the width of the parameter space). Table 1 also contains the optimal sample sizes obtained using the Average Length Criterion ALC [13], given a threshold for the interval width as small as 0.1, for both exact ($n_L^\star$) and approximate intervals ($n_{\tilde{L}}^\star$).

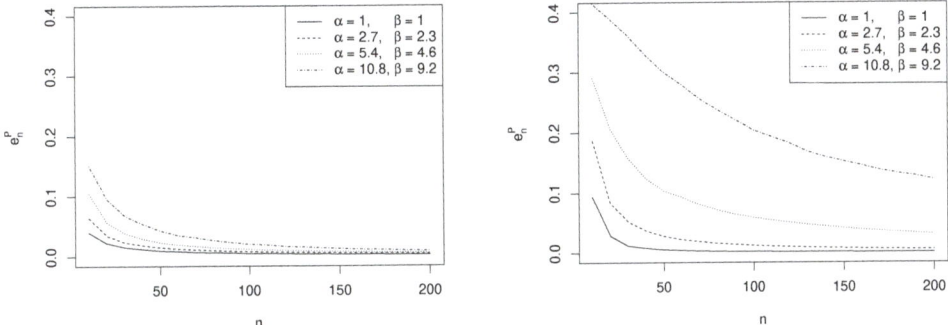

Figure 2. Plots of e_n^P as a function of n for several values of the prior hyperparameters (α, β), with $\theta_d = 0.45$ (**left column**) and $\theta_d = 0.8$ (**right column**).

The most relevant comments are the following.

1. *Effect of sample size.* As expected, the values of e_n^P decrease as n increases and depend on the specific choices of α, β and θ_d as commented in the following remarks.
2. *Effect of prior sample size.* For each value of n, the larger $\alpha + \beta$, the greater the values of e_n^P. In fact, as the prior becomes more and more concentrated around the prior mean 0.54, the weight of the prior in the posterior distribution increases with respect to the role of the likelihood. This makes the discrepancy between Bayesian exact intervals and their likelihood approximation more striking. Moreover, when the uniform non-informative prior is considered, the smallest values of e_n^P are observed (see solid line in Figure 2). As a consequence, larger values of the prior sample size imply greater values of $n_P^\star$, as shown in Table 1.
3. *Effect of the difference between design value and prior mean.* When the distance between θ_d and the prior mean $\alpha/(\alpha+\beta)$ is relatively large and, at the same time, the prior

sample size $\alpha + \beta$ dominates n, the posterior mode and the maximum likelihood estimate are well separated. In other words, Equation (4) does not provide a good approximation of the posterior density of θ. This explains the larger values of e_n^P, in the right panel of Figure 2, where $|\theta_d - \mathbb{E}(\theta)| = 0.35$, with respect to those observed in the left panel, where $|\theta_d - \mathbb{E}(\theta)| = 0.09$. As before, the effect of the difference between design value and prior mean on e_n^P also reflects on the values of the optimal sample sizes reported in Table 1. For instance, under the most informative prior, if $|\theta_d - \mathbb{E}(\theta)| = 0.09$, then $n_P^\star = 182$; conversely, when $|\theta_d - \mathbb{E}(\theta)| = 0.35$, a huge number of experimental units (e.g., $n_P^\star = 2911$) is required to have a sufficiently small expected discrepancy.

4. Comparison with $n_B^\star$. As expected, the trend of $n_B^\star$ w.r.t. to (α, β) and θ_d is consistent with that of $n_P^\star$.
5. Comparison with ALC. For each θ_d, $n_L^\star$ becomes slightly smaller when the prior sample size gets larger and the corresponding posterior is more concentrated (see Table 1). Conversely, since approximate intervals do not depend on the prior, $n_{\tilde{L}}^\star$ is not affected by the choice of prior hyperparameters. Furthermore, when the design value is closer to the boundary of the parameter space, the posterior distribution and, consequently, its approximation, become more concentrated, yielding shorter intervals. Hence the values of $n_L^\star$ and of $n_{\tilde{L}}^\star$ are uniformly smaller for $\theta_d = 0.80$ than for $\theta_d = 0.45$.

It is interesting to note the opposite impact of the prior sample size $\alpha + \beta$ on $n_P^\star$ and $n_B^\star$ on the one hand, and on $n_L^\star$ on the other hand. In fact, larger values of $\alpha + \beta$ determine shorter intervals and smaller values of $n_L^\star$. On the contrary, when $\theta_d \neq \mathbb{E}(\theta)$, a more concentrated prior implies a more remarkable discrepancy between the posterior and its likelihood approximation and, consequently, yields greater values of $n_P^\star$ and $n_B^\star$.

Table 1. Optimal sample sizes for several choices of the prior hyperameters and of the design values, given $\epsilon_P = \epsilon_B = 0.01$ and $\epsilon_L = 0.1$.

θ_d	(α, β)	$(1, 1)$	$(2.7, 2.3)$	$(5.4, 4.6)$	$(10.8, 9.2)$
0.45	$n_P^\star$	49	80	119	182
	$n_B^\star$	42	96	180	347
	$n_L^\star$	265	262	257	247
	$n_{\tilde{L}}^\star$	267	267	267	267
0.80	$n_P^\star$	35	118	646	2911
	$n_B^\star$	91	228	482	992
	$n_L^\star$	170	169	169	167
	$n_{\tilde{L}}^\star$	172	172	172	172

One of the drawbacks of approximate intervals for θ is that it is not guaranteed that $(\tilde{\ell}, \tilde{u}) \subseteq [0, 1]$. A common solution in the applications is to trasform the parameter into the log odds scale so that the normal approximation of the posterior improves. As an example we implemented the credible intervals introduced in Section 3.2. Figure 3 shows the behavior of e_n^P as a function of n for the same choices of hyperparameters and design values used in the previous example. Similar remarks apply.

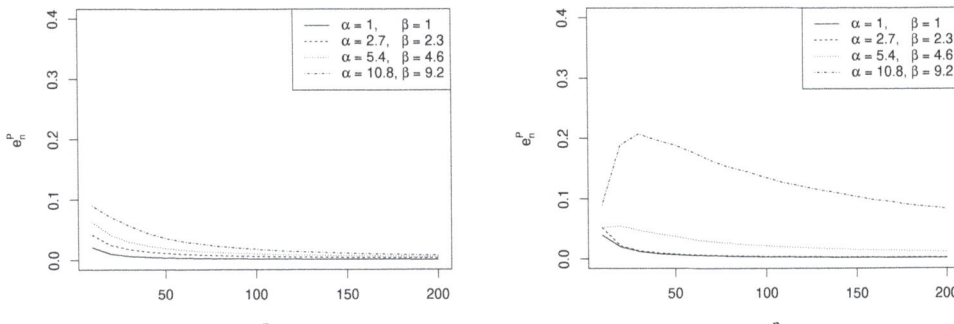

Figure 3. Plots of e_n^P as a function of n for several values of the prior hyperparameters (α, β) with $\theta_d = 0.45$ (**left panel**) and $\theta_d = 0.8$ (**right panel**), when the logodds ψ is the parameter of interest.

5. Conclusions

The control of relevant aspects of interval estimates is the starting point for the definition of several SSD criteria both from the frequentist and from the Bayesian perspective. For instance, in the Bayesian side, traditional criteria rely on the pre-posterior control of length and position of credible intervals. In this article we focus on a different request: we look for a sample size sufficiently large so that the approximate likelihood interval provides an accurate approximation to the HPD interval determined from the exact posterior distribution of the parameter of interest. Since the likelihood normal approximation does not depend on the prior distribution, another way to interpret the criterion is that it provides the smallest sample size such that the role of the prior in the posterior distribution is made negligible by the information provided by the data. This kind of analysis can be read in two different ways. On the one side, one can know the number of units needed to use safely closed-form and handy formulas (those provided by the normal approximation) in the place of exact Bayesian intervals. On the other hand, a data analyst who uses approximate intervals instead of exact Bayesian intervals can know the price of this choice in terms of expected discrepancy.

From another perspective this kind of preposterior analysis allows one to know what the study dimension should be for a consensus between a Bayesian interval and a frequentist interval, i.e., a non-informative analysis.

In general, the criterion we propose does not control the main goal of a clinical trial, that can be, for instance, accuracy of estimation or efficacy/inefficacy of a given treatment. For this reason, our criterion should be put beside additional criteria specifically related to the main goal of the trial. For instance in our examples of Section 4 we consider the optimal sample sizes based on ALC. Then, taking the maximum between the two sample sizes obtained using the two criteria, one can control both interval length and accuracy of approximation.

Possible extensions of this work are listed below.

1. Other models. The methodology proposed in the paper can be easily extended to other models and setups relevant to clinical trials applications. A natural extension is to two-arms designs for the comparison of two proportions (difference or log odds ratio), in which the additional issue of units allocation arises [32]. For a predictive approach to allocation based on the control of posterior variances, see for instance [33]. See also [5] for related ideas in the Poisson model.
2. Probability vs Expectation. In Section 2.2 we propose to summarize the predictive distribution of the discrepancy using the expected value w.r.t. $f_n(\cdot|\theta_d)$. An alternative is to take into account the whole probability distribution of P and to determine the smallest n such that $\mathbb{P}[P(X_n) > \epsilon_P]$ is sufficiently small.

3. Design prior. For simplicity in this article we have performed preposterior calculations using the sampling distribution $f_n(\cdot|\theta_d)$. An alternative is to consider the so-called *two–priors approach* [23,24,30,34]) which avoids local optimality by replacing the design value with the design prior.
4. Decision-theoretic approach. The approach proposed in the paper is performance-based. Alternatively one could follow some previous works and rephrase the problem in a decision-theoretic framework and define a measure of discrepancy based on the posterior expected loss of C and $\widetilde{C}$. We will elaborate on this in the future.

Author Contributions: Conceptualization, F.D.S.; Data curation, S.G.; Formal analysis, F.D.S. and S.G.; Methodology, F.D.S. and S.G.; Software, S.G.; Visualization, S.G.; Writing—original draft, F.D.S. and S.G.; Writing—review and editing, F.D.S. and S.G. All authors have read and agreed to the published version of the manuscript.

Funding: This research received no external funding.

Institutional Review Board Statement: Not applicable.

Informed Consent Statement: Not applicable.

Data Availability Statement: No new data were created or analyzed in this study. Data sharing is not applicable to this article.

Acknowledgments: The authors would like to thank the guest editors of this Special Issue and the reviewers.

Conflicts of Interest: The authors declare no conflict of interest.

References

1. Lee, J.; Chu, C.T. Bayesian clinical trials in action. *Stat. Med.* **2012**, *31*, 2955–2972. [PubMed]
2. Yin, G.; Lam, C.K.; Shi, H. Bayesian randomized clinical trials: From fixed to adaptive design. *Contemp. Clin. Trials* **2017**, *59*, 77–86. [CrossRef] [PubMed]
3. Bittl, J.A.; He, Y. Bayesian analysis. A practical approach to interpret clinical trials and create clinical practice guidelines. *Circ. Cardiovasc. Qual. Outcomes* **2017**, *10*, e003563. [CrossRef] [PubMed]
4. Spiegelhalter, D.J.; Abrams, K.R.; Myles, J.P. *Bayesian Approaches to Clinical Trials and Health-Care Evaluation*; Statistics in Practice; Wiley: Chichester, UK, 2004.
5. De Santis, F.; Gubbiotti, S. A note on the progressive overlap of two alternative Bayesian intervals. *Commun. Stat. Theory Methods* **2019**, 1–18. [CrossRef]
6. Lesaffre, E.; Lawson, A.B. *Bayesian Biostatistics*; Wiley:Chichester, UK, 2012.
7. Gelman, A.; Carlin, J.B.; Stern, H.S.; Dunson, D.B.; Vehtari, A.; Rubin, D.B. *Bayesian Data Analysis*, 3rd ed.; Chapman & Hall/CRC Texts in Statistical Science; Taylor & Francis: Boca Raton, FL,USA, 2013.
8. Kalbfleisch, J.G. *Probability and Statistical Inference. Volume 2: Statistical Inference*, 2nd ed.; Springer: New York, NY, USA, 1985.
9. Robert, C.P. *The Bayesian Choice: From Decision-Theoretic Foundations to Computational Implementation*, 2nd ed.; Springer: New York, NY, USA, 2007.
10. Meeker, W.Q.; Hahn, G.J.; Escobar, L.A. *Statistical Intervals: A Guide for Practitioners and Researchers*; Wiley: Hoboken, NJ, USA, 2017.
11. Brutti, P.; De Santis, F.; Gubbiotti, S. Bayesian—Frequentist sample size determination: A game of two priors. *Metron* **2014**, *72*, 133–151. [CrossRef]
12. Adcock, C.J. Sample size determination: A review. *J. R. Stat. Soc. Ser. D Stat.* **1997**, *46*, 261–283. [CrossRef]
13. Joseph, L.; du Berger, R.; Belisle, P. Bayesian and mixed Bayesian/likelihood criteria for sample size determination. *Stat. Med.* **1997**, *16*, 769–781. [CrossRef]
14. Joseph, L.; Wolfson, D. Interval-based versus decision theoretic criteria for the choice of sample size. *J. R. Stat. Soc. Ser. Stat.* **1997**, *46*, 145–149. [CrossRef]
15. Brutti, P.; De Santis, F. Robust Bayesian sample size determination for avoiding the range of equivalence in clinical trials. *J. Stat. Plan. Inference* **2008**, *138*, 1577–1591. [CrossRef]
16. Cao, J.; Lee, J.J.; Alber, S. Comparison of Bayesian sample size criteria: ACC, ALC, and WOC. *J. Stat. Plan. Inference* **2009**, *139*, 4111–4122. [CrossRef]
17. Gubbiotti, S.; De Santis, F. A Bayesian method for the choice of the sample size in equivalence trials. *Aust. New Zealand J. Stat.* **2011**, *53*, 443–460. [CrossRef]
18. Joseph, L.; Wolfson, D.B.; Berger, R.D. Sample Size Calculations for Binomial Proportions via Highest Posterior Density Intervals. *J. R. Stat. Soc. Ser. D Stat.* **1995**, *44*, 143–154. [CrossRef]

19. M'Lan, C.E.; Joseph, L.; Wolfson, D.B. Bayesian sample size determination for binomial proportions. *Bayesian Anal.* **2008**, *3*, 269–296.10.1214/08-BA310. [CrossRef]
20. De Santis, F.; Fasciolo, M.C.; Gubbiotti, S. Predictive control of posterior robustness for sample size choice in a Bernoulli model. *Stat. Methods Appl.* **2013**, *22*, 319–340. [CrossRef]
21. De Santis, F. Sample size determination for robust Bayesian analysis. *J. Am. Stat. Assoc.* **2006**, *101*, 278–291. [CrossRef]
22. Brutti, P.; De Santis, F.; Gubbiotti, S. Robust Bayesian sample size determination in clinical trials. *Stat. Med.* **2008**, *27*, 2290–2306. [CrossRef] [PubMed]
23. Joseph, L.; Belisle, P. Bayesian consensus-based sample size criteria for binomial proportions. *Stat. Med.* **2019**.10.1002/sim.8316. [CrossRef] [PubMed]
24. Brutti, P.; De Santis, F.; Gubbiotti, S. Predictive measures of the conflict between frequentist and Bayesian estimators. *J. Stat. Plan. Inference* **2014**, *148*, 111–122.10.1016/j.jspi.2013.12.009. [CrossRef]
25. De Santis, F.; Gubbiotti, S. A decision-theoretic approach to sample size determination under several priors. *Appl. Stoch. Model. Bus. Ind.* **2017**, *33*, 282–295. [CrossRef]
26. Casella, G.; Berger, R. *Statistical Inference*; Duxbury: Belmont, CA, USA, 2001.
27. R Core Team. *R: A Language and Environment for Statistical Computing*; R Foundation for Statistical Computing: Vienna, Austria, 2018.
28. Sacchi, S.; Marcheselli, R.; Bari, A.; Buda, G.; Molinari, A.L.; Baldini, L.; Vallisa, D.; Cesaretti, M.; Musto, P.; Ronconi, S.; et al. Safety and efficacy of lenalidomide in combination with rituximab in recurrent indolent non-follicular lymphoma: final results of a phase II study conducted by the Fondazione Italiana Linfomi. *Haematologica* **2016**, *101*, e196–e199. [CrossRef]
29. Zhou, H.; Lee, J.J.; Yuan, Y. BOP2: Bayesian optimal design for phase II clinical trials with simple and complex endpoints. *Stat. Med.* **2017**, *36*, 3302–3314. [CrossRef] [PubMed]
30. Sambucini, V. Bayesian predictive monitoring with bivariate binary outcomes in phase II clinical trials. *Comput. Stat. Data Anal.* **2019**, *132*, 18–30. [CrossRef]
31. Morita, S.; Thall, P.F.; Muller, P. Determining the effective sample size of a parametric prior. *Biometrics* **2008**, *64*, 595–602.10.1111/j.1541-0420.2007.00888.x. [CrossRef] [PubMed]
32. M'Lan, C.E.; Joseph, L.; Wolfson, D.B. Bayesian Sample Size Determination for Case-Control Studies. *J. Am. Stat. Assoc.* **2006**, *101*, 760–772.10.1198/016214505000001023. [CrossRef]
33. De Santis, F.; Perone Pacifico, M.; Sambucini, V. Optimal predictive sample size for case-control studies. *Appl. Stat.* **2004**, *53*, 427–441. [CrossRef]
34. Wang, F.; Gelfand, A.E. A simulation-based approach to Bayesian sample size determination for performance under a given model and for separating models. *Statist. Sci.* **2002**, *17*, 193–208. [CrossRef]

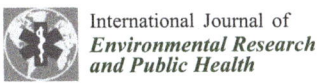

Article

Bayesian Meta-Analysis for Binary Data and Prior Distribution on Models

Miguel-Angel Negrín-Hernández *, María Martel-Escobar and Francisco-José Vázquez-Polo

Department of Quantitative Methods & TiDES Institute, University of Las Palmas de Gran Canaria, E-35017 Las Palmas de Gran Canaria, Spain; maria.martel@ulpgc.es (M.M.-E.); francisco.vazquezpolo@ulpgc.es (F.-J.V.-P.)
* Correspondence: miguel.negrin@ulpgc.es; Tel.: +34-928-451-800

Abstract: In meta-analysis, the structure of the between-sample heterogeneity plays a crucial role in estimating the meta-parameter. A Bayesian meta-analysis for binary data has recently been proposed that measures this heterogeneity by clustering the samples and then determining the posterior probability of the cluster models through model selection. The meta-parameter is then estimated using Bayesian model averaging techniques. Although an objective Bayesian meta-analysis is proposed for each type of heterogeneity, we concentrate the attention of this paper on priors over the models. We consider four alternative priors which are motivated by reasonable but different assumptions. A frequentist validation with simulated data has been carried out to analyze the properties of each prior distribution for a set of different number of studies and sample sizes. The results show the importance of choosing an adequate model prior as the posterior probabilities for the models are very sensitive to it. The hierarchical Poisson prior and the hierarchical uniform prior show a good performance when the real model is the homogeneity, or when the sample sizes are high enough. However, the uniform prior can detect the true model when it is an intermediate model (neither homogeneity nor heterogeneity) even for small sample sizes and few studies. An illustrative example with real data is also given, showing the sensitivity of the estimation of the meta-parameter to the model prior.

Keywords: bayesian meta-analysis; clustering; binary data; priors; frequentist validation

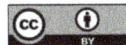

1. Introduction

Meta-analysis has been widely applied in many research areas and is of particular importance in healthcare studies. When there exist different randomized controlled clinical trials (or studies) of a particular medical treatment, a meta-analysis may be conducted to determine what final conclusion can be drawn from each study, the effectiveness of the treatment.

One of the cases that has received more attention in the literature is the meta-analysis for binary data [1]. On the one hand, because it is very common for effectiveness to be measured through a binary variable according to whether or not a certain objective has been achieved (to survive, do not relapse or to reach a low viral load). Charles et al. [2] found that half of trials calculated their sample size based on a binary outcomes. On the other hand, binary outcomes have different statistical considerations to using continuous outcomes. The Bayesian random-effects model for meta-analysis given by Sutton and Abrams [3] would not be suitable for modeling binary data:

$$x_i \sim \mathcal{N}(\theta_i, \tau_i), \ i = 1, \ldots, k$$
$$\theta_i \sim \mathcal{N}(\theta, \tau),$$
$$\theta \sim [-,-] \ \tau \sim [-,-],$$

(1)

where x_i denotes an observed effect for each of k studies, θ the estimated pooled effect, and τ^2 is an estimate of the between-study variance. For binary data, the preceding normal hierarchical model has been applied to the logit transformation $y_i = \log[x_i/(n_i - x_i)]$ with the reparametrization $\log[\theta_i/(1-\theta_i)]$, where x_i denotes the number of successes at the ith study [4–7]. However, this normal approximation does not work properly when the samples sizes (n_i) are small or when the number of successes is zero, even if a continuity correction is applied to the original data, as it was shown by Sweeting et al. [8].

Moreno et al. [9] proposed an objective Bayesian meta-analysis model for binary data in which no continuity correction is required. The Bayesian model proposed for the study i is based on the binomial distribution $\{M_i : \text{Bin}(x_i, \theta_i, n_i), \pi(\theta_i)\}$, and the linking distribution between the parameters of each study θ_i and the meta-parameter θ, $\pi(\theta_i, \theta)$, belongs to the Fréchet class of bidimensional distributions with fixed marginals $\pi(\theta_i)$ and $\pi(\theta)$. The objective Bayesian analysis assumes that these marginals are uniform priors, $\text{Unif}(\theta_i|0,1)$ and $\text{Unif}(\theta|0,1)$.

The model parameters will therefore be the parameters for the k studies, $\theta_1, \ldots, \theta_k$, and the meta-parameter θ. However, if some of the $\theta_i's$ are equal the dimension of the model would be reduced. In [10], the authors proposed to study the between-sample heterogeneity as a model selection problem, clustering the parameters $\theta_1, \ldots, \theta_k$ based on the samples $(x_1, n_1), \ldots, (x_k, n_k)$. They adopted a Bayesian approach based on product partition models proposed in [11,12]. Bayesian model selection process requires the definition of a specific model prior.

In the absence of information about the models, the uniform prior is the most common prior assumed in a Bayesian model selection problem. However, this prior does not consider the structure of the cluster problem and other alternative model priors are possible such as considering the uniform distribution in each of the hierarchy levels of the clusters, or even considering the Poisson-Intrinsic prior proposed by Casella et al. [13] which penalizes the number of clusters. Although all these priors can be considered as not informative as they do not add new information to that provided by the data, the prior probabilities assigned to each partition vary. Due to the sensitivity of the estimation of the meta-parameter to the chosen cluster, we analyze in this paper the characteristics of these model priors and in which cases each one my be preferable.

A frequentist evaluation is carried out with simulated data, where different number of studies, sample sizes, and real clusters are considered. The rest of the paper is organized as follows. The binomial Bayesian model is presented in Section 2, where the Bayesian procedure for clustering the samples and the likelihood of the meta-parameter are also given. In this section, the four model priors to be compared will be presented. The simulated data and the results of the frequentist validation are described in Section 3. Section 4 provides one illustrative example with a real dataset. Finally, Section 5 summarizes the main conclusions drawn and presents some concluding remarks.

2. The Bayesian Binomial Model

Assume a meta-analysis involving k studies that provide k independent discrete samples which follow a binomial distribution $\{\text{Bin}(x_i|n_i, \theta_i), i = 1, \ldots, k\}$, where θ_i represents the treatment effectiveness, n_i the number of patients, and x_i the number of successful treatments, conditional on the study i. We assume weak prior information on the conditional treatment effectiveness θ_i. Accordingly, the uniform prior $\text{Unif}(\theta_i|0,1)$ is used [14,15]. The Bayesian sampling model (M_i) for $i = 1, \ldots, k$ studies is then given by

$$M_i : \left\{\text{Bin}(x_i|n_i, \theta_i), \ \pi(\theta_i) \propto \mathbf{1}_{(0,1)}(\theta_i)\right\}, \tag{2}$$

where

$$\text{Bin}(x_i|n_i, \theta_i) = \binom{n_i}{x_i}\theta_i^{x_i}(1-\theta_i)^{n_i-x_i}, \quad x_i = 0, 1, \ldots, n_i, \tag{3}$$

and $\mathbf{1}_A$ is the indicator function that takes a value of 1 to all elements of A, and 0 elsewhere.

The meta-model is defined by a patient in a virtual study, which is not affected by between-study variability. The variable x is a binary latent variable and the meta-parameter θ defines the probability of success for this virtual patient. The distribution of this meta-variable x is the Bernoulli meta-model $\text{Ber}(x|\theta)$, where the meta–parameter θ represents the true (unconditional) treatment effect. The objective Bayesian meta-model M is then given by

$$M : \left\{ \Pr(x|\theta) = \theta^x (1-\theta)^{1-x}, \ \pi(\theta) = \mathbf{1}_{(0,1)}(\theta) \right\}. \tag{4}$$

2.1. The Linking Distribution

A distribution $\pi(\theta_i|\theta)$ is needed to link the experimental parameters θ_i and the meta-parameter θ. This linking distribution should ensure there is coherence between the conditional and marginal distributions of the experimental parameters and the meta-parameter. This requires that the corresponding bivariate distribution belongs to the class of bivariate distributions with given marginals. The class of bivariate distributions solving this problem is called the Frèchet class:

$$\int_0^1 \pi(\theta_i, \theta) d\theta_i = \pi(\theta) \ \text{ and } \ \int_0^1 \pi(\theta_i, \theta) d\theta = \pi(\theta_i). \tag{5}$$

Following Moreno et al. [9], a candidate $\pi(\theta_i, \theta)$ is constructed using the intrinsic priors for model selection [16]. The conditional intrinsic linking distributions $\{\pi^I(\theta_i|\theta, t), \ t = 1, 2, \ldots\}$ arises from the model comparison between the meta-model M and the experimental model M_i. For any positive integer t, the intrinsic method gives the conditional intrinsic prior as a Beta-Binomial mixture,

$$\pi^I(\theta_i|\theta) = \sum_{z=0}^{t} \text{Bin}(z|t, \theta) \times \text{Beta}(\theta_i|z+1, t-z+1). \tag{6}$$

In general, the bivariate intrinsic prior $\pi^I(\theta_i, \theta|t)$ enjoys two interesting properties. One is that it belongs to the Frèchet class with marginals $\pi(\theta_i)$ and $\pi(\theta)$ following a uniform distribution. A second one is that the concentration degree of $\pi^I(\theta_i|\theta, t)$ around θ is controlled by the training sample size t, the larger the t the larger the concentration degree. Note that the correlation coefficient between θ_i and θ is $\rho = t/(t+1)$. In practice, the hyperparameter t is fixed, assuming a large enough correlation between θ_i and θ. We assume in our examples a correlation of 0.98, which implies that $t = 48$. Hence, for the sake of simplicity in notation, we refer to the linking distribution $\pi^I(\theta_i|\theta)$ rather than $\pi^I(\theta_i|\theta, t)$.

As it is assumed that θ_i, $i = 1, \ldots, k$ are conditional independent given θ, the linking distribution of $\theta_1, \ldots, \theta_k$ conditional on θ is given by

$$\pi^I(\theta_1, \ldots, \theta_k|\theta) = \prod_{i=1}^{k} \pi^I(\theta_i|\theta). \tag{7}$$

2.2. Clusters

The previous section assumes that there are k experimental parameters θ_i, $i = 1, \ldots, k$ to be estimated. However the dimension of the experimental model can be reduced if some of the θ_i's are equal. Following Moreno et al. [10], model estimation in this parametric setting is a problem of clustering the parameters $\theta_1, \ldots, \theta_k$, based on the samples $x_1, \ldots, x_k$ from the experiments. We first define what is meant by cluster. The samples x_i and x_j, $i \neq j$, from $f(x|\theta_i, n)$ and $f(x|\theta_j, n)$, respectively, are said to be in the same cluster if $\theta_i = \theta_j$. The between-sample heterogeneity is then determined by the number of clusters and by the location of the samples $(x_1, n_1), \ldots, (x_k, n_k)$ within these clusters.

To cluster the samples we adopt the product partition model approach proposed by Barry and Hartigan [12], together with a Bayesian model selection procedure based on Bayes factors for the intrinsic priors for the model parameters.

We employ the following notations and expressions in the meta-analysis conducted [13]. For a given p, we define a partition of the samples into p clusters by the vector $\mathbf{r}_p = (r_1, \ldots, r_k)$, where r_i, $i = 1, \ldots, k$, is an integer between 1 and p denoting the cluster to which x_i is assigned. Figure 1 shows the possible clustering structures for $k = 3$, and their corresponding $\mathbf{r}_p$.

$x_1 x_2 x_3$	$x_1 \| x_2 x_3$ $x_2 \| x_1 x_3$ $x_3 \| x_1 x_2$	$x_1 \| x_2 \| x_3$
Homogeneity	Type 2–Heterogeneity	Heterogeneity
$\mathbf{r}_1 = (1,1,1)$	$\mathbf{r}_2 = (1,2,2)$ $\mathbf{r}_2 = (1,2,1)$ $\mathbf{r}_2 = (1,1,2)$	$\mathbf{r}_3 = (1,2,3)$

Figure 1. Clustering structure and different heterogeneity structures with $k = 3$ studies.

2.3. The Likelihood of θ for a Particular Partition

The likelihood of θ will depend on the partition of the samples. Given a partition $\mathbf{r}_p = (r_1, \ldots, r_k)$, the sampling distribution of $x = (x_1, \ldots, x_k)$ given in (2) is

$$f(x|p, \mathbf{r}_p, \boldsymbol{\theta}_p) = \prod_{j=1}^{p} \binom{m_j}{s_j} \theta_j^{s_j} (1 - \theta_j)^{m_j - s_j}, \quad (8)$$

where $\boldsymbol{\theta}_p = (\theta_1, \ldots, \theta_p)$ is an unknown parameter of dimension p, the component θ_j in (8) corresponds to $r_i = j$, and $m_j = \sum_{i: r_i = j} n_i$ and $s_j = \sum_{i: r_i = j} x_i$ are the sample size and number of success of the cluster j. The likelihood of a particular partition, for example, $\mathbf{r}_2 = (1, 2, 2)$, is

$$f(x|2, \mathbf{r}_2 = (1,2,2), \boldsymbol{\theta}_2) = \binom{n_1}{x_1} \theta_1^{x_1} (1-\theta_1)^{n_1 - x_1} \binom{n_2 + n_3}{x_2 + x_3} \theta_2^{x_2 + x_3} (1-\theta_2)^{(n_2 + n_3) - (x_2 + x_3)}.$$

The heterogeneity partition $\mathbf{r}_k = (1, 2, 3, \ldots, k)$ has the corresponding likelihood function given by

$$f(x|k, \mathbf{r}_k, \boldsymbol{\theta}_k) = \prod_{i=1}^{k} \binom{n_i}{x_i} \theta_i^{x_i} (1 - \theta_i)^{n_i - x_i},$$

and the homogeneity partition $\mathbf{r}_1 = (1, 1, \ldots, 1)$ has the corresponding likelihood function given by

$$f(x|1, \mathbf{r}_1, \theta_1) = \binom{\sum_{i=1}^{k} n_i}{\sum_{i=1}^{k} x_i} \theta_1^{\sum_{i=1}^{k} x_i} (1 - \theta_1)^{\sum_{i=1}^{k}(n_i - x_i)}.$$

Now, integrating out $\boldsymbol{\theta}_p$ with the intrinsic prior $\pi(\boldsymbol{\theta}_p | p, \mathbf{r}_p) = \int \pi^I(\theta_1, \ldots, \theta_p | \theta) \mathbf{1}_{(0,1)}(\theta) d\theta$, we obtain the likelihood of θ, conditional on the cluster model $(p, \mathbf{r_p})$ given by

$$f(x|p, \mathbf{r}_p, \theta) = \prod_{j=1}^{p} \int_0^1 f(x|p, \mathbf{r}_p, \boldsymbol{\theta}_p) \pi(\theta_j | \theta) \, d\theta_j =$$

$$= (1 + t)^p (1 - \theta)^{tp} \prod_{j=1}^{p} \frac{\Gamma(s_j + 1) \Gamma(m_j + t - s_j + 1)}{\Gamma(m_j + t + 2)} \, {}_3F_2\left(\mathbf{a}_j, \mathbf{b}_j, \frac{\theta}{\theta - 1}\right), \quad (9)$$

where ${}_3F_2(\mathbf{v}, \mathbf{w}, z)$ denotes the generalized hypergeometric function with argument z and vector parameters $\mathbf{v}$ and $\mathbf{w}$ of dimensions 3 and 2. In this case, the parameters $\mathbf{a}_j = (-t, -t, s_j + 1)$ and $\mathbf{b}_j = (1, -m_j - t + s_j)$ are related with the number of 1's and 0's in cluster j, respectively.

2.4. The Likelihood of θ the Prior Distribution over the Partitions

To derive the likelihood function of θ we need to integrate out (9) with respect to a discrete prior on $(p, \mathbf{r}_p)$. The (unconditional) likelihood of θ for the data x is given by

$$f(x|\theta) = \sum_{p=1}^{k} \left(\sum_{\mathbf{r}_p} f(x|p, \mathbf{r}_p, \theta) \pi(p, \mathbf{r}_p|k) \right). \tag{10}$$

The prior distribution on the partitions $\pi(p, \mathbf{r}_p|k)$ plays an important role in the estimation of the parameter θ [13]. We consider here four priors on $(p, \mathbf{r}_p)$ which are motivated by reasonable but different assumptions. The four selected prior distribution assume the absence of prior information about the models, but ranges from the assignment of high prior probability at the boundary $p = 1$ and $p = 4$ (homogeneity and heterogeneity structures, respectively) to other intermediate situations that moderate the a priori assignment to these two clusters or considers them all equally probable.

- The Uniform prior.
  The first prior proposed is the uniform prior (U), which gives the same probability to every model, that is,

$$\pi^U(p, \mathbf{r}_p|k) = \frac{1}{\mathcal{B}_k}, \tag{11}$$

  where $\mathcal{B}_k$, the Bell number, is the number of subsets a set of size k can be partitioned into. Figure 2 shows the prior probabilities for each partition when four studies are considered. In this example, the Bell number is 15. This choice does not take into account the level of complexity of each partition.

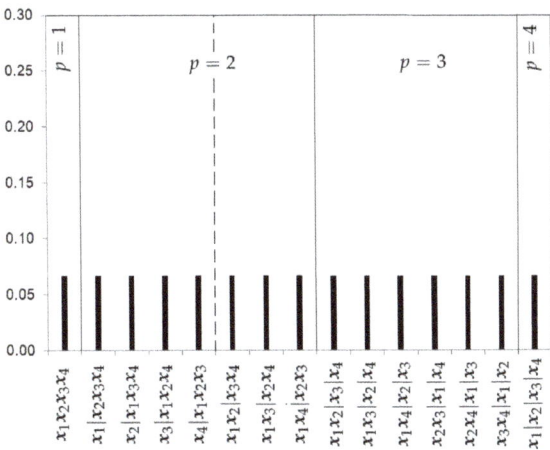

Figure 2. Uniform prior probabilities for the partitions with $k = 4$ studies.

- The Hierarchical Uniform Prior with 2 levels (HU2).
  As recommended by Casella et al. [13], a hierarchical uniform prior can be appropriate to take into account the different levels of complexity of the partitions. This prior distribution distinguishes two levels of complexity in the partitions. The first level is given by the number of clusters p in which the k samples are grouped. The second level will be given by the number of possible partitions of the k samples into p clusters. Let $\mathcal{R}_p$ represent this set of partitions into p clusters, which we call the cluster class. The number of partitions in $\mathcal{R}_p$ is given by the Stirling number of the second kind $\mathcal{S}(k, p)$ and can be written as

$$S(k,p) = \sum_{1\leq k_1\leq\ldots\leq k_p} \binom{k_1+\ldots+k_p}{k_1\cdots k_p} \frac{1}{R(k_1,\ldots,k_p)}, \tag{12}$$

where $\binom{k_1+\ldots+k_p}{k_1\cdots k_p}$ is the multinomial coefficient and $R(k_1,\ldots,k_p) = \prod_{i=1}^{k}[\sum_{j=1}^{p} I(k_j = i)]!$ corrects the count by considering the redundant strings corresponding to the vector $(k_1,\ldots,k_p)$. For instance, to calculate the Stirling number $S(4,2)$, there are two possible vectors (k_1,k_2), the vector $(1,3)$, and the vector $(2,2)$, and the Stirling number would be

$$S(4,2) = \binom{4}{1,3}\frac{1}{R(1,3)} + \binom{4}{2,2}\frac{1}{R(2,2)} = \frac{4!}{1!3!}\frac{1}{1!1!} + \frac{4!}{2!2!}\frac{1}{2!} = 4 + 3 = 7, \tag{13}$$

which is the number of possible partitions for $p = 2$ and $k = 4$.

The hierarchical uniform distribution for 2 levels will be given by the decomposition

$$\pi^{HU2}(p, \mathbf{r}_p|k) = \pi(\mathbf{r}_p|p,k)\pi(p|k) = \frac{1}{S(k,p)}\frac{1}{k}. \tag{14}$$

Figure 3 shows the prior probabilities for each partition using the hierarchical uniform prior with 2 levels with 4 studies. Note that this hierarchical distribution assigns a higher prior probability to cases of homogeneity and heterogeneity.

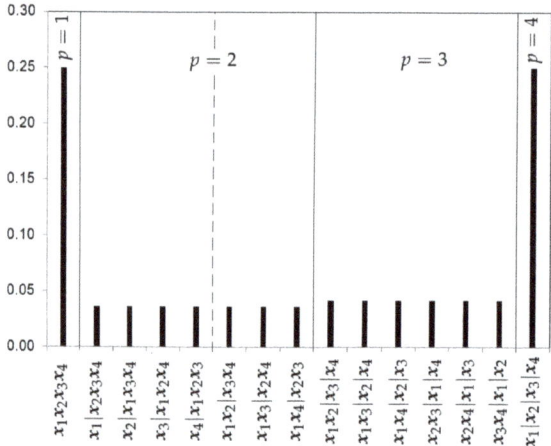

Figure 3. Hierarchical Uniform prior with 2 levels probabilities for the partitions with $k = 4$ studies.

- The Hierarchical Uniform Prior with 3 levels (HU3).
  Following Casella et al. [13] and Moreno et al. [10], the prior specification for $(p, \mathbf{r}_p)$ can be decomposed in three levels:

$$\pi^{HU3}(p, \mathbf{r}_p|k) = \pi(p, \mathbf{r}_p|\mathcal{R}_{p;k_1,\ldots,k_p}, k)\pi(\mathcal{R}_{p;k_1,\ldots,k_p}|p,k)\pi(p|k). \tag{15}$$

Unlike the previous prior distribution, the hierarchical uniform prior with 3 levels considers the number of ways the integer k can be partitioned into p clusters. We will call it the number of configuration classes within each $\mathcal{R}_p$ and it will be denoted by $b(k,p)$. In our illustrative example with $k = 4$, this value is equal to 1 for $p = 1, 3, 4$ ($b(4,1) = b(4,3) = b(4,4) = 1$), and only for the cluster class $p = 2$ there are two configuration classes, corresponding to the configurations $x|xxx$ and $xx|xx$, so $b(4,2) = 2$.

The hierarchical uniform prior with 3 levels is given by the expression

$$\pi^{HU3}(p, \mathbf{r}_p|k) = \frac{k_1! \cdot \ldots \cdot k_p!}{k!} \frac{R(k_1, \ldots, k_p)}{b(k, p)} \frac{1}{k}. \quad (16)$$

Figure 4 shows the prior probabilities for each partition using the hierarchical uniform prior with 3 levels and 4 studies.

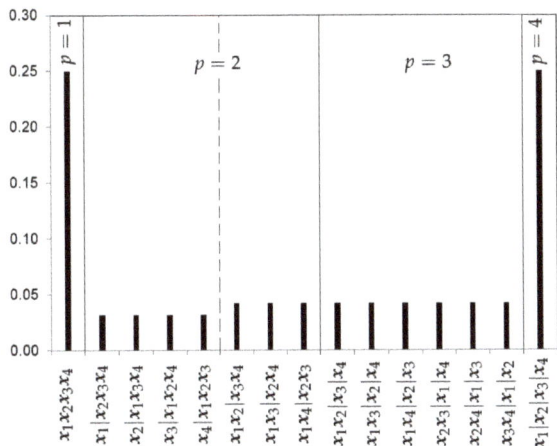

Figure 4. Hierarchical Uniform prior with 3 levels probabilities for the partitions with $k = 4$ studies.

- The Hierarchical Poisson Prior with 3 levels (HP3).
  Casella et al. [13] argue that when analyzing a cluster problem of a sample size k, the extreme case of having k clusters should be given *a priori* a smaller probability than that given to any other case. Extending this argument for any k, it might be reasonable that the prior distribution on the number of clusters $\pi(p|k)$ might be a truncated Poisson distribution $\mathcal{P}(p|\lambda)$, where λ is an unknown parameter. We can assume an intrinsic prior $\pi^I(\lambda|\lambda_0 = 1)$ for λ, constructed by testing the Poisson null hypothesis $H_0 : \lambda = \lambda_0$ versus $H_1 : \lambda \in R^+$ [17],

$$\pi^I(\lambda|\lambda_0 = 1) = \frac{\lambda^{-1/2}}{\Gamma(1/2)} e^{-(\lambda+1)} {}_0F_1(1/2, \lambda), \quad (17)$$

where ${}_0F_1(1/2, \lambda)$ denotes the confluent hypergeometric function. The reason for taking $\lambda_0 = 1$ is that the one cluster model is the reference model throughout the analysis. The resulting marginal intrinsic distribution for p is

$$\pi^I(p|k) = \frac{m^I(p)}{\sum_{p=1}^{k} m^I(p)}, p = 1, \ldots, k, \quad m^I(p) = \int_0^{+\infty} \frac{\lambda^p e^{-\lambda}}{p!} \pi^I(\lambda|\lambda_0 = 1) d\lambda. \quad (18)$$

We cannot assume a Poisson distribution for the other two levels of the hierarchical structure because there is no a clear order in relation to complexity. For this reason, a uniform distribution is assumed for the other two levels. The hierarchical Poisson prior will be given by

$$\pi^{HP3}(p, \mathbf{r}_p|k) = \frac{k_1! \cdot \ldots \cdot k_p!}{k!} \frac{R(k_1, \ldots, k_p)}{b(k, p)} \pi^I(p|k). \quad (19)$$

Figure 5 shows the prior probabilities for each partition using the hierarchical Poisson prior with 4 studies. The prior probability for the homogeneity cluster is more than four times higher than the prior probability of the heterogeneity case.

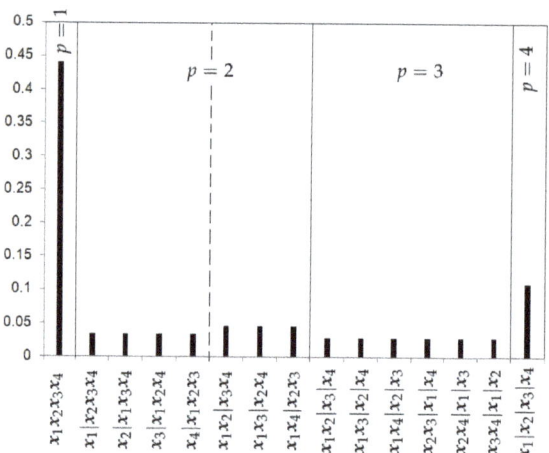

Figure 5. Hierarchical Poisson prior with 3 levels probabilities for the partitions with $k = 4$ studies.

Finally, from (10) and the priors defined in (11), (14), (16) and (19), the (unconditional) likelihood of θ for the data x is given by

$$f(x|\theta) = \sum_{p=1}^{k} \left(\sum_{\mathbf{r}_p} f(x|p, \mathbf{r}_p, \theta) \pi(p, \mathbf{r}_p) \right). \quad (20)$$

2.5. Bayesian Model Averaging in the Meta-Analysis

The BMA approach to meta-analysis involves averaging over all the possible models (heterogeneity structures or partitions) when making inferences about the parameter of interest θ.

In this case, the posterior probabilities correspond to those of any heterogeneity structure given by a pair $(p, \mathbf{r}_p)$, which is represented by

$$\Pr(p, \mathbf{r}_p | x, k) = \frac{m_{\mathbf{r}_p}(x|p, \mathbf{r}_p) \pi(p, \mathbf{r}_p)|k}{\sum_{p=1}^{k} \left(\sum_{\mathbf{r}_p} m_{\mathbf{r}_p}(x|p, \mathbf{r}_p) \pi(p, \mathbf{r}_p|k) \right)}, \quad (21)$$

where $m_{\mathbf{r}_p}(x|p, \mathbf{r}_p) = \int f(x|p, \mathbf{r}_p, \theta_p) \pi(\theta_p|p, \mathbf{r}_p) d\theta_p$ is the marginal of the data x conditional on model $(p, \mathbf{r}_p)$, with $f(x|p, \mathbf{r}_p, \theta_p)$ and $\pi(\theta_p|p, \mathbf{r}_p)$. These posterior model probabilities $\Pr(p, \mathbf{r}_p|x)$ are the weights for the meta inference.

The posterior distribution for the parameter of interest θ becomes

$$\pi(\theta|x) = \sum_{\mathbf{r}_p} \pi(\theta|x, p, \mathbf{r}_p) \Pr(p, \mathbf{r}_p|x, k), \quad (22)$$

where

$$\pi(\theta|x, p, \mathbf{r}_p) = \frac{f(x|p, \mathbf{r}_p, \theta)}{\int_0^1 f(x|p, \mathbf{r}_p, \theta) d\theta}, \quad 0 < \theta < 1. \quad (23)$$

The posterior distribution in (22) is computed numerically using Wolfram Mathematica (see code in the Supplementary Material Section).

3. Simulated Data and Frequentist Validation

3.1. Simulated Data

This section presents the simulated data used in the frequentist validation. The data have been simulated from binomial distributions, where the number of studies included in the meta-analysis (k), the partition for the data ($\mathbf{r}_p$), and the sample size within each study (n) vary between simulations.

The values for the number of studies (k) in the meta-analysis are 3, 5. Other greater values of k are obviously possible. For instance, we developed the case $k = 8$ (see supplementary material Section) where the conclusions obtained are similar to that in the cases $k = 3$ and 5. Therefore, in order to facilitate the reading of the Table 1 we only present the cases $k = 3$ and $k = 5$. These numbers of studies are manageable to do this simulation exercise. In this respect, Davey et al. [18] conducted an extensive review of the Cochrane Database of Systematic Reviews (CDSR) and pointed out that just under 75% of the meta-analyses contained five or fewer studies.

The sample size within each study is also a crucial parameter of the simulation. For simplicity we assume a common sample size for the k studies and this sample size takes values of 10, 30, 100, and 300. Finally different "true" partitions are considered for each k, where the heterogeneity and homogeneity cases are always included and one or two intermediate cases are also analyzed. Table 1 shows the parameters of the simulated data.

Table 1. Parameters for the simulation data.

True Model ($\mathbf{r}_p$)	Parameters (θ_i's)	Sample Sizes (n_i)
$k = 3$		
1, 1, 1	(0.5, 0.5, 0.5)	(10, 30, 100, 300)
1, 1, 2	(0.5, 0.5, 0.2)	(10, 30, 100, 300)
1, 2, 3	(0.7, 0.5, 0.2)	(10, 30, 100, 300)
$k = 5$		
1, 1, 1, 1, 1	(0.5, 0.5, 0.5, 0.5, 0.5)	(10, 30, 100, 300)
1, 1, 1, 2, 2	(0.5, 0.5, 0.5, 0.2, 0.2)	(10, 30, 100, 300)
1, 1, 2, 2, 3	(0.7, 0.7, 0.5, 0.5, 0.2)	(10, 30, 100, 300)
1, 2, 3, 4, 5	(0.9, 0.7, 0.5, 0.3, 0.1)	(10, 30, 100, 300)

The θ_i parameters used in the simulation are sufficiently disparate between clusters to expect that with moderate sample sizes, the Bayesian selection process will be able to detect the true model. For all simulation scenarios, 500 simulations were performed. To analyze the properties of the prior distributions over posterior probabilities of the partitions we show the proportion of times the true model is found as the model with the highest posterior probability and the mean posterior probability in those cases in which the true model is found as the most probable. We also show the number of cases the homogeneity cluster ($\mathbf{r}_1 = (1, 1, \ldots, 1)$) and the heterogeneity case ($\mathbf{r}_k = (1, 2, 3, \ldots, k)$) are found as the most probable model.

3.2. Frequentist Evaluation

Figures 6 and 7 show the results of the frequentist validation for the case $k = 3$ and true partitions $\mathbf{r}_1 = (1, 1, 1)$, $\mathbf{r}_2 = (1, 1, 2)$ and $\mathbf{r}_3 = (1, 2, 3)$ corresponding to a situation of homogeneity, intermediate heterogeneity, and heterogeneity, respectively. As expected, for the true case of homogeneity $\mathbf{r}_1$, the uniform prior shows worse performance as it is the only one that does not assume an a priori preference for the homogeneity. However, the results show how the uniform prior reaches a proportion of correct choices close to 70% with sample sizes greater than 100. The mean posterior probabilities reach values greater than 30% and 40% for sample sizes of 100 and 300, respectively. Observe that $b(3, p) = 1$, $1 \leq p \leq 3$, thus the results from HU2 and HU3 priors are identical. The hierarchical Poisson prior, which assigns a higher prior probability to the homogeneity case, reaches a proportion of correct choices higher than 95% even with sample sizes of 10, and posterior probabilities higher than 50%. All the prior distributions show a good performance for high sample sizes.

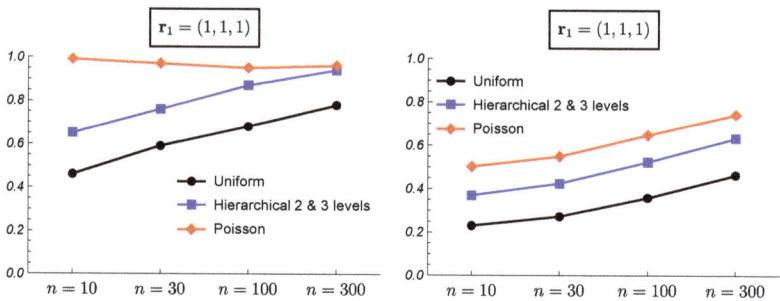

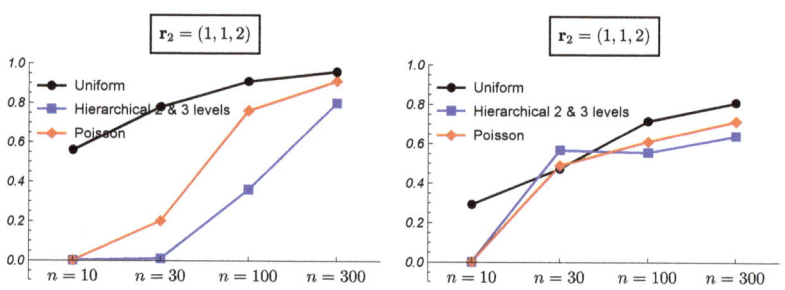

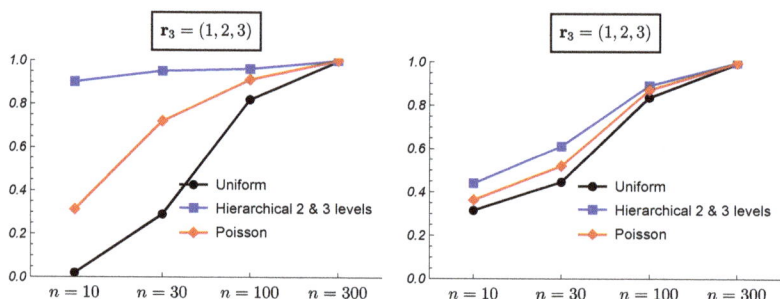

Figure 6. Frequentist validation for the case $k = 3$ and true partitions $\mathbf{r}_1 = (1, 1, 1), \mathbf{r}_2 = (1, 1, 2)$ and $\mathbf{r}_3 = (1, 2, 3)$. (**Left column**) proportion of times the true partition is found as the most probable. (**Right column**) mean of the posterior probability for the true partition when it is found as the most probable.

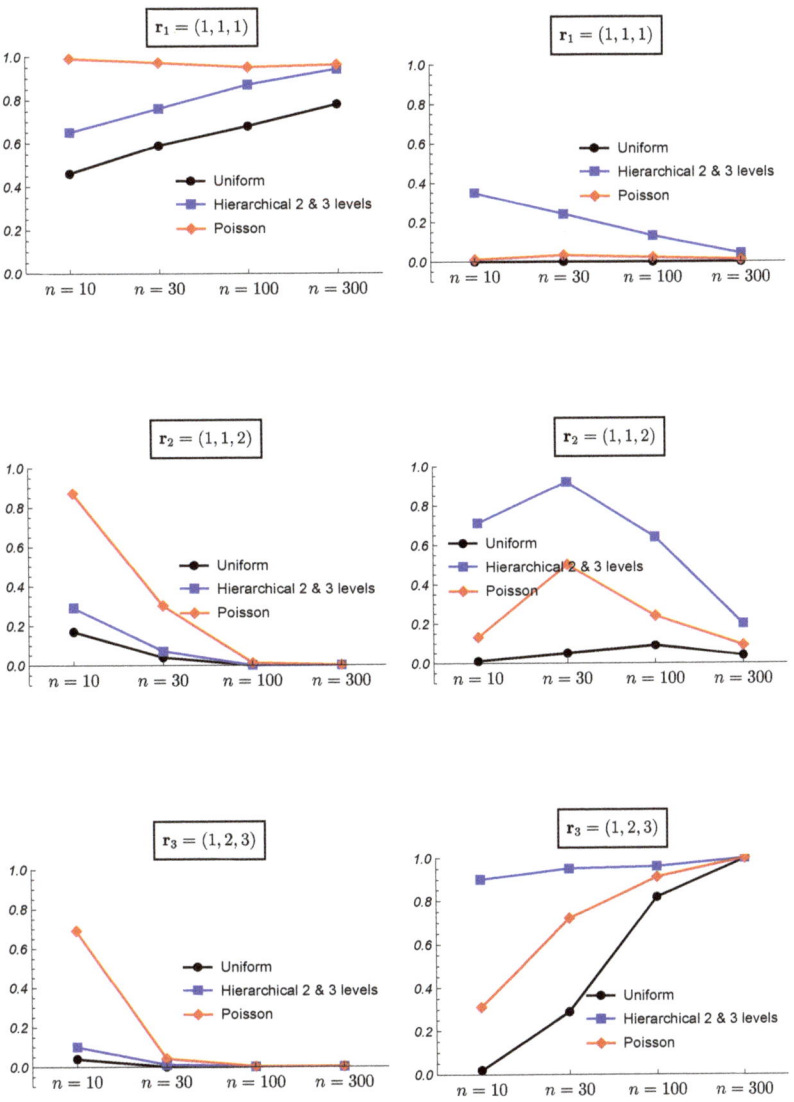

Figure 7. Frequentist validation for the case $k = 3$ and true partitions $r_1 = (1, 1, 1)$, $r_2 = (1, 1, 2)$ and $r_3 = (1, 2, 3)$. (**Left column**) proportion of times the homogeneity case is found as the most probable. (**Right column**) proportion of times the heterogeneity case is found as the most probable.

When the true partition is an intermediate one, the results vary. Figure 6 shows the results for the true case $r_2 = (1, 1, 2)$. The uniform prior shows the best performance although the proportion of right choices is smaller than 50% for $n = 10$. The mean posterior probability reaches a value of 80% with a sample size of 300. With the hierarchical Uniform priors the true model is never chosen as the most probable for a sample size of $n = 10$. In this case, the mean of the posterior probability for the true partition when it is found as the most probable does not exist and it is shown as 0 in the figure. For small sample sizes these prior distributions found the heterogeneity case as the most probable (Figure 7). The hierarchical Uniform priors only achieve the 50% of right choices for a sample size of 300. The hierarchical Poisson prior improves the behavior of the hierarchical Uniform priors although for a small sample size of $n = 10$, it chooses the homogeneity case more than 85% of the simulations (Figure 7).

When the true model is the heterogeneity case, i.e., $r_3 = (1, 2, 3)$, the hierarchical Uniform priors (HU2 and HU3) show the best performance even with small sample sizes. Surprisingly, the uniform prior shows worse results than those of the hierarchical Poisson prior. This can be explained by the higher prior probabilities assigned to intermediate partitions by the uniform prior, which hinder the identification of the heterogeneity case as the true model. The proportion of right choices and the mean posterior probabilities for the true model are near to 100% for all the prior models when the sample size is 300.

Figures 8 and 9 show the results of the frequentist validation for the case $k = 5$ and true partitions $r_1 = (1, 1, 1, 1, 1)$, homogeneity case, $r_2 = (1, 1, 1, 2, 2)$ and $r_3 = (1, 1, 2, 2, 3)$, intermediate situations and $r_5 = (1, 2, 3, 4, 5)$, heterogeneity case.

The analysis of the homogeneity case with $k = 5$ shows a bad performance of the uniform prior, even worse than observed for $k = 3$. The proportion of right choices only exceed 50% for a sample size of 300. As it is shown in the Figure 9, the uniform prior found as the most probable model some intermediate models as the proportion of cases in which the heterogeneity case is chosen is 0. As it was found with $k = 3$, the hierarchical Poisson prior shows a better performance than the HU2 and HU3 which becomes similar as the sample size increases. Some results obtained for the HU2 and HU3 priors are quite similar, showing an overlapping behavior in some cases.

Once again, the analysis of the intermediate cases with $k = 5$ shows a similar behavior to that observed with $k = 3$. The uniform prior reaches a higher proportion of correct choices, although for the case of two clusters ($p = 2$), the hierarchical Poisson improves it for sample sizes greater than 100. With a moderate number of clusters ($p = 3$), all the prior models show difficulties to choose the true model with small sample sizes. In the case of the hierarchical Poisson prior, it chooses the homogeneity case for small sample sizes, while the uniform prior chooses other intermediate models (Figure 9). The hierarchical uniform priors never choose the true model with sample sizes smaller than 300, showing preference for the heterogeneity case.

For the heterogeneity case $r_5 = (1, 2, 3, 4, 5)$, the proportion of right choices show a U-shape for all model priors except the Uniform prior. For small sample sizes, the greater prior probability assigned to the extreme cases leads to a preference for the heterogeneity case (the homogeneity case is never chosen as it is shown in Figure 9). As the sample size increases, the importance of the prior information is reduced and other intermediate partitions are chosen, probably due to the small difference in the true probability of success between the 5 studies (see Table 1). Finally, with a sample size of 300, all model prior distributions choose the true model.

An additional analysis for the case $k = 8$ is shown in the Supplementary Material Section. The results are very similar to those obtained for the case $k = 5$.

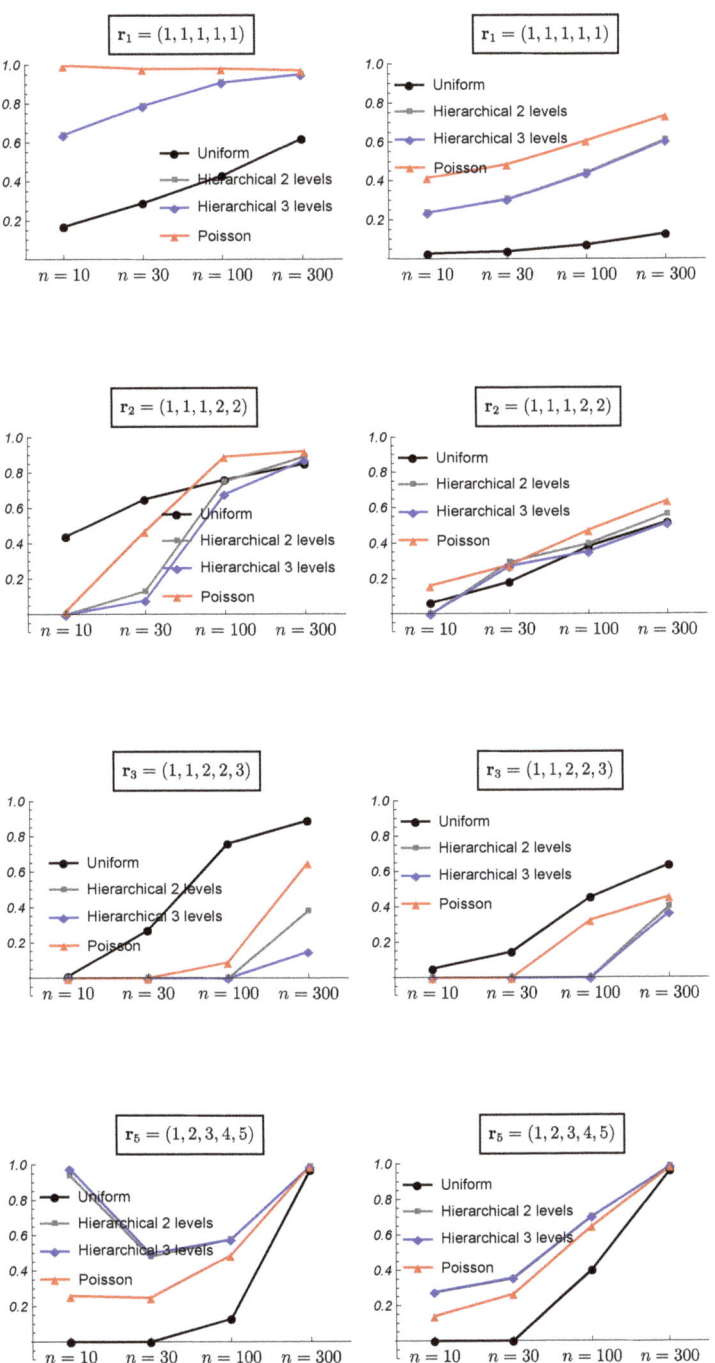

Figure 8. Frequentist validation for the case $k = 5$ and true partitions $\mathbf{r}_1 = (1,1,1,1,1)$, $\mathbf{r}_2 = (1,1,1,2,2)$, $\mathbf{r}_3 = (1,1,2,2,3)$, and $\mathbf{r}_5 = (1,2,3,4,5)$. (**Left column**) proportion of times the true partition is found as the most probable. (**Right column**) mean of the posterior probability for the true partition when it is found as the most probable.

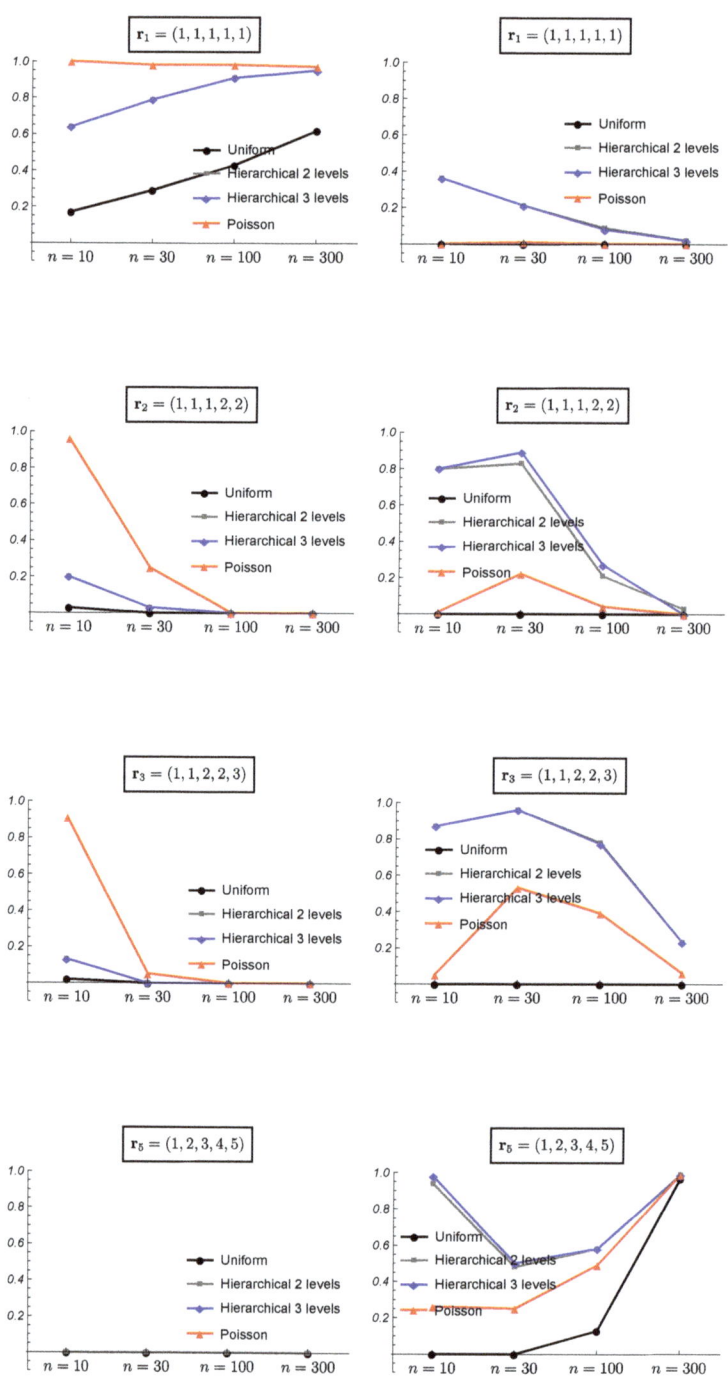

Figure 9. Frequentist validation for the case $k = 5$ and true partitions $\mathbf{r}_1 = (1,1,1,1,1)$, $\mathbf{r}_2 = (1,1,1,2,2)$, $\mathbf{r}_3 = (1,1,2,2,3)$, and $\mathbf{r}_5 = (1,2,3,4,5)$. (**Left column**) proportion of times the homogeneity case is found as the most probable. (**Right column**) proportion of times the heterogeneity case is found as the most probable.

4. An Illustrative Example with Real Data

In this section, we show an illustrative example with real data to analyze the impact of the prior models over the estimation of the meta-parameter θ. With the objective to determine the effectiveness of granulocyte transfusions compared to no granulocyte transfusions for treating infections in patients with neutropenia or disorders of neutrophil function in reducing mortality, Stanworth et al. [19] conducted a meta-analysis. The dataset in Table 2 is extracted from Stanworth et al. [19] and corresponds to the mortality analysis in four studies ($k = 4$, subgroup analysis for studies transfusing greater than 1×10^{10} granulocytes at days 20–22) for granulocyte transfusions for treating infections in patients with neutropenia or neutrophil dysfunction treated with transfusion (Treatment).

Table 2. Data in Stanworth et al. [19].

Study	Treatment	
	Events	Total
Herzig 1977 (x_1)	1	16
Higby 1975 (x_2)	2	17
Scali 1978 (x_3)	0	13
Vogler 1977 (x_4)	7	17

This is a good example to apply the model proposed by Moreno et al. [9] as the number of cases is small and there are even no cases in one study. For $k = 4$, there are 15 possible partitions and the estimation of the meta-parameter θ will depend on the partition considered. Figure 10 shows the posterior mean conditioned on each partition. The posterior mean varies from the 0.1929 obtained for the partition $\mathbf{r}_2 = (1,1,1,2)$ to 0.1344 for the partition $\mathbf{r}_3 = (1,2,3,2)$.

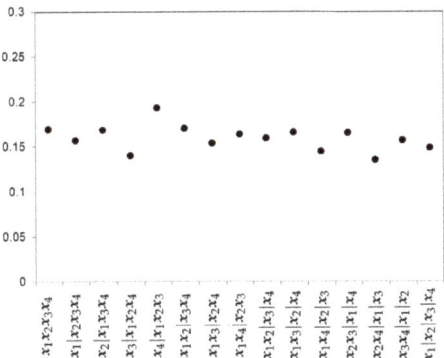

Figure 10. Posterior mean of the meta–parameter θ for each partition.

The four prior models are applied to this dataset. The prior probabilities assigned to each partition can be shown in Figures 2–5. To include into the analysis the model uncertainty, the posterior distributions for θ are all averaged in the BMA posterior distribution, and this BMA posterior distribution depends on the model priors assumed. Table 3 shows the top cluster models for the four model priors.

Table 3. Top cluster models in Stanworth et al. for treatment data.

Prior # 1: Uniform		Prior # 2: HU with 2 levels		Prior # 3: HU with 3 Levels		Prior # 4: HP with 3 Levels	
Cluster Model	Post. Prob.	Cluster Model	Post. Prob.	Cluster Model	Post. Prob.	Cluster Model	Post. Prob.
$x_1x_2x_3\|x_4$	0.19	$x_1\|x_2\|x_3\|x_4$	0.37	$x_1\|x_2\|x_3\|x_4$	0.37	$x_1\|x_2\|x_3\|x_4$	0.21
$x_1x_3\|x_2\|x_4$	0.14	$x_1x_2x_3\|x_4$	0.11	$x_1x_2x_3\|x_4$	0.10	$x_1x_2x_3x_4$	0.18
$x_1x_2\|x_3\|x_4$	0.11	$x_1x_3\|x_2\|x_4$	0.09	$x_1x_3\|x_2\|x_4$	0.09	$x_1x_2x_3\|x_4$	0.14
$x_1\|x_2x_3\|x_4$	0.11	$x_1x_2x_3x_4$	0.08	$x_1x_2x_3x_4$	0.08	$x_1x_3\|x_2\|x_4$	0.8
$x_1\|x_2\|x_3\|x_4$	0.09	$x_1x_2\|x_3\|x_4$	0.08	$x_1x_2\|x_3\|x_4$	0.08	$x_1x_3\|x_2x_4$	0.08
the rest	<0.09	the rest	<0.07	the rest	<0.07	the rest	<0.07
BMA estimates of the meta-parameter θ							
Posterior mean: 0.164		Posterior mean: 0.159		Posterior mean: 0.159		Posterior mean: 0.163	
95% HDI: 0.050–0.317		95% HDI: 0.049–0.312		95% HDI: 0.049–0.311		95% HDI: 0.048–0.327	

Top cluster models and their posterior probabilities are sensitive to the model prior. For the uniform prior model, the most probable model is $\{x_1x_2x_3|x_4\}$, with a posterior probability of 0.19. However, this model is found as the second most probable model for the hierarchical uniform priors, and reaches the third position for the Poisson prior. These last models found the heterogeneity case as the most probable model.

Table 2 shows a different mortality rate between studies, where study 4 stands out with a mortality rate of 41.18%, while the mortality rate for the other studies do not exceed 12%. The uniform prior is the only model capable of detecting this structure as the most probable model. The other prior models discard the homogeneity case but cannot detect the intermediate model, showing preference for the heterogeneity case. In this example, the uniform prior would be the best choice.

This analysis also points out the importance of the BMA estimation as it allows the model uncertainty to be included in the estimation of the meta-parameter. As can be seen, the estimation of the meta-parameter by BMA is less sensitive to the choice of the prior distribution for the models, ranging from 0.159 for the hierarchical Uniform priors to 0.164 for the Uniform prior.

5. Conclusions

Bayesian methods for the design, analysis, and synthesis of clinical trials have been developed in several areas including meta-analysis where the structure of the between-sample heterogeneity is essential in estimating the meta-parameter. As part of the design of the Bayesian framework, we address the question from a different standpoint, arguing that between-sample heterogeneity is a clustering problem and that model uncertainty can be incorporated into the inference using a Bayesian procedure. Under this procedure, the posterior probabilities of the cluster models are computed and the definition of the prior distribution over the models takes on special importance.

Meta-analysis for binary data is an increasingly used tool for estimating the effectiveness of a certain treatment. Meta-analysis for binary data presents interesting statistical challenges that have been addressed in the literature, such as the presence of zeros, that make it difficult to apply logit transformations to the data [20,21]. The definition of an objective Bayesian meta-analysis for binary data that does not require transformations to the data represented an advance in literature [9].

The objectivity of this analysis is given by the prior distribution assumed for the experimental parameters (θ_i) and the meta-parameter (θ) [22]. However, when the between-sample heterogeneity is considered in the analysis as a problem of clustering the experimental parameters (θ_i), the objectivity remains in doubt since the Bayesian model selection requires the definition of the prior distributions over the models. The hierarchical structure of the clusters does not allow to conclude that the Uniform prior distribution is the best or unique option. Moreno et al. [10] proposed to use the hierarchical Uniform prior with three levels, but other options are possible.

In this paper we analyze the properties of four model priors assuming the absence of prior information about the cluster model: the Uniform prior, the hierarchical Uniform prior with two and three levels and the hierarchical Poisson prior. There are other priors proposed by the literature for the problem of clustering, such as the Ewens–Pitman prior [23–25] or the Jensen–Liu prior [26]. However, these prior distributions require the assessing of a hyperparameter that reflects the a priori information about the models.

A first conclusion achieved from the frequentist validation is that none of the prior distributions is completely non-informative. The posterior probabilities for the models are very sensitive to the model priors, even with moderately large sample sizes. A useful guideline for daily practice could be as follows. If you consider that the homogeneity case is probable, the hierarchical Poisson prior for small samples sizes, or the hierarchical Uniform prior for moderately large sample sizes are the best options. If you consider that the heterogeneity case is probable, the hierarchical Uniform priors are preferable. Finally, if you consider that the real cluster is not the homogeneity or heterogeneity cases, the Uniform prior can be used for small number of studies and sample sizes.

A second conclusion is that carrying out a meta-analysis based on a single partition (even if it is the partition with the maximum posterior probability) can obtain biased results as it ignores a very important part of the uncertainty around the estimation of the meta-parameter. The BMA procedure offers a natural way to incorporate this model uncertainty into the estimation of θ [27].

As the BMA procedure implies estimating the meta-parameter for all possible partitions, computational difficulties arise when the number of studies k is moderately large due to time required for estimation. In that case, a set of good cluster models can certainly by found using a stochastic algorithm [13].

Supplementary Materials: The following are available at https://www.mdpi.com/1660-4601/18/2/809/s1.

Author Contributions: Conceptualization, M.-A.N.-H. and F.-J.V.-P.; methodology, M.-A.N.-H., F.-J.V.-P. and M.M.-E.; software, M.-A.N.-H. and F.-J.V.-P.; investigation, M.-A.N.-H., F.-J.V.-P. and M.M.-E.; writing—original draft preparation, M.-A.N.-H. and F.-J.V.-P.; writing—review and editing, M.-A.N.-H., F.-J.V.-P. and M.M.-E.; project administration, F.-J.V.-P.; funding acquisition, F.-J.V.-P. All authors have read and agreed to the published version of the manuscript.

Funding: Financial support for this study was provided in part by grant ECO2017–85577–P (Ministerio de Ciencia, Innovación y Universidades, Agencia Estatal de Investigación, Spain).

Institutional Review Board Statement: Not applicable.

Informed Consent Statement: Not applicable.

Data Availability Statement: Mathematica codes implementing the simulate and real data experiment are available on the supplementary material section.

Acknowledgments: The authors thank the Associate Editor and three referees for their suggestions which have improved the original manuscript.

Conflicts of Interest: The authors declare no conflict of interest.

References

1. Thomas, D.; Radji, S.; Benedetti, A. Systematic review of methods for individual patient data meta- analysis with binary outcomes. *BMC Med. Res. Methodol.* **2014**, *14*, 79. [CrossRef]
2. Charles, P.; Giraudeau, B.; Dechartres, A.; Baron, G.; Ravaud, P. Reporting of sample size calculation in randomised controlled trials: Review. *BMJ* **2009**, *338*, b1732. [CrossRef]
3. Sutton, A.J.; Abrams, K.R. Bayesian methods in meta–analysis and evidence synthesis. *Stat. Methods Med. Res.* **2001**, *10*, 277–303. [CrossRef]
4. Morris, C.N.; Norm, S.L. Hierarchical models for combining information and for meta–analyses. In *Bayesian Statistics 4*; Bernardo, J.M., Berger, J.O., Dawid, A.P., Smith, A.F.M., Eds.; Clarendon Press: Oxford, UK, 1992; pp. 321–344.
5. Carlin, J.B. Meta–analysis for 2x2 tables: A Bayesian approach. *Stat. Med.* **1992**, *11*, 141–159. [CrossRef]

6. Sutton, A.J.; Abrams, K.R.; Jones, D.R.; Sheldon, T.A.; Song, F. *Methods for Meta–Analysis in Medical Research*; Wiley: New York, NY, USA, 2000.
7. Bhaumik, D.K.; Amatya, A.; Norm, S.L.T.; Greenhouse, J.; Kaizar, E.; Neelon, B.; Gibbons, R.D. Meta–Analysis of rare binary adverse event. *J. Am. Stat. Assoc.* **2012**, *107*, 555–567. [CrossRef]
8. Sweeting, M.J.; Sutton, A.J.; Lambert, P.C. What to add to nothing? Use and avoidance of continuity corrections in meta–analysis of sparse data. *Stat. Med.* **2004**, *23*, 1351–1375. [CrossRef]
9. Moreno, E.; Vázquez–Polo, F.J.; Negrín, M.A. Objective Bayesian meta–analysis for sparse discrete data. *Stat. Med.* **2014**, *33*, 3676–3692. [CrossRef]
10. Moreno, E.; Vázquez–Polo, F.J.; Negrín, M.A. Bayesian meta–analysis: The role of the between–sample heterogeneity. *Stat. Methods Med. Res.* **2018**, *27*, 3643–3657. [CrossRef]
11. Hartigan, J. Partition models. *Commun. Stat. Theory Met.* **1990**, *19*, 2745–2756. [CrossRef]
12. Barry, D.; Hartigan, J.A. Product partition models for change point problems. *Ann. Stat.* **1992**, *20*, 260–279 [CrossRef]
13. Casella, G.; Moreno, E.; Girón, F.J. Cluster analysis, model selection, and prior distributions on models. *Bayesian Anal.* **2014**, *9*, 613–658. [CrossRef]
14. Tuyl, F.; Gerlach, R.; Mengersen, K. A comparison of Bayes–Laplace, Jeffreys, and other priors: The case of zero events. *Am. Stat.* **2008**, *62*, 40–44. [CrossRef]
15. Tuyl, F.; Gerlach, R.; Mengersen, K. Posterior predictive arguments in favor of the Bayes–Laplace prior as the consensus prior for binomial and multinomial parameters. *Bayesian Anal.* **2009**, *4*, 151–158. [CrossRef]
16. Berger, J.O.; Pericchi, L.R. The intrinsic Bayes factor for model selection and prediction. *J. Am. Stat. Assoc.* **1996**, *91*, 109–122. [CrossRef]
17. Moreno, E. Objective Bayesian methods for one–sided testing. *Test* **2005**, *14*, 181–198. [CrossRef]
18. Davey, J.; Turner, R.M.; Clarke, M.J.; Higgins, J.P. Characteristics of meta–analyses and their component studies in the Cochrane Database of Systematic Reviews: A cross–sectional, descriptive analysis. *BMC Med. Res. Methodol.* **2011**, *11*, 160. [CrossRef]
19. Stanworth, S.; Massey, E.; Hyde, C.; Brunskill, S.J.; Navaretter, C.; Lucas, G.; Marks, D.; Paulus, U. Granulocyte transfusions for treating infections in patients with neutropenia or neutrophill dysfunction (Review). *Cochrane Libr.* **2010**, *8*, 1–32.
20. Friede, T.; Röver, C.; Wandel, S.; Neuenschwander B. Meta–analysis of few small studies in orphan diseases. *Res. Syn. Methods* **2017**, *8*, 79–91. [CrossRef]
21. Pateras, K.; Nikolakopoulos, S.; Mavridis, D.; Roes, K.C.B. Interval estimation of the overall treatment effect in a meta–analysis of a few small studies with zero events. *Contemp. Clin. Trials Comm.* **2018**, *9*, 98–107. [CrossRef]
22. Berger, J. The case for objective Bayesian analysis *Bayesian Anal.* **2006**, *1*, 385–402. [CrossRef]
23. Crowley EM. Product partition models for normal means. *J. Am. Stat. Assoc.* **1997**, *92*, 192–198. [CrossRef]
24. Quintana, F.A.; Iglesias, P.L. Bayesian clustering and product partition models. *J. R. Stat. Soc. Ser. B Stat. Methodol.* **2003**, *65*, 557–574. [CrossRef]
25. McCullagh, P.; Yang, J. Stochastic classification models. In *Proceedings of the International Congress of Mathematicians*; Springer: Berlin/Heidelberg, Germany, 2006; pp. 669–686.
26. Jensen, S.T.; Liu, J.S. Bayesian Clustering of Transcription Factor Binding Motifs. *J. Am. Stat. Assoc.* **2008**, *103*, 188–200. [CrossRef]
27. Negrín, M.A.; Vázquez–Polo, F.J. Incorporating model uncertainty in cost–effectiveness analysis: A Bayesian model averaging approach. *J. Health Econ.* **2008**, *27*, 1250–1259. [CrossRef]

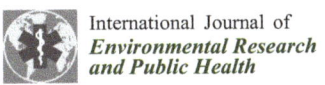

Review

Bayesian Approaches for Confirmatory Trials in Rare Diseases: Opportunities and Challenges

Moreno Ursino [1,2,*] and Nigel Stallard [3]

1. Inserm, Centre de Recherche des Cordeliers, Sorbonne Université, USPC, Université de Paris, F-75006 Paris, France
2. F-CRIN PARTNERS Platform, AP-HP, Université de Paris, F-75010 Paris, France
3. Statistics and Epidemiology, Division of Health Sciences, Warwick Medical School, University of Warwick, Coventry CV4 7AL , UK; n.stallard@warwick.ac.uk
* Correspondence: moreno.ursino@inserm.fr

Abstract: The aim of this narrative review is to introduce the reader to Bayesian methods that, in our opinion, appear to be the most important in the context of rare diseases. A disease is defined as rare depending on the prevalence of the affected patients in the considered population, for example, about 1 in 1500 people in U.S.; about 1 in 2500 people in Japan; and fewer than 1 in 2000 people in Europe. There are between 6000 and 8000 rare diseases and the main issue in drug development is linked to the challenge of achieving robust evidence from clinical trials in small populations. A better use of all available information can help the development process and Bayesian statistics can provide a solid framework at the design stage, during the conduct of the trial, and at the analysis stage. The focus of this manuscript is to provide a review of Bayesian methods for sample size computation or reassessment during phase II or phase III trial, for response adaptive randomization and of for meta-analysis in rare disease. Challenges regarding prior distribution choice, computational burden and dissemination are also discussed.

Keywords: Bayesian; rare disease; prior distribution; meta-analysis; sample size

1. Introduction

A disease is defined as rare depending on the prevalence of the affected patients in the considered population. In the United States, a disease is rare if it affects fewer than 200,000 people in the U.S. [1] (or about 1 in 1500 people); in Japan, if it affects fewer than 50,000 patients in Japan (or about 1 in 2500 people); and in the European Union if the prevalence is no more than 5 per 10,000 (that is, fewer than 1 in 2000 people), but the definition excludes diseases that are not also life-threatening, chronically debilitating, or inadequately treated [2]. There are between 6000 and 8000 rare diseases [3], 71.9% of which are genetic and 69.9% which exclusively affect paediatric populations, and it is estimated that the global population prevalence of rare diseases is of 3.5–5.9%, which implies that 263–446 million persons are affected at any stage in their life [4]. The usual level of rigorous clinical trial evaluation of treatments is required in rare diseases just as much as in more common ones. Although in some cases, particularly in phase II trials, single-arm trials might be considered (see, for example, Grayling et al. [5]), randomized controlled trials are to be preferred when this is possible. For example, the European regulatory guidance [2] affirms that "patients with [rare] conditions deserve the same quality, safety and efficacy in medicinal products as other patients; orphan medicinal products should therefore be submitted to the normal evaluation process"; this is also in agreement with U.S. guidance [6].

The main issue in drug development for rare diseases is linked to the challenge of achieving robust evidence from clinical trials in small populations when trial sample sizes are necessarily limited [7]. Even if for some rare diseases the population size is

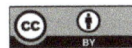

relatively large (for instance, Friedreich Ataxia in the EU) [8], the majority of rare diseases are less frequent [9]. Small population clinical trials have been the focus of much methodological research activity in the last two decades. From a regulatory perspective, the European Medicines Agency (EMA) described a methodological framework, summarizing several possible approaches, in the guidance "Guideline on Clinical Trials in Small Populations" [10] and the Food and Drug Administration (FDA) in the draft guidance on rare disease [6]. The European Union's Seventh Framework Programme for Research, Technological development and Demonstration (EU FP7), acknowledging the need for additional methodological research work, funded three projects in 2013; the Integrated Design and Analysis of Small Populations Group Trials (IDeAl) project (www.ideal.rwth-aachen.de), the Innovative Methodology for Small Populations Research (InSPiRe) project (www.warwick.ac.uk/inspire), and the Advances in Small Trials Design for Regulatory Innovation and Excellence (Asterix) project (www.asterix-fp7.eu) [8,11–13].

The drug development process involves on-going learning as data are observed through the series of clinical trials, and, above all in rare diseases, there is a considerable effort to optimize this learning process [14,15]. A better use of all available information can help the process and Bayesian statistics provides an opportunity to do this in a formal way (at the design stage, during the conduct of the trial, and at the analysis stage) [16,17]. Like drug development, the Bayesian approach can be seen as an on-going learning process: it starts with a prior belief (quantified as a prior distribution for the unknown model parameters), which is then updated with the new evidence (likelihood data from the new trial/experiment) to yield a posterior belief (expressed as a posterior probability distribution for the unknown model parameters). In this way, Bayesian statistics provides a mathematical method for calculating the predictive probabilities of future events, given the actual trial and the knowledge from prior trials. Moreover, a formal Bayesian analysis can incorporate different utilities or prior beliefs coming from different stakeholders and quantify how these could impact potential decision-making.

Bayesian methods and designs are well established and mostly accepted, by both clinicians and regulatory agencies, in early phase clinical trials. Due to the greater flexibility, in both design and analysis, of the Bayesian paradigm with respect to the frequentist one and since type I and II errors do not have to be controlled at this stage, Bayesian adaptive designs are mostly chosen for these stages [18]. As early phase trials in all diseases use small sample sizes, designs, specifically developed for rare diseases are unnecessary. Thus, in this manuscript we will focus on novel Bayesian approaches firstly developed for confirmatory/randomized trials in the rare disease setting, where more conventional approaches may be unfeasible.

The aim of this narrative review is to show to the reader Bayesian methods that, in our opinion, appear to be the most important in the context of rare diseases. Its purpose is not to present a comprehensive compendium of Bayesian statistics in rare diseases, but to give a starting point for the reader on some uses of novel Bayesian methods in this field. All methods are presented in a general way, without mathematical formalism, so that a reader who already have a basis of Bayesian statistics can understand the general idea, along with the corresponding principal(s) reference(s), in such a way the reader can find the details for methods they wish to explore in more detail. In the following sections, three specific topics dealing with the application of a Bayesian design are introduced. The first topic, in Section 2, regards methods for sample size computation or reassessment during randomized phase II or phase III trial. The second topic, a recent method proposed for response adaptive randomization, is presented in Section 3. Section 4 presents the fourth topic of Bayesian meta-analysis methods developed for evidence combination in rare diseases. Finally, we discuss frequent challenges faced when choosing a Bayesian design; in particular, the priors distributions choice, which include the issue of the quantity of information and commensurability between prior information and actual data; the computational burden required; and dissemination issues.

2. Sample Size Determination/Re-Estimation

Usual sample size determination approach focus on frequentist properties, that is, type I error and study power. However, in a rare disease setting, accruing the number of patients required to perform a fully-powered significance test after the trial may be infeasible. Increasing the allowed type I error can be a solution to reduce the required sample size. However, as recalled in the introduction, this practice is not generally supported by regulatory agencies. As an alternative, some authors have proposed the use of a Bayesian decision-theoretic framework [19]. A Bayesian decision-theoretic approach can be applied when we would like a treatment recommendation not based on type I error but on maximizing an expected gain for the total population. According this approach, we can compare the costs of clinical trial evaluation with the potential benefits to current and future patients, assessing how the cost-benefit balance differs between large and small patient populations when, in the latter, patients recruited to a clinical trial could be a substantial proportion of the population. The design of the study, including the sample size, can then be chosen on the basis of the expected gain, with the sample size that maximizes the expected gain chosen for the clinical study. Here the concept of a "gain" is interpreted very broadly and can be defined from the patient, sponsor, regulatory, public health, or society perspective, or from a combined perspective. Stallard et al. [20] have shown that for a wide range of distributions, including those for continuous, binary or count responses, and gain function forms, the optimal trial sample size is proportional to the square root of the population size, with the constant of proportionality depending on the gain function form and prior distribution of the parameters of the distribution of the data. A smaller sample size may thus be appropriate for a trial in a rare disease than in a more common one.

Bayesian statistics can also be adopted to overcome some challenges in the calculation of sample sizes from the frequentist perspective. For example, for normally distributed outcomes, values for variances need to be specified, but, especially in the case of small populations, may be based on very little information, for example, that from only one very small pilot study. When using a Bayesian approach, the aggregation of prior information on the variance with newly collected data is more formalized. Brakenhoff et al. [21] proposed a framework incorporating the employment of power priors in order for operational characteristics to be controlled in case of prior-new data conflict.

Bayesian group sequential designs could also be used to provide interim stopping criteria, based on efficacy and/or futility. Even if the frequentist operating characteristics of these designs are usually checked, they are not designed to optimize them. A practical guide for their implementation and reference for software can be found in Gsponer et al. [22].

3. Response Adaptive Randomization

While randomization is the established method for obtaining scientifically valid treatment comparisons in clinical trials, as the trial progresses, increasing evidence may suggest that one study group is responding or doing much better than another. As a consequence, novel randomization methods, such as response adaptive randomization [23] (RAR), have been proposed to address this ethical question continuously updating assignment probabilities based on response of the different groups to their respective treatments so as to allocate more patients to better-performing treatments. Both, frequentist and Bayesian approach can be applied, however, the latter one has gained more popularity due to its flexibility [24,25]. In the same manner as the previous decision theoretic idea, this approach could be considered in rare disease setting, where future patients in the general population is limited, to balance the benefits to current trial patients and future ones. Nonetheless, standard adaptive randomization may lead to estimation bias [26], with the potential for the trial to reach an erroneous conclusion. Therefore, novel and calibrated RAR approaches should be preferred. The small sample sizes in trials in rare diseases may also mean that it is possible to calibrate RAR methods in a way that would be infeasible in larger trials.

A recent paper suggests a novel randomized response-adaptive design specifically developed for a rare disease trial [27]. It uses the framework of finite-horizon Markov decision processes and dynamic programming (DP) to recruit more patients to the more beneficial arms while guaranteeing a minimum sample size to each treatment arm. The authors show that the design has good operating characteristics, in term of (i) the percentage of patients allocated to the superior arm, which is much higher than in the traditional fixed randomized design; (ii) the power, which is higher than optimal DP; and (iii) bias and mean square error of the treatment effect estimator, which are small.

4. Meta-Analysis

Meta-analyses are used to combine evidence from multiple studies. Differences in study characteristics, such as trial design and study populations, can bring to heterogeneous treatment effects and these must be accounted for in the meta-analysis formulation. To deal with the between-trial heterogeneity, random-effects meta-analysis has become the gold standard, and the most used method is the normal–normal hierarchical model (NNHM) [28]. In a rare disease, the limited number of trials and their small sample size may impact the validity of usual frequentist meta-analysis methods. A Bayesian approach offers another way to perform random-effect meta-analyses within the NNHM framework. One of the advantages is that the solution remains coherent for small numbers of studies, although careful prior specification is required. Friede et al. [29] showed that, when doing meta-analysis with only two studies, Bayesian random-effects meta-analyses with priors covering plausible heterogeneity values offer a good compromise. They compared the Bayesian method to the NNHM, to the Hartung-Knapp-Sidik-Jonkman method (HKSJ) and to the modified Knapp-Hartung method (mKH). On one hand, the coverage of the standard method, based on normal quantiles, was unsatisfactory; on the other hand, very large (therefore uncertain) confidence intervals resulted from the HKSJ and mKH. An acceptable trade-off between these two extremes was achieved, in general, by Bayesian intervals that showed suitable characteristics. Usually, the Bayesian approach is computationally more demanding. However, optimized free software are available, such as the bayesmeta R package, which uses a general semi-analytical approach to solve the meta-analysis problem via the DIRECT approach [30] and provides an efficient and user-friendly interface to Bayesian random-effects meta-analysis [31].

When dealing with binary outcomes, the binomial-normal hierarchical model is usually preferred to the NNHM, which then relies on asymptotic approximations. A challenge in this setting in rare diseases is that we could face the probability to have no events due to the small sample sizes. Frequentist approaches are known to induce bias and to result in improper interval estimation of the overall treatment effect in a meta-analysis with zero events [13]. On the other hand, Bayesian models are known for being sensitive to the choice of heterogeneity prior distributions in sparse settings, therefore, the need to identify priors with robust properties is crucial. Pateras et al. [32] proposed a general way to set prior distributions. Via simulations, they showed that a uniform heterogeneity prior, bounded between -10 and 10, on the log heterogeneity parameter scale shows appropriate 95% coverage and induces relatively acceptable under/over estimation of both the overall treatment effect and heterogeneity, across a wide range of heterogeneity levels.

The Bayesian meta-analysis approach also allows implementation of a number of more advanced analysis strategies. A series of studies may be used to inform the analysis when the focus is not on an overall synthesis, but rather on a particular study that is to be viewed in the light of previously accumulated evidence. For example, Wandel et al. [33] used a Bayesian meta-analytic approach to inform a phase III study with phase II data. They investigated the use of shrinkage estimates to support data from a single trial in the light of external information. The method allows quantifying and discounting the phase II data through the predictive distribution relevant for phase III. Bayesian meta-analysis approach can also be adapted to incorporate external information from historical controls [34] or borrow information from other arms in a randomized control trial, for example, in a basket design [35,36]. Such approaches could prove very valuable in the setting of rare diseases where trials are necessarily small.

5. Challenges

As stated above, the Bayesian approach can be more flexible than the frequentist counterpart. However, the flexibility comes along with a number of possible challenges. Even if Bayesian methods can bring substantial benefits, their validity and effectiveness require expertise and care. In the following, we will describe some points that should be addressed when planning a Bayesian analysis.

5.1. Prior Distributions Choices

In Bayesian statistics, external information can be easily incorporated into the prior distributions. An informative prior distribution for the unknown parameters could be determined through elicitation of expert knowledge, from data from other trials or from a search of the literature to identify results obtained in trials of similar drugs, or the same drug in a different population, via the so called "extrapolation". Extrapolation approaches are well known in paediatrics, where the proper dosage for children is estimated starting from adults' data, and in bridging studies, where the drug is tested in a new geographical population, for example, in Asian, given the results in a previous one, for example, Caucasian. This concept can be translated in rare disease, since rare diseases prevalence may vary by continent (i.e., IgA nephropathy is rather rare in the EU but more frequent in Asia and Africa) and we can be to adopt proofs of efficacy from the larger populations to the smaller one [8].

However the prior distribution is obtained, the use of an informative prior to make inferences about medical treatments based on small sample size trials remains inherently controversial, however. Choice of a prior distribution must therefore be done carefully, since the use of informative priors may be seen as introducing bias into posterior inferences and inflating type I error rates. This is a general problem common in many different fields, and several authors have addressed the issue of eliciting experts' opinions, building priors upon the elicited values, and performing Bayesian analyses using the resulting priors. See O'Hagan et al. [37] for a complete review. The elicitation needs to be made as meticulous and objective as possible to catch expert expertise. One way is to follow a recognized protocol that is designed to address and minimize the cognitive biases [38]. In the following, we summarize two approaches that have already been used in the context of rare disease.

The first approach describes how to obtain a consensus between experts. This research was motivated by the design of the MYPAN trial, a multicentre RCT comparing mycophenolate mofetil (MMF) with cyclophosphamide (CYC) for the treatment of polyarteritis nodosa, a rare and serious inflammatory blood vessel disease in children [39]. The authors proposed to add priors on the probability of success of one arm and on the log-odds ratio of the probabilities. Then, a behavioral aggregation process, by which experts interact to reach a mutually agreeable consensus through constructive discussions, was chosen for systematic elicitation from clinicians of their beliefs concerning treatment efficacy. In particular, experts' individual prior beliefs were obtained at the beginning of the process; then, the full group was asked to reach a consensus. The results are then used to establish Bayesian priors for unknown model parameters and the authors have also considered the possibility of considering results from related trials. A similar strategy was used in a trial of adalimumab versus pamidronate for children with CNO/CRMO [40].

The second approach focuses on reflecting, when eliciting experts' opinions, how these depend on differences in experience, training and medical practice [41]. Motivating by a 70-patient randomized trial to compare two treatments (the same described in the first approach) for idiopathic nephrotic syndrome in children (NCT 01092962), the authors proposed a Bayesian methodology for constructing a bivariate parametric prior starting from elicited graphical information. The method involves four steps: (i) each physician builds manually two histograms, one for each treatment parameter using the "bins-and-chips" graphical method of Johnson et al. [42]; (ii) then, for each physician and each treatment parameter, a marginal prior, characterized by location and precision hyperparameters, is fitted to the elicited histogram; (iii) a bivariate prior is built by averaging the marginals over a latent bivariate distribution; (iv) finally, an overall prior is obtained as a mixture of the individual physicians' priors. The approach also suggests a framework for performing a sensitivity analysis of posterior inferences to prior location and precision.

Incorporating external information, whatever the source type (other trial, experts' elicitation, etc.), has to be done properly, as the information can be in conflict with the actual data or the amount of information can overwhelm trial data. Several methods that allow prior information to be incorporated if it is in accordance with the trial data and otherwise to be down-weighted have been proposed [34,43,44]. Moreover, the effective sample size allows to quantify the information in the prior to be specified in term of the number of hypothetical patients used to build the prior [45]. Different prior building approaches may be used for different parameters; for example, historical control can be included via a power prior approach and experts' opinion can be used for the new treatment effect. An adaptation of the power prior approach, that is useful particularly for borrowing evidence from a single historical study, was proposed in rare disease setting [46]. Borrowing information from a historical trial is often related the type I error inflation. By determining the amount of similarity between the new and historical data, this method uses predictive probabilities and is parameterized in order to control the type I error.

5.2. Computational Burden

Estimation of posterior distributions can be challenging when prior distributions do not have simple conjugate forms. Specific Markov chain Monte Carlo algorithms, such as the Gibbs sampling or the Hamiltonian Monte Carlo, can be used to obtain an approximation of posteriors. Even if freely available software and the increasing computational power of computers may help the Bayesian implementation, writing, coding and testing the models usually requires a bigger effort than choosing a frequentist approach. In general, the more complex the model or the prior distribution, the longer the computational time to obtain the result. Validation of the method via simulation is one of the common way used in Bayesian setting. Simulating several possible scenarios can allow the user to calibrate model parameters (i.e., the quantity of information in the prior distribution) to obtain desired operational characteristics, such as the type I error control or the power. Choosing a fast and reliable approximation method is, however, crucial when simulations are required.

5.3. Dissemination

Even if the Bayesian approach has been shown to capture the thinking behavior of clinicians [41], Bayesian methods and results are sometimes still viewed with suspicion by clinicians and traditional statisticians. The influence of the prior distribution may be considered disturbing and the lack of p-values can give the feeling that regulatory agencies will not consider the results obtained. In effect, Bayesian methodologies are usually less discussed in public regulatory guidelines than the frequentist counterpart. However, the FDA Guidance for the Use of Bayesian Statistics in Medical Device Clinical Trials [47] shows the regulatory agencies efforts in this direction. The guidance gives several Bayesian insights that could be used in general, not only in medical device field. Several sections explain how to well plan a Bayesian clinical trial, what to consider when choosing prior distributions, and how to analyze the data. Then, in the technical details sections, the FDA points out the importance of simulations to obtain operating characteristics of the planned design, to assess the type one error rate, power, etc. While also other recommendations for Bayesian analyses have been developed [17,48,49], they were primarily addressed to researchers, not to readers unfamiliar with Bayesian approaches [50]. Therefore, efforts are needed to well explain the Bayesian philosophy to non-statisticians. An example is given in Ferreira et al. [51] and Ferreira et al. [50], where the authors help clinicians interpretation of Bayesian clinical trial though a side-by-side comparison with the frequentist approach. On one hand, they teach how to transfer frequentist ideas, such as the p-values or hypotheses testing, to the Bayesian framework, such as posterior probabilities and Bayes factor, and, on the other hand, they give insights on what to check when reading a Bayesian report.

6. Conclusions

The aim of this article has been to review the use of Bayesian methods in confirmatory trials in rare diseases, though many of the approaches described could also be applied in clinical trials in other more common disease areas.

The formal Bayesian approach permits the incorporation of accumulating information into the analysis of the actual trial and, therefore, the updating of belief. This feature is extremely attractive in rare disease setting, where usually sample sizes and the opportunities to performs clinical trials are limited. Incorporation of previous information should be strongly considered and the Bayesian approach, with its flexibility, could be seen as a future gold standard in this field. As shown in the manuscript, the accumulated information can be used in the prior distribution settings, in sample size optimization and/or in randomization. Depending on the trial, where and when using this kind of information is used has to be carefully chosen and simulations are strongly suggested to evaluate method performances.

Author Contributions: Conceptualization, M.U.; writing—original draft preparation, M.U.; writing—review and editing, N.S. All authors have read and agreed to the published version of the manuscript.

Funding: This research received no external funding.

Institutional Review Board Statement: Not applicable.

Informed Consent Statement: Not applicable.

Acknowledgments: We would like to thank the anonymous reviewers for their constructive feedback.

Conflicts of Interest: The authors declare no conflict of interest.

Abbreviations

The following abbreviations are used in this manuscript:

CYC	cyclophosphamide
CNO/CRMO	chronic recurrent multifocal osteomyelitis
DP	dynamic programming
EMA	European Medicines Agency
FDA	Food and Drug Administration
HKSJ	Hartung-Knapp-Sidik-Jonkman method
mKH	modified Knapp-Hartung method
MMF	mycophenolate Mofetil
NNHM	normal-normal hierarchical model
RAR	response adaptive randomization

References

1. Rare Diseases Act of 2002. Available online: https://www.congress.gov/107/plaws/publ280/PLAW-107publ280.pdf (accessed on 15 November 2020).
2. European Union. Regulation (EC) No 141/2000 of the European Parliament and of the Council of 16 December 1999 on Orphan Medicinal Products. 2015. Available online: http://eur-lex.europa.eu/LexUriServ/LexUriServ.do?uri=OJ:L:2000:018:0001:0005:en:PDF (accessed on 15 November 2020).
3. Stephens, J.; Blazynski, C. Rare disease landscape: Will the blockbuster model be replaced? *Expert Opin. Orphan Drugs* **2014**, *2*, 797–806. [CrossRef]
4. Wakap, S.N.; Lambert, D.M.; Olry, A.; Rodwell, C.; Gueydan, C.; Lanneau, V.; Murphy, D.; Le Cam, Y.; Rath, A. Estimating cumulative point prevalence of rare diseases: analysis of the Orphanet database. *Eur. J. Hum. Genet.* **2020**, *28*, 165–173. [CrossRef] [PubMed]
5. Grayling, M.J.; Dimairo, M.; Mander, A.P.; Jaki, T.F. A review of perspectives on the use of randomization in phase II oncology trials. *JNCI J. Natl. Cancer Inst.* **2019**, *111*, 1255–1262. [CrossRef] [PubMed]

6. Food and Drug Administration. Rare Diseases: Common Issues in Drug Development—Guidance for Industry. 2019. Available online: https://www.fda.gov/regulatory-information/search-fda-guidance-documents/rare-diseases-common-issues-drug-development-guidance-industry (accessed on 15 November 2020).
7. Hee, S.W.; Willis, A.; Smith, C.T.; Day, S.; Miller, F.; Madan, J.; Posch, M.; Zohar, S.; Stallard, N. Does the low prevalence affect the sample size of interventional clinical trials of rare diseases? An analysis of data from the aggregate analysis of clinicaltrials. gov. *Orphanet J. Rare Dis.* **2017**, *12*, 44. [CrossRef] [PubMed]
8. Hilgers, R.D.; König, F.; Molenberghs, G.; Senn, S. Design and analysis of clinical trials for small rare disease populations. *J. Rare Dis. Res. Treat.* **2016**, *1*, 53–60. [CrossRef]
9. Orphanet. Orphanet Report Series—Rare Disease Registries in Europe. [Online]. 2015. Available online: http://www.orpha.net/orphacom/cahiers/docs/GB/Registries.pdf (accessed on 15 November 2020).
10. Committee for Medicinal Products for Human Use. Guideline on Clinical Trials in Small Populations. 2007. Available online: https://www.ema.europa.eu/en/documents/scientific-guideline/guideline-clinical-trials-small-populations_en.pdf (accessed on 15 November 2020).
11. Hilgers, R.; Roes, K.; Stallard, N. Directions for new developments on statistical design and analysis of small population group trials. *Orphanet J. Rare Dis.* **2016**, *11*, 78. [CrossRef]
12. Friede, T.; Posch, M.; Zohar, S.; Alberti, C.; Benda, N.; Comets, E.; Day, S.; Dmitrienko, A.; Graf, A.; Günhan, B.K.; et al. Recent advances in methodology for clinical trials in small populations: The InSPiRe project. *Orphanet J. Rare Dis.* **2018**, *13*, 186. [CrossRef]
13. Mitroiu, M.; Rengerink, K.O.; Pontes, C.; Sancho, A.; Vives, R.; Pesiou, S.; Fontanet, J.M.; Torres, F.; Nikolakopoulos, S.; Pateras, K.; et al. Applicability and added value of novel methods to improve drug development in rare diseases. *Orphanet J. Rare Dis.* **2018**, *13*, 200. [CrossRef]
14. Racine, A.; Grieve, A.; Fluhler, H.; Smith, A.M. Bayesian Methods in Practice: Experiences in the Pharmaceutical Industry. *J. R. Stat. Soc. Ser. C (Appl. Stat.)* **1986**, *35*, 93–120. [CrossRef]
15. Gupta, S. Use of Bayesian statistics in drug development: Advantages and challenges. *Int. J. Appl. Basic Med. Res.* **2012**, *2*, 3–6. [CrossRef]
16. Spiegelhalter, D.; Myles, J.; Jones, D.; Abrams, K. An introduction to bayesian methods in health technology assessment. *BMJ* **1999**, *319*, 508–512. [CrossRef] [PubMed]
17. Spiegelhalter, D.; Myles, J.; Jones, D.; Abrams, K. Bayesian methods in health technology assessment: A review. *Health Technol. Assess.* **2000**, *4*, 1–130. [CrossRef] [PubMed]
18. Yuan, Y.; Nguyen, H.Q.; Thall, P.F. *Bayesian Designs for Phase I-II Clinical Trials*; CRC Press: Boca Raton, FL, USA, 2016.
19. Miller, F.; Zohar, S.; Stallard, N.; Madan, J.; Posch, M.; Hee, S.W.; Pearce, M.; Vågerö, M.; Day, S. Approaches to sample size calculation for clinical trials in rare diseases. *Pharm. Stat.* **2018**, *17*, 214–230. [CrossRef]
20. Stallard, N.; Miller, F.; Day, S.; Hee, S.W.; Madan, J.; Zohar, S.; Posch, M. Determination of the optimal sample size for a clinical trial accounting for the population size. *Biom. J.* **2017**, *59*, 609–625. [CrossRef] [PubMed]
21. Brakenhoff, T.B.; Roes, K.C.; Nikolakopoulos, S. Bayesian sample size re-estimation using power priors. *Stat. Methods Med. Res.* **2019**, *28*, 1664–1675. [CrossRef]
22. Gsponer, T.; Gerber, F.; Bornkamp, B.; Ohlssen, D.; Vandemeulebroecke, M.; Schmidli, H. A practical guide to Bayesian group sequential designs. *Pharm. Stat.* **2014**, *13*, 71–80. [CrossRef]
23. Hu, F.; Rosenberger, W.F. *The Theory of Response-Adaptive Randomization in Clinical Trials*; John Wiley & Sons: Hoboken, NJ, USA, 2006; Volume 525.
24. Thall, P.F.; Wathen, J.K. Practical Bayesian adaptive randomisation in clinical trials. *Eur. J. Cancer* **2007**, *43*, 859–866. [CrossRef]
25. Lin, J.; Lin, L.A.; Sankoh, S. A general overview of adaptive randomization design for clinical trials. *J. Biom. Biostat.* **2016**, *7*, 294. [CrossRef]
26. Wathen, J.K.; Thall, P.F. A simulation study of outcome adaptive randomization in multi-arm clinical trials. *Clin. Trials* **2017**, *14*, 432–440. [CrossRef]
27. Williamson, S.F.; Jacko, P.; Villar, S.S.; Jaki, T. A Bayesian adaptive design for clinical trials in rare diseases. *Comput. Stat. Data Anal.* **2017**, *113*, 136–153. [CrossRef]
28. Spiegelhalter, D.J.; Abrams, K.R.; Myles, J.P. *Bayesian Approaches to Clinical Trials and Health-Care Evaluation*; John Wiley & Sons: Chichester, UK, 2004; Volume 13, Chpater 8.
29. Friede, T.; Röver, C.; Wandel, S.; Neuenschwander, B. Meta-analysis of two studies in the presence of heterogeneity with applications in rare diseases. *Biom. J.* **2017**, *59*, 658–671. [CrossRef] [PubMed]
30. Röver, C.; Friede, T. Discrete approximation of a mixture distribution via restricted divergence. *J. Comput. Graph. Stat.* **2017**, *26*, 217–222. [CrossRef]
31. Röver, C. Bayesian random-effects meta-analysis using the bayesmeta R package. *J. Stat. Softw.* **2020**, *93*, 1–51. [CrossRef]
32. Pateras, K.; Nikolakopoulos, S.; Roes, K.C. Prior distributions for variance parameters in a sparse-event meta-analysis of a few small trials. *Pharm. Stat.* **2021**, *20*, 39–54. [CrossRef]
33. Wandel, S.; Neuenschwander, B.; Röver, C.; Friede, T. Using phase II data for the analysis of phase III studies: An application in rare diseases. *Clin. Trials* **2017**, *14*, 277–285. [CrossRef]

34. Schmidli, H.; Gsteiger, S.; Roychoudhury, S.; O'Hagan, A.; Spiegelhalter, D.; Neuenschwander, B. Robust meta-analytic-predictive priors in clinical trials with historical control information. *Biometrics* **2014**, *70*, 1023–1032. [CrossRef]
35. Chu, Y.; Yuan, Y. A Bayesian basket trial design using a calibrated Bayesian hierarchical model. *Clin. Trials* **2018**, *15*, 149–158. [CrossRef]
36. Hobbs, B.P.; Landin, R. Bayesian basket trial design with exchangeability monitoring. *Stat. Med.* **2018**, *37*, 3557–3572. [CrossRef]
37. O'Hagan, A.; Buck, C.E.; Daneshkhah, A.; Eiser, J.R.; Garthwaite, P.H.; Jenkinson, D.J.; Oakley, J.E.; Rakow, T. *Uncertain Judgements: Eliciting Experts' Probabilities*; John Wiley & Sons: Chichester, UK, 2006.
38. O'Hagan, A. Expert knowledge elicitation: Subjective but scientific. *Am. Stat.* **2019**, *73*, 69–81. [CrossRef]
39. Hampson, L.V.; Whitehead, J.; Eleftheriou, D.; Brogan, P. Bayesian methods for the design and interpretation of clinical trials in very rare diseases. *Stat. Med.* **2014**, *33*, 4186–4201. [CrossRef]
40. Ramanan, A.; Hampson, L.; Lythgoe, H.; Jones, A.; Hardwick, B.; Hind, H.; Jacobs, B.; Vasileiou, D.; Wadsworth, I.; Ambrose, N.; et al. Defining consensus opinion to develop randomised controlled trials in rare diseases using Bayesian design: An example of a proposed trial of adalimumab versus pamidronate for children with CNO/CRMO. *PLoS ONE* **2019**, *14*, e0215739. [CrossRef] [PubMed]
41. Thall, P.F.; Ursino, M.; Baudouin, V.; Alberti, C.; Zohar, S. Bayesian treatment comparison using parametric mixture priors computed from elicited histograms. *Stat. Methods Med. Res.* **2019**, *28*, 404–418. [CrossRef] [PubMed]
42. Johnson, S.R.; Tomlinson, G.A.; Hawker, G.A.; Granton, J.T.; Grosbein, H.A.; Feldman, B.M. A valid and reliable belief elicitation method for Bayesian priors. *J. Clin. Epidemiol.* **2010**, *63*, 370–383. [CrossRef] [PubMed]
43. Ibrahim, J.G.; Chen, M.H.; Gwon, Y.; Chen, F. The power prior: Theory and applications. *Stat. Med.* **2015**, *34*, 3724–3749. [CrossRef]
44. Hobbs, B.P.; Carlin, B.P.; Mandrekar, S.J.; Sargent, D.J. Hierarchical commensurate and power prior models for adaptive incorporation of historical information in clinical trials. *Biometrics* **2011**, *67*, 1047–1056. [CrossRef]
45. Morita, S.; Thall, P.F.; Müller, P. Determining the effective sample size of a parametric prior. *Biometrics* **2008**, *64*, 595–602. [CrossRef]
46. Nikolakopoulos, S.; van der Tweel, I.; Roes, K.C. Dynamic borrowing through empirical power priors that control type I error. *Biometrics* **2018**, *74*, 874–880. [CrossRef]
47. Food and Drug Administration. Guidance for the Use of Bayesian Statistics in Medical Device Clinical Trials—Guidance for Industry and FDA Staff. 2010. Available online: https://www.fda.gov/regulatory-information/search-fda-guidance-documents/guidance-use-bayesian-statistics-medical-device-clinical-trials (accessed on 15 November 2020).
48. Sung, L.; Hayden, J.; Greenberg, M.L.; Koren, G.; Feldman, B.M.; Tomlinson, G.A. Seven items were identified for inclusion when reporting a Bayesian analysis of a clinical study. *J. Clin. Epidemiol.* **2005**, *58*, 261–268. [CrossRef]
49. Zhai, J.; Cao, H.; Ren, M.; Mu, W.; Lv, S.; Si, J.; Wang, H.; Chen, J.; Shang, H. Reporting of core items in hierarchical Bayesian analysis for aggregating N-of-1 trials to estimate population treatment effects is suboptimal. *J. Clin. Epidemiol.* **2016**, *76*, 99–107. [CrossRef]
50. Ferreira, D.; Barthoulot, M.; Pottecher, J.; Torp, K.D.; Diemunsch, P.; Meyer, N. Theory and practical use of Bayesian methods in interpreting clinical trial data: A narrative review. *Br. J. Anaesth.* **2020**, *125*, 201–207. [CrossRef]
51. Ferreira, D.; Barthoulot, M.; Pottecher, J.; Torp, K.D.; Diemunsch, P.; Meyer, N. A consensus checklist to help clinicians interpret clinical trial results analysed by Bayesian methods. *Br. J. Anaesth.* **2020**, *125*, 208–215. [CrossRef] [PubMed]

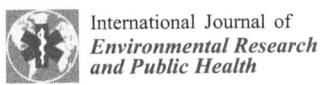

Article

Estimating Similarity of Dose–Response Relationships in Phase I Clinical Trials—Case Study in Bridging Data Package

Adrien Ollier [1], Sarah Zohar [1,*], Satoshi Morita [2] and Moreno Ursino [1,3]

[1] INSERM, Centre de Recherche des Cordeliers, Sorbonne Université, USPC, Université de Paris, F-75006 Paris, France; adrien.ollier@inserm.fr (A.O.); moreno.ursino@inserm.fr (M.U.)
[2] Department of Biomedical Statistics and Bioinformatics, Kyoto University Graduate School of Medicine, Kyoto 606-8501, Japan; smorita@kuhp.kyoto-u.ac.jp
[3] F-CRIN PARTNERS Platform, Assistance Publique-Hôpitaux de Paris, Université de Paris, F-75010 Paris, France
* Correspondence: sarah.zohar@inserm.fr

Abstract: Bridging studies are designed to fill the gap between two populations in terms of clinical trial data, such as toxicity, efficacy, comorbidities and doses. According to ICH-E5 guidelines, clinical data can be extrapolated from one region to another if dose–reponse curves are similar between two populations. For instance, in Japan, Phase I clinical trials are often repeated due to this physiological/metabolic paradigm: the maximum tolerated dose (MTD) for Japanese patients is assumed to be lower than that for Caucasian patients, but not necessarily for all molecules. Therefore, proposing a statistical tool evaluating the similarity between two populations dose–response curves is of most interest. The aim of our work is to propose several indicators to evaluate the distance and the similarity of dose–toxicity curves and MTD distributions at the end of some of the Phase I trials, conducted on two populations or regions. For this purpose, we extended and adapted the commensurability criterion, initially proposed by Ollier et al. (2019), in the setting of completed phase I clinical trials. We evaluated their performance using three synthetic sets, built as examples, and six case studies found in the literature. Visualization plots and guidelines on the way to interpret the results are proposed.

Keywords: bridging studies; distribution distance; oncology; phase I; dose-finding; dose–response; bayesian inference

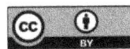

1. Introduction

Bridging studies are designed to fill the gap between two populations in terms of clinical trial data, such as toxicity, efficacy, comorbidities and doses. A bridging data package consists of selected data from the Clinical Data Package of the population in the new region, including pharmacokinetic, any pharmacodynamic, dose–toxicity or dose–efficacy data, and if appropriate, a bridging study to extrapolate the foreign dose–response data to the new region [1].

According to the International Council for Harmonisation of Technical Requirements for Pharmaceuticals for Human Use E5 (ICH-E5) guidelines, data can be extrapolated from one region to another if "a bridging study [...] indicates that a different dose in the new region results in a safety and efficacy profile that is not substantially different from the one derived from the original region; it will often be possible to extrapolate the foreign data to the new region, with an appropriate dose adjustment, if this can be adequately justified (e.g., by pharmacokinetic and/or pharmacodynamic data)" [1]. This is the reason why proposing a statistical tool evaluating the similarity between two foreign dose–response curves is of great interest. If this is proven, then, other clinical trials data can be used and extrapolated for the new region.

In Japan, the Pharmaceuticals and Medical Devices Agency (PMDA) recommends the re-evaluation of a drug if there are insufficient data from Japanese patients [2]. Indeed, Phase I clinical trials in oncology, which aim to estimate the maximum tolerated dose (MTD), are often repeated. Ogura et al. [3] pointed out that MTD differences between populations could be due to the different distribution of genetic polymorphisms in enzymes involved in drug metabolism or of biomarker incidences in different populations. In particular, in Japan, Phase I trials are repeated based on a physiological/metabolic paradigm: MTDs for Japanese patients are often lower than the ones of for Caucasian patients [4]. Based on this assumption, Maeda and Kurokawa [5] have performed an intensive study comparing the MTD of 21 molecularly targeted cancer drugs in Japanese versus Caucasian populations. They found out that this assumption does not hold well: in their study, the MTD was lower for Japanese patients in only two cases, there were no differences between the two populations with 10 drugs and MTD was incommensurable as the evaluated dose range acted different with nine drugs. Moreover, Mizugaki et al. [6] have analyzed data of single-agent Phase I trials at the National Cancer Center Hospital between 1995 and 2012, comparing the dose-limiting toxicity (DLT) profiles and MTDs of Japanese trials with the trials from Caucasian populations.

Recently, methods for bridging dose-finding design have been proposed where previous population data were used to either calibrate the prior distribution of the Bayesian model parameter(s) or to choose the "working model" of the design for prospective trials [7]. Liu et al. [8] proposed using a Bayesian model to average the dose-finding method where the previous trial data were used to build three different skeletons which would then be averaged during the study. Moreover, Takeda and Morita recently defined an "historical-to-current" parameter that could describe the degree of borrowing from one population to the other [9]. Ollier et al. [10] proposed a bridging method where a borrowing parameter was estimated sequentially in a response adaptive design which quantifies the amount of reasonable borrowing according to the similarity between the two populations' estimates. Usually, the proposed methods focus on one parameter, strictly related to the MTD and not on the full dose–toxicity response curve. All these methods were proposed with the purpose of using the foreign data to plan and conduct the future Phase I trial in the new region. Indeed, at this stage, the idea is to use the foreign data to calibrate model-based priors to be used in the new region trial. However, in most cases, the trial in the new region will not be planned this way, but rather by using the MTD information from the foreign region only, if available. The sophisticated statistical approach will not be used.

Another option is to compare the two dose–response curves estimated from each region and to evaluate how similar they are. In this case, the overall purpose is different from before; if the curves prove to be similar (under the uncertainty estimation), the new purpose will be to extrapolate other trial data—such as that of Phase II—to the new region and to avoid further repetition of clinical investigations. For dose–response curves, Bretz et al. [11] introduced an asymptotic test to evaluate the difference of the *minimum efficient dose* among several groups of subjects, according to a threshold. However, this method was built for later clinical phases and presents weaknesses when applied to a small sample size. By contrast, Bayesian methods could mitigate the issue of estimation based on a small sample size setting, since they do not rely on asymptotic approximations and prior distributions can be used to ensure more stability in computation. Thereafter, the degree of similarity could be considered directly at the posterior distributions level. Therefore, methods proposing to estimate the similarity between dose–toxicity curves should be proposed when there is the need to evaluate if the safety data can be extrapolated or not.

The aim of our work is to propose some Bayesian indicators that evaluate the distance and the similarity of (1) dose–toxicity curves, taking into account the variability, (2) the MTD posterior distributions, by extending and adapting the commensurability criterion initially proposed by Ollier et al. [10]. These indicators were applied to several Phase I trials presented in Maeda and Kurokawa [5] and Mizugaki et al. [6], evaluating the similarity between Western dose–toxicity data to Eastern ones. The proposed tools should be used by trial stakeholders in order to decide if other trials data could be extrapolated from the new region, and, if so, to avoid the repetition of multiple clinical trials. In the next section, the original commensurability parameter is summarized along with the proposed extensions and the dose–toxicity model used. The case studies are described in Section 3, while Section 4 details the computational settings. The results are given in Section 5, followed by a Discussion section.

2. Methods

In this section, we briefly recall the Bayesian commensurability measure used in Ollier et al. [10], which was originally adopted into a power prior setting [12]; we then propose extensions and modifications to this measure to be applied at the end of the study. We also introduce the Bayesian dose–toxicity model, which will be used for retrospective data analyses.

Let $\mathbf{D}_c$ denote the Caucasian data, $\mathbf{D}_c = \{(y_j, x_j)\}_{n_c}$, n_c the sample size of $\mathbf{D}_c$, and y_j the binary outcome of the j-th patient which received dose x_j. In a similar way, we can define $\mathbf{D}_a$, the Japanese data and associated parameters. Let us also set a model for the probability of toxicity vs dose; $p_T(x) = f(x, \beta)$, where $f(.)$ denotes a convenient monotonous link function parametrized by β. The likelihood function for each population can be written as $L(\beta | \mathbf{D}_m) = \prod_{j=1}^{n_m} f(x, \beta)^{y_j} (1 - f(x, \beta))^{1-y_j}$, for $m = c, a$.

2.1. Commensurability Distances

Ollier et al. [10] suggested to consider the likelihood function as a distribution, divided by a normalization constant. This type of normalized likelihood can also be seen as the resulting Bayesian posterior distribution when constant (probably improper) priors are used for the analysis. Then, the authors defined a measure of "commensurability" between the two data-sets through a distance $d(\mathbf{D}_c, \mathbf{D}_a)$, the Hellinger one, in the parameters space via the following relation

$$d^2(\mathbf{D}_c, \mathbf{D}_a) = \frac{1}{2} \int \left(\sqrt{\frac{L(\beta|\mathbf{D}_c)^{\min(1, \frac{n_a}{n_c})}}{\int L(\beta|\mathbf{D}_c)^{\min(1, \frac{n_a}{n_c})} d\beta}} - \sqrt{\frac{L(\beta|\mathbf{D}_a)^{\min(1, \frac{n_c}{n_a})}}{\int L(\beta|\mathbf{D}_a)^{\min(1, \frac{n_c}{n_a})} d\beta}} \right)^2 d\beta. \quad (1)$$

The commensurability measure, denoted by γ, is then defined as $\gamma = d^q(\mathbf{D}_c, \mathbf{D}_a)$, with $q \in R^+$. Values of q higher than 1 will reduce the computed distance, while values lower than 1 will lead to a more conservative method, increasing the computed distance. In case of sequential trials, the authors proved that, when coupled with the power prior approach, a conservative value of γ leads to a better result in terms of operating characteristics, as a percentage of the right MTD selection. However, at the end of the trial, we are interested in comparing the achieved results, without any discount in the resulting distance. Therefore, in this paper, we will focus on the original Hellinger distance, which is $q = 1$. This computed distance is a positive number between 0 and 1, it tends towards the maximum value when the two datasets are quite different, and towards zero when they are close to each other. Each likelihood is divided by a normalization constant in order to ensure that it can be viewed as a probability distribution. The variance of the likelihood density depends on the sample size of the trial. To make the two likelihoods comparable in terms of precision (variance), if $n_c > n_a$, $L(\beta|\mathbf{D}_c)$ is raised to a power of less than 1, otherwise, $L(\beta|\mathbf{D}_a)$ is raised to a power of less than 1. Following this method, the variance of likelihood density of the trial with more patients is increased to almost fit the one of the trial with fewer patients. Practical examples are given in Ollier et al. [10].

A straightforward modification of the distance in Equation (1) was performed by changing the underlying flat prior into a proper one. The posterior distribution obtained with the weighted likelihood is then used in the Hellinger formula. Thus, denoted by

$\pi_{post,c}(\boldsymbol{\beta}|\mathbf{D}_c) \propto L(\boldsymbol{\beta}|\mathbf{D}_c)^{\min(1,\frac{n_a}{n_c})} \pi_{prior}(\boldsymbol{\beta})$ and by $\pi_{post,a}(\boldsymbol{\beta}|\mathbf{D}_a) \propto L(\boldsymbol{\beta}|\mathbf{D}_a)^{\min(1,\frac{n_c}{n_a})} \pi_{prior}(\boldsymbol{\beta})$ the posterior distribution of $\boldsymbol{\beta}$ given D_c and D_a, respectively, we have

$$d_{mod}^2(\mathbf{D}_c, \mathbf{D}_a) = \frac{1}{2} \int \left(\sqrt{\pi_{post,c}(\boldsymbol{\beta}|\mathbf{D}_c)} - \sqrt{\pi_{post,a}(\boldsymbol{\beta}|\mathbf{D}_a)} \right)^2 d\boldsymbol{\beta}. \qquad (2)$$

This modification will ensure more stability in computation when the likelihoods involve more than one parameter. When flat/constant priors are used for $\pi_{prior}(\boldsymbol{\beta})$, Equation (2) is equivalent to Equation (1). Even if, theoretically, two different priors can be chosen for the two trials, we suggest using a single one for the sake of comparability.

Both previous distances work at the parameter level. They check if the whole dose–toxicity curve is similar or not. Using a single parameter model for the dose–toxicity relationship, as a one parameter logistic model used in the continual reassessment method (CRM) [13], is also equivalent to check the MTD distance. However, in models with more parameters, such as the Bayesian Logistic Regression Model (BLRM) [14] where we have two parameters, intercept and slope, we check if the bivariate distribution of $\boldsymbol{\beta}$ is the same. Since the distance is difficult to interpret in case of the multidimensional parameters space, we propose a summary distance using the resulting posterior MTD distribution. In our setting, the MTD, x^*, is estimated as the dose linked to a pre-specified toxicity target τ, that is, $x^* = f^{-1}(\tau|\boldsymbol{\beta})$, where $f^{-1}(.)$ is the inverse function of $f(.)$. The posterior MTD distribution, $\pi_{MTD,m}(x^*|\mathbf{D}_m)$, is obtained evaluating x^* through the posterior distribution of the parameter, $\pi_{post,m}(\boldsymbol{\beta}|\mathbf{D}_m)$, for $m = c, a$. Therefore, we can define

$$d_{MTD}^2(\mathbf{D}_c, \mathbf{D}_a) = \frac{1}{2} \int \left(\sqrt{\pi_{MTD,c}(x^*|\mathbf{D}_c)} - \sqrt{\pi_{MTD,a}(x^*|\mathbf{D}_a)} \right)^2 dx^*. \qquad (3)$$

Note that this distance always involves a one dimensional integral.

Previous distances focused on understanding the similarity of the whole dose–toxicity curve between two populations. However, even with different slopes and intercepts, two populations can still have the same MTD. Those differences should generally indicate a difference in responsiveness to a drug and it is important to know when MTDs are similar but not the underlying curves. Therefore, we propose to couple the distances, previously described, with a measure denoting the difference in MTD point estimations. We can build this measure as a percentage using the median of the posterior MTD distributions, such as

$$d_{p1}(\mathbf{D}_c, \mathbf{D}_a) = \left(\frac{\text{med}_c}{\text{med}_a} \right)^{1-2I(\text{med}_c < \text{med}_a)} - 1, \qquad (4)$$

where $I(.)$ is the indicator function, which assumes the value 1 if the statement in parentheses is true and zero otherwise, and med_i with $i = c, a$, is the median of the posterior MTD distribution of Caucasians and Japanese, respectively. This formulation was chosen for its easy interpretation, indeed, we check how much the highest MTD differs in percentage in respect to the lowest one. For this reason, the formula implies the exponent $1 - 2I(\text{med}_c < \text{med}_a)$, which allows us to always have the highest estimate at the numerator, and the -1 term. Similarly to the three previous measures, Equation (4) tends to zero when the two MTDs are very similar. However, this measure does not have an upper bound. We propose the use of the median since it is less impacted by outliers than the mean. The *maximum a posteriori* is another possible candidate, that is

$$d_{p2}(\mathbf{D}_c, \mathbf{D}_a) = \left(\frac{\tilde{x}_c^*}{\tilde{x}_a^*} \right)^{1-2I(\tilde{x}_c^* < \tilde{x}_a^*)} - 1, \qquad (5)$$

where

$$\tilde{x}_i^* = \arg\max_{x^*} \pi_{MTD,i}(x^*|\mathbf{D}_i).$$

To summarize, the first three measures d, d_{mod}, and d_{MTD} are bounded between 0 and 1. Even if they are not built as percentages, their interpretation could be strictly linked to the percentage. Otherwise, the last two measures d_{p1} and d_{p2} have a ratio-like measure, lower bounded at 0. In practice, they give the information on the number of times the maximum MTD is higher than the lowest one.

2.2. Dose–Toxicity Model

In this section, we describe the model selected for the link function $f(.)$. Instead of the CRM, originally used in Ollier et al. [10], which is better suited to prospective trials than retrospective analyses (retrospective CRM requires special techniques), we opted for a more flexible BLRM model, with two parameters, the intercept β_0 and the (logarithm of the) slope β_1 [14]. The dose–toxicity relationship is represented by

$$\text{logit}\{p_T(x)\} = \beta_0 + \exp(\beta_1) \log\left(\frac{x}{x_r}\right)$$

where $\beta \in \mathbb{R}^2$, x_r denotes a reference dose and $\exp(\beta_1)$ assures a positive final slope in the model. In this case, $f^{-1}(.)$ is equal to the logit function and the BLRM formulation is similar to the one of Zheng and Hampson [15]. To close the Bayesian model, we suggest a bivariate normal distribution as prior for (β_0, β_1).

Following the described model, the final MTD is estimated as $x^* = x_r \exp \frac{\text{logit}(\tau) - \beta_0}{\exp(\beta_1)}$. In order to minimize the overdispersion generated by this formula, we compared the distribution of the log ratio of the MTD and the reference dose, $x^{**} = \log(x^*/x_r)$ (instead of the real MTD). Therefore, we have also changed Equations (4) and (5), accordingly, to the new formulation (x^{**}) in order to preserve the original distance meaning, that is $d_{p1}(\mathbf{D}_c, \mathbf{D}_a) = \exp|\text{med}_c - \text{med}_a| - 1$ and $d_{p2}(\mathbf{D}_c, \mathbf{D}_a) = \exp|\tilde{x}_c^* - \tilde{x}_a^*| - 1$.

Finally, in a previous sensitivity analysis (not shown), even when comparing the distribution of the log ratio of the MTD and the reference dose, we faced instability in computation due to the issue of outliers. We have found that truncating the posterior distribution of x^{**} between the 10 and 90 percentiles gives a good compromise between preserving trial information and computation stability.

3. Case Studies

To show the results and the interpretation of the proposed measures, we first introduce four different synthetic datasets (1 for Caucasian and 3 for Japanese), to check the results when two datasets are similar or not. We fixed the Caucasian dataset first: setting τ equal to 0.3, the MTD at dose 600 mg/day. The same setting was used for the Japanese synthetic-1 set. Moreover, the two datasets were generated to have the same dose–toxicity shape. Japanese synthetic-2 set shares the same MTD with the Caucasian set, but has a different dose–toxicity shape: the Japanese dose–toxicity is steeper at the MTD than the Caucasian one. The Japanese synthetic-3 set has a different dose–toxicity curve and MTD (200 mg/day). The data are summarized in Table 1.

Then, we applied our methods to eight examples found in the literature. Our research started by looking at the drugs presented in Maeda and Kurokawa [5] and Mizugaki et al. [6]. We selected only drugs for which both Caucasian and Japanese trial data were available. We then extracted the number of toxicities and the number of allocated patients to the administered doses in each trial. All those data are shown in Table 2, each time with the reference article. The MTD declared at the end of the trial is shown in a box. As we can see from Table 2, Caucasians and Japanese trials were not usually used with the same set of doses.

Table 1. Number of dose-limiting toxicity and total number of patients accrued at each dose for 1 Caucasian trial and 3 Japanese synthetic trials. In the first column, the trial population is specified. A dash (-) means that the dose was not tested in the specified population. A box denotes the dose that has been defined as maximum tolerated dose (MTD).

	Doses					
Example (mg/day)	100	200	400	500	600	800
Caucasian (DLTs/nb pt)	0/3	0/3	0/6	-	[3/9]	2/3
Japanese Synthetic-1 (DLTs/nb pt)	-	-	-	1/10	[2/8]	2/2
Synthetic-2 (DLTs/nb pt)	-	-	0/3	0/9	[4/12]	3/3
Synthetic-3 (DLTs/nb pt)	0/3	[1/6]	3/3	-	-	-

Table 2. Value of dose-limiting toxicity and total number of patients accrued at each dose for all trials analysed in this manuscript. In the first column, the trial population is specified. A dash (-) means that the dose was not tested in the specified population. A box denotes the dose that has been defined as MTD, if the MTD was reached in the trial. For Sorafenib, the doses were given twice daily (bid).

Investigated Drug	Doses							
Erilubin (mg/m^2)	0.25	0.5	0.7	1.0	1.4	2	2.8	4
Caucasian [16] (DLTs/nb pt)	0/1	0/4	-	0/3	-	[1/7]	2/3	3/3
Japanese [17] (DLTs/nb pt)	-	-	0/3	0/3	2/6	[3/3]	-	
Lapatinib (mg/day)	500	650	900	1000	1200	1600	1800	
Caucasian [18] (DLTs/nb pt)	0/13	1/15	0/11	1/3	1/12	1/13	-	
Japanese [19] (DLTs/nb pt)	-	-	0/6	-	0/6	1/6	[1/6]	
Sorafenib (mg bid)	100	200	400	600				
Caucasian [20] (DLTs/nb pt)	0/3	1/6	[0/8]	3/7				
Japanese [21] (DLTs/nb pt)	0/3	1/12	[0/6]	1/6				
Ixabepilone (mg/m^2)	7.4	15	30	40	50	57	65	
Caucasian [22] (DLTs/nb pt)	0/3	0/3	0/3	-	[3/22]	3/3	2/3	
Japanese [23] (DLTs/nb pt)	-	0/3	0/3	1/6	[2/2]	-	-	
Edotecarin (mg/m^2)	6	8	11	13	15			
Caucasian [24] (DLTs/nb pt)	0/3	0/3	0/6	1/9	[4/9]			
Japanese [25] (DLTs/nb pt)	-	0/3	1/6	1/9	[2/6]			
E7070 (mg/m^2)	50	100	200	400	600	700	800	900	1000
Caucasian [26] (DLTs/nb pt)	0/4	0/3	0/3	0/3	0/4	[2/7]	2/4	-	3/3
Japanese [27] (DLTs/nb pt)	-	-	-	0/3	0/3	0/6	1/6	[2/3]	-

4. Settings

We chose τ, the target toxicity probability, to be used to define the MTD, which equals 0.3 for the three synthetic set examples, while it equals 0.25 for the real case studies. Most of real case studies followed an algorithm base allocation; therefore, it seemed more natural to have a threshold lower than 0.3, which is more frequently used when model based designs are adopted in oncology.

A non-informative bivariate prior distribution, commonly used in this setting, was chosen for the BLRM model as follows:

$$\begin{pmatrix} \beta_0 \\ \beta_1 \end{pmatrix} \sim \mathcal{N}\left(\begin{pmatrix} \text{logit}(0.1) \\ \log 1 \end{pmatrix}, \begin{bmatrix} 4 & 0 \\ 0 & 4 \end{bmatrix} \right).$$

The hyperprior parameters of the bivariate prior were chosen after a preliminary sensitivity analysis (not shown) in order to ensure computational stability. In detail, this prior choice suggests a mean prior probability of toxicity at the reference dose, x_r, of 0.1 and that the slope has the prior median centered at zero. Therefore, x_r was chosen in the first half of the total dose panel for each example. In detail, 400 mg/day was set for the three synthetic examples, 1 mg/m² for Erilubin, 900 mg/day for Lapatinib, 200 mg/day for Sorafenib, 30 mg/m² for Ixabepilone, 8 mg/m² for Edotecarin and 700 mg/m² for E7070.

All distances were computed with $q = 1$, which is why we focus on the square root of Equation (1)–(3) and on the original value for Equation (4) and (5). The reference doses selected are reported along with the results in Table 3. All computations were performed in R, version 3.5.2. Monte Carlo approximations were adopted for all integrals involved, and uniform prior distribution on compact supports was set to approximate weighted likelihoods (as posterior distributions) in Equation (4). Details can be found in R scripts in the Supplementary Materials.

Table 3. Results in terms of d, d_{mod}, d_{MTD}, d_{p1} and d_{p2} for the synthetic examples and the real case studies. x_r denotes the reference dose selected for the Bayesian Logistic Regression Model (BLRM).

Drug	d	d_{mod}	d_{MTD}	d_{p1}	d_{p2}
Synthetic-1	0.23	0.18	0.19	0	0
Synthetic-2	0.53	0.37	0.41	0.02	0.02
Synthetic-3	0.91	0.83	1.00	1.50	1.27
Erilubin	0.92	0.83	0.91	0.47	0.43
Lapatinib	0.58	0.39	0.50	7.29	0.35
Sorafenib	0.45	0.43	0.57	10.07	0.75
Ixabepilone	0.77	0.56	0.62	0.34	0.26
Edotecarin	0.38	0.24	0.32	0.32	0.04
E7070	0.63	0.63	0.88	0.59	0.23

5. Results

The computed distances under all the proposed methods are shown in Table 3. When the MTD and the dose–toxicity curves are similar, like in synthetic-1 data, d, d_{mod}, d_{MTD} are lower than 0.23 and $d_{p1} = d_{p2} = 0$. When only the MTDs are similar (synthetic-2 data) but not the dose–toxicity curves, $d_{p1} = d_{p2} = 0.02$ but d, d_{mod}, d_{MTD} are higher than 0.37. Finally, when both curves and MTDs (synthetic-3 data) differ $d_{p1} = 1.50$, $d_{p2} = 1.27$ and d, d_{mod}, d_{MTD} are higher than 0.83.

Taking these cases' studies as reference, we then analyse the data from published papers with Caucasian and Japanese datasets. Erilubin has the highest values of d, d_{mod} and d_{MTD}, greater than 0.80, which suggests differences between the dose–toxicity curves. It is also shown in Figure 1. Its values of d_{p1} and d_{p2} are around 0.45. Ixabepilone and E7070 have quite large d, d_{mod} and d_{MTD}, greater than 0.56 and they also have similar results in term of d_{p2}. The value of d_{p1} is different in these two examples and reflects the presence of unbalanced heavy tails in the E7070 case. The heavy tail concern is observed, in at least one population, in all examples except for Erilubin. The results obtained in Table 3 show that d_{p1} is directly impacted by this phenomenon. For example, Lapatinbib and Sorafenb have a very high value of d_{p1}, greater than 7.29, whereas the maximum a posteriori, d_{p1}, has more stable and usual results. Edotecarin has close values of d, d_{mod} and d_{MTD}, around 0.3, representing similar dose–toxicity curves.

Figure 2 and Figure A1, in the Appendix A, show how the Caucasian posterior distribution is different in the three synthetic examples even if it comes from the same

Caucasian dataset. This behaviour is due to the variance adjustment given by $\min\left(1, \frac{n_a}{n_c}\right)$. In general, the posterior peak is preserved and the variance increases when the exponent is less than 1 (as in the synthetic-3 example).

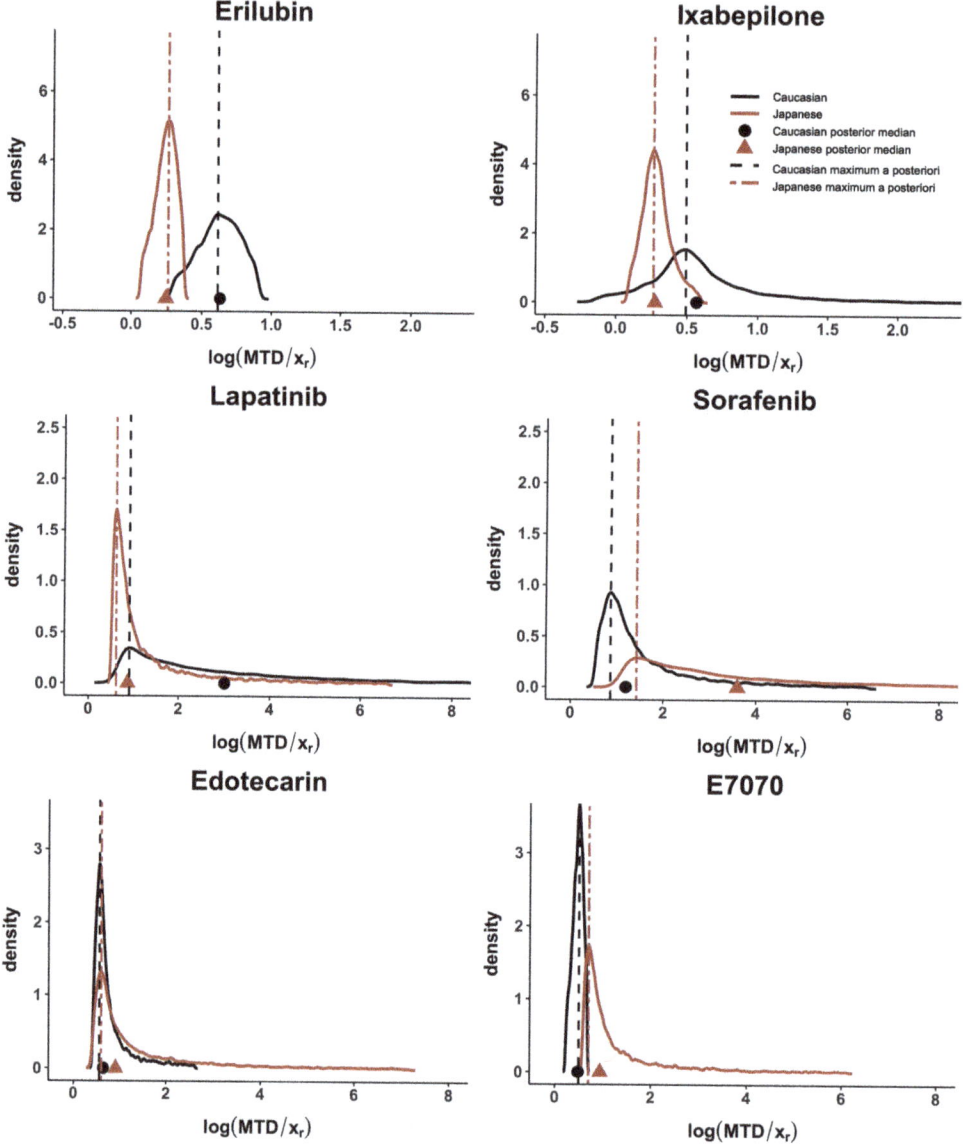

Figure 1. MTD posterior distributions for Erilubin, Ixabepilone, Lapatinib, Sorafenib, Edotecarin and E7070 case studies. Posterior medians are represented by a circle for Caucasian and a triangle for Japanese, while *maximum a posteriori* is represented by a dashed line for Caucasian and a two-dash line for Japanese.

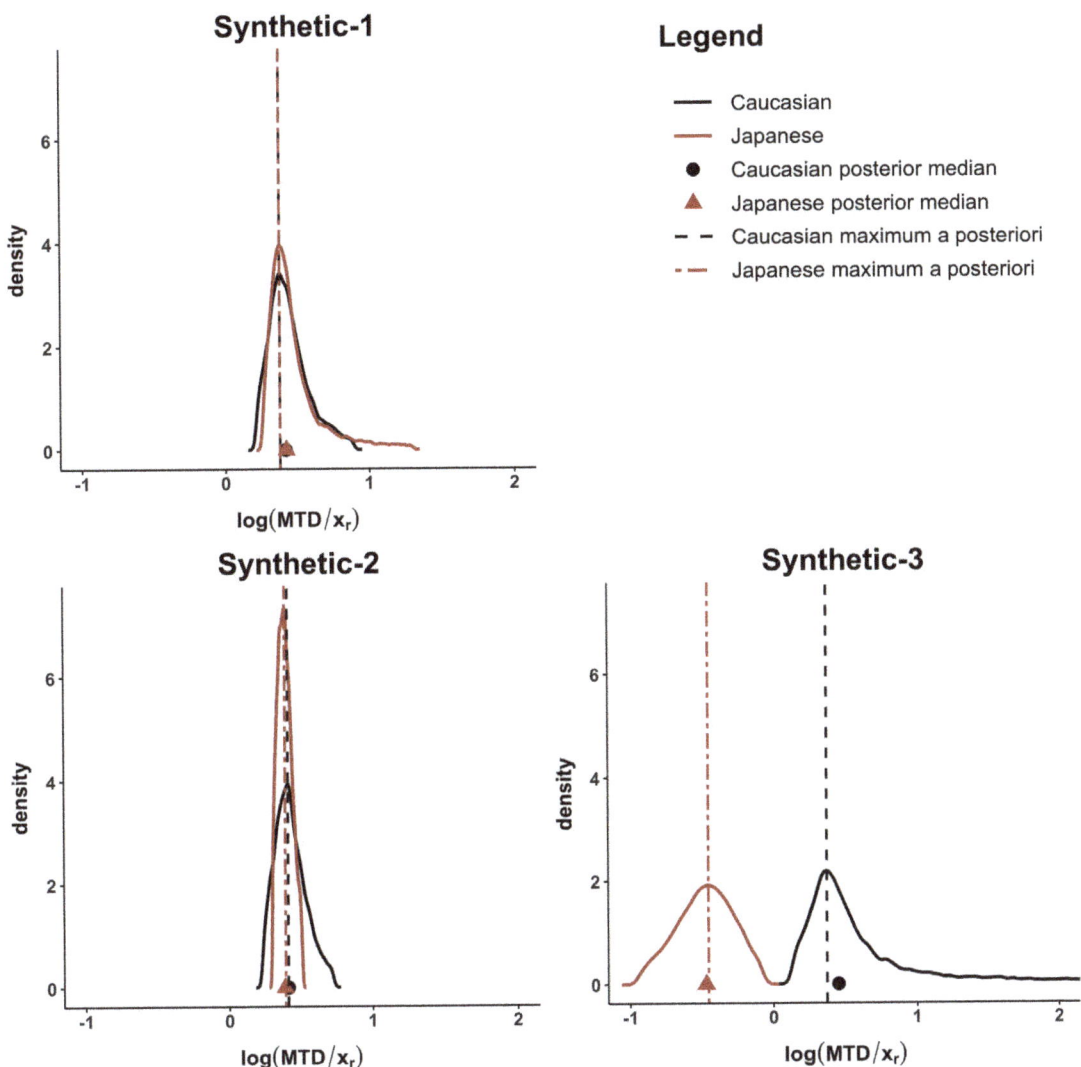

Figure 2. MTD posterior distributions for the Synthetic-1, Synthetic-2 and Synthetic-3 examples. Posterior medians are represented by a circle for Caucasian and a triangle for Japanese, while *maximum a posteriori* by a dashed line for Caucasian and a two-dash line for Japanese.

Figure 3 represents the distance between dose–toxicity curves, d_{mod}, and maximum of the posterior MTD distribution, d_{p2}. For the sake of interpretability, we have equally divided the axes into three parts, each one denoting a small, moderate or high distance, respectively. In this plot, Sorafenib has moderate distances between curves and high difference between MTDs. This is the opposite for Erilubin, where there is a moderate difference between MTD and a large distance between curves. When MTDs are similar or close (first column of the gradient), Edotecarin has similar dose–toxicity curves, while the distance between curves of Ixabepilone and E7070 is moderate. Lapatinib shows a moderate distance of both dose–toxicity curve and estimated MTDs.

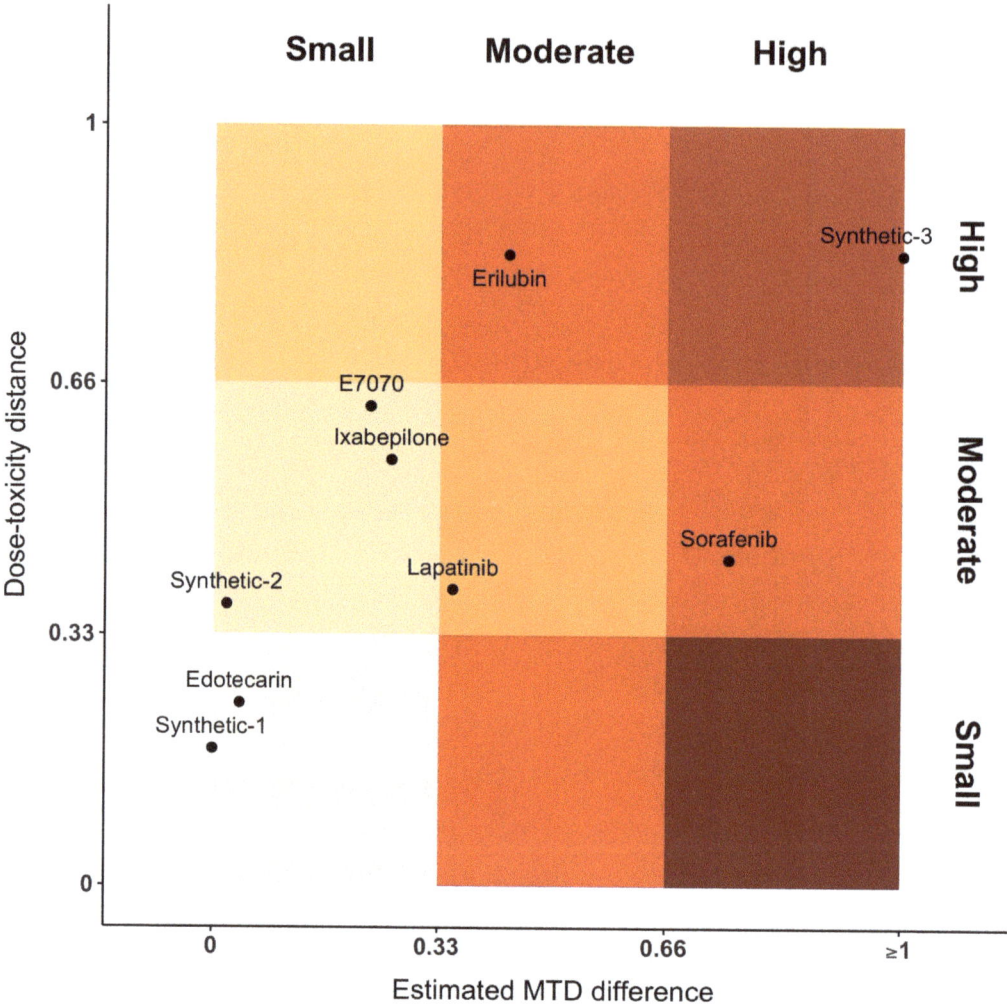

Figure 3. Gradient plot representing the distance between dose–toxicity curves, d_{mod} (y-axis), and maximum of the posterior MTD distribution, d_{p2} (x-axis). The intensity of the color varies along with the increasing distance value and coherence. Small dose–toxicity distance and high MTD distance is incoherent, as such it is plotted in a darker color.

6. Discussion

The aim of our work was to propose several Bayesian indicators to support further decisions when using a bridging data package [1]. Bayesian methods permit the definition of a similarity degree based on posterior distribution, which do not rely on asymptotic approximations and can be used also in small sample size settings. Specifically, we proposed Bayesian indicators which evaluate the distance and the similarity of dose–toxicity curves and MTD. When evaluating a drug among different populations, assessing the dose–response curves similarity is of most importance, since, if it is proved, other clinical trial data can be used, as well as extrapolation from one population to the other. Maeda and Kurokawa [5] pointed out the difficulty of defining a commensurability measure for different populations.

We presented and studied five criteria, where three of them, d, d_{mod} and d_{MTD}, measure the similarity between dose–toxicity curves, and two of them, d_{p1} and d_{p2}, measure the distance between the median and the *maximum a posteriori* of the MTD posterior distributions. The first three measures are bounded between 0 and 1 and their interpretation could be linked to a proportion. The second ones, d_{p1} and d_{p2} have a ratio-like value with a lower bound at 0. In practice, they represent a relative risk measure.

Our approach allows for the identification and discussion of similarities and differences between dose–toxicity curves and MTDs. However, as small samples were used in these studies, estimation of the entire dose–toxicity curve, when only part of the doses in the panel were evaluated, is complex and leads to an estimation with high variability. This is reflected in the values of d, d_{mod} and d_{MTD}, which in our real case studies were above 0.2. When high differences between d and d_{mod} are observed, this is probably due to computational difficulties in Equation (1), especially in computing the weighted likelihood without a stabilization term. In general, d_{mod} is lower than d_{MTD}. This could be expected for two reasons: (i) d_{MTD} introduces, via the transformation, more variability (increased in the density estimation step); (ii) d_{MTD} is computed after truncating the posterior induced distribution of the MTD. Moreover, we showed that d_{p2}, based on the maximum a posteriori, is more stable than d_{p1}, which is based on the median, in the presence of unbalanced heavy tails. Therefore, d_{p2} could be suggested as a more reliable measure in this setting. We have attempted the analysis while varying the variance matrix of the bivariate normal prior distribution and d_{p1} was less stable (results not shown).

The MTD definition can vary according to the trial and to the population. Therefore, even if the same MTD is claimed in both Caucasian and Japanese populations, our analysis can identify differences. For instance, in the Japanese trial of Sorafenib, 400 mg/day is defined in the clinical trial as the MTD, but at the closest higher dose level, 600 mg/day, only one patient experienced toxicities (16.7%). Otherwise, in the Caucasian trial, three patients out of seven experienced toxicity at 600 mg/day (42.6%). Even if the two trials find the same MTD, the toxicity probability associated with each one differs. That is the reason why our results showed otherwise. Indeed, in the published clinical trials, there is a discrepancy between the method section defining the MTD and the real given MTD at the end of the trial. Our methods are based on data only and allow for evaluation of the actual similarity.

We decided to present the plot of the posterior densities (of the parameters and of the MTD) as it shows the super-position (or not) of the information. Plotting directly one-dimensional dose–response curves could, instead, be misleading and give hazardous interpretation.

A first limitation of our work is that we used published data, where the reporting can be sometimes incomplete in terms of DLTs and doses. For instance, in the paper of Burris et al. [18], we had to re-compose the DLT table and the dose-allocation sequence. Therefore, some interpretation discrepancy can be found in our Table 2. The issue of poor reporting in cancer trials was already raised by Zohar et al. [28] and Comets and Zohar [29]. As a second limitation, we did not provide fixed cut-offs for each criterion. In our opinion, the choice of the cut-offs depends on the application and on the quantity of information in the two trials. The more information we have, the more stringent cut-offs can be considered. Figure 3 only represents a proposition on the way to display the results.

The criteria proposed in this manuscript may be extended to be used in other settings. For example, when several trials are available, a meta-analysis of the dose–toxicity curves or of the MTDs can be considered [30–32]. In this case, pairwise distances can be previously estimated, in an empirical Bayes approach, and then be used to model the heterogeneity parameter(s) or to set prior distribution(s). Other extensions, which do not involve necessarily Phase I studies, could be considered: (i) in adults–children extrapolation; (ii) when we are interested to jointly evaluate efficacy and toxicity [33]; (iii) when comparing outcomes (efficacy or toxicity) of the same drug in different indications; (iv) when dealing with similarities in subgroups; (v) in comparing historical control data with respect to the actual trial in randomized Phase III trials.

Being able to quantify distance and bridging between two populations at the end of early Phase I trials can be useful to better characterize the dose–toxicity relationship and differences. In case of small or acceptable differences, the extrapolation process can be considered, as suggested in the ICH-E5.

Supplementary Materials: The following are available at https://www.mdpi.com/1660-4601/18/4/1639/s1.

Author Contributions: Conceptualization, A.O., M.U. and S.Z.; methodology, A.O. and M.U.; validation, S.Z. and S.M.; writing—original draft preparation, A.O.; writing—review and editing, M.U., S.Z and S.M. All authors have read and agreed to the published version of the manuscript.

Funding: The research of Adrien Ollier and Moreno Ursino was funded by the Institut National Du Cancer, grant numbers INCa_11324 and INCa_9539, respectively.

Institutional Review Board Statement: Not applicable.

Informed Consent Statement: Not applicable.

Data Availability Statement: R scripts are given as Supplemental Materials.

Conflicts of Interest: The authors declare no conflict of interest.

Abbreviations

The following abbreviations are used in this manuscript:

bid	*bis in die*: twice a day
BLRM	Bayesian Logistic Regression Model
CRM	Continual reassessment method
DLT	dose-limiting toxicity
ICH	International Conference on Harmonisation of Technical Requirements for Registration of Pharmaceuticals for Human Use
MTD	maximum tolerated dose
PMDA	Pharmaceuticals and Medical Devices Agency

Appendix A. Bivariate Posterior Plots

Figures A1 and A2 show the bivariate posterior distributions of β_0 and β_1 when using d_{mod}.

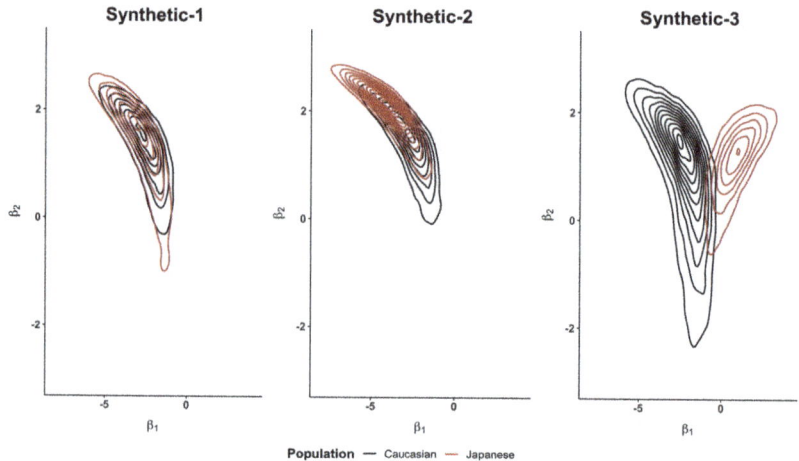

Figure A1. Bivariate posterior distributions of β_0 and β_1 when using d_{mod} for the three synthetic examples.

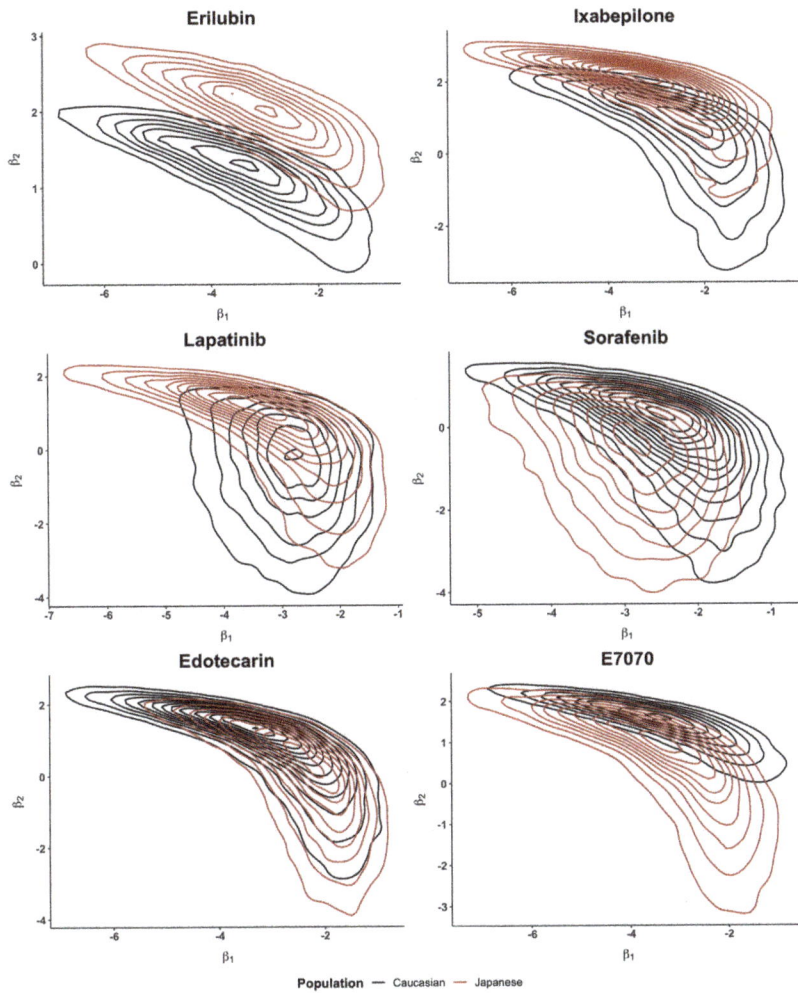

Figure A2. Bivariate posterior distributions of β_0 and β_1 when using d_{mod} for the real case studies shown in Table 2.

References

1. ICH E5 (R1). *Ethnic Factors in the Acceptability of Foreign Clinical Data E5 (R1)*; International Conference on Harmonisation of Technical Requirements for Registration of Pharmaceuticals for Human Use: Geneva, Switzerland, 1998.
2. Pharmaceuticals and Medical Devices Agency. Basic Principles for Conducting Phase I Trials in the Japanese Population Prior to Global Clinical Trials. 2015. Available online: https://www.pmda.go.jp/files/000157777.pdf (accessed on 26 September 2019).
3. Ogura, T.; Morita, S.; Yonemori, K.; Nonaka, T.; Urano, T. Exploring Ethnic Differences in Toxicity in Early-Phase Clinical Trials for Oncology Drugs. *Ther. Innov. Regul. Sci.* **2014**, *48*, 644–650. [CrossRef] [PubMed]
4. Malinowski, H.J.; Westelinck, A.; Sato, J.; Ong, T. Same drug, different dosing: Differences in dosing for drugs approved in the United States, Europe, and Japan. *J. Clin. Pharmacol.* **2008**, *48*, 900–908. [CrossRef]
5. Maeda, H.; Kurokawa, T. Differences in maximum tolerated doses and approval doses of molecularly targeted oncology drug between Japan and Western countries. *Investig. New Drugs* **2014**, *32*, 661–669. [CrossRef]
6. Mizugaki, H.; Yamamoto, N.; Fujiwara, Y.; Nokihara, H.; Yamada, Y.; Tamura, T. Current status of single-agent phase I trials in Japan: toward globalization. *J. Clin. Oncol.* **2015**, *33*, 2051–2061. [CrossRef]
7. O'Quigley, J.; Iasonos, A. Bridging Solutions in Dose Finding Problems. *Stat. Biopharm. Res.* **2014**, *6*, 185–197. [CrossRef] [PubMed]

8. Liu, S.; Pan, H.; Xia, J.; Huang, Q.; Yuan, Y. Bridging continual reassessment method for phase I clinical trials in different ethnic populations. *Stat. Med.* **2015**, *34*, 1681–1694. [CrossRef] [PubMed]
9. Takeda, K.; Morita, S. Incorporating Historical Data in Bayesian Phase I Trial Design: The Caucasian-to-Asian Toxicity Tolerability Problem. *Ther. Innov. Regul. Sci.* **2015**, *49*, 93–99. [CrossRef] [PubMed]
10. Ollier, A.; Morita, S.; Ursino, M.; Zohar, S. An adaptive power prior for sequential clinical trials—Application to bridging studies. *Stat. Methods Med. Res.* **2020**, *29*, 2282–2294. [CrossRef]
11. Bretz, F.; Möllenhoff, K.; Dette, H.; Liu, W.; Trampisch, M. Assessing the similarity of dose response and target doses in two non-overlapping subgroups. *Stat. Med.* **2016**. [CrossRef] [PubMed]
12. Ibrahim, J.G.; Chen, M.H.; Gwon, Y.; Chen, F. The power prior: Theory and applications. *Stat. Med.* **2015**, *34*, 3724–3749. [CrossRef]
13. O'Quigley, J.; Pepe, M.; Fisher, L. Continual reassessment method: A practical design for phase 1 clinical trials in cancer. *Biometrics* **1990**, 33–48. [CrossRef]
14. Neuenschwander, B.; Branson, M.; Gsponer, T. Critical aspects of the Bayesian approach to phase I cancer trials. *Stat. Med.* **2008**, *27*, 2420–2439. [CrossRef]
15. Zheng, H.; Hampson, L.V. A Bayesian decision-theoretic approach to incorporate preclinical information into phase I oncology trials. *Biom. J.* **2020**, *62*, 1408–1427. [CrossRef] [PubMed]
16. Tan, A.R.; Rubin, E.H.; Walton, D.C.; Shuster, D.E.; Wong, Y.N.; Fang, F.; Ashworth, S.; Rosen, L.S. Phase I study of eribulin mesylate administered once every 21 days in patients with advanced solid tumors. *Clin. Cancer Res. Off. J. Am. Assoc. Cancer Res.* **2009**, *15*, 4213–4219. [CrossRef]
17. Mukohara, T.; Nagai, S.; Mukai, H.; Namiki, M.; Minami, H. Eribulin mesylate in patients with refractory cancers: A Phase I study. *Investig. New Drugs* **2011**, *30*, 1926–1933. [CrossRef]
18. Burris, H.A.; Hurwitz, H.I.; Dees, E.C.; Dowlati, A.; Blackwell, K.L.; O'Neil, B.; Marcom, P.K.; Ellis, M.J.; Overmoyer, B.; Jones, S.F.; et al. Phase I Safety, Pharmacokinetics, and Clinical Activity Study of Lapatinib (GW572016), a Reversible Dual Inhibitor of Epidermal Growth Factor Receptor Tyrosine Kinases, in Heavily Pretreated Patients With Metastatic Carcinomas. *J. Clin. Oncol. Off. J. Am. Soc. Clin. Oncol.* **2005**, *23*, 5305–5313. [CrossRef]
19. Nakagawa, K.; Minami, H.; Kanezaki, M.; Mukaiyama, A.; Minamide, Y.; Uejima, H.; Kurata, T.; Nogami, T.; Kawada, K.; Mukai, H.; et al. Phase I Dose-escalation and Pharmacokinetic Trial of Lapatinib (GW572016), a Selective Oral Dual Inhibitor of ErbB-1 and -2 Tyrosine Kinases, in Japanese Patients with Solid Tumors. *Jpn. J. Clin. Oncol.* **2009**, *39*, 116–123. [CrossRef]
20. Moore, M.; Hirte, H.; Siu, L.; Oza, A.; Hotte, S.; Petrenciuc, O.; Cihon, F.; Lathia, C.; Schwartz, B. Phase I study to determine the safety and pharmacokinetics of the novel Raf kinase and VEGFR inhibitor BAY 43-9006, administered for 28 days on/7 days off in patients with advanced, refractory solid tumors. *Ann. Oncol.* **2005**, *16*, 1688–1694. [CrossRef] [PubMed]
21. Minami, H.; Kawada, K.; Ebi, H.; Kitagawa, K.; Kim, Y.i.; Araki, H.; Mukai, H.; Tahara, M.; Nakajima, H.; Nakajima, K. Phase I and pharmacokinetic study of sorafenib, an oral multikinase inhibitor, in Japanese patients with advanced refractory solid tumors. *Cancer Sci.* **2008**, *99*, 1492–1498. [CrossRef]
22. Aghajanian, C.; Burris, H.A.; Jones, S.; Spriggs, D.R.; Cohen, M.B.; Peck, R.; Sabbatini, P.; Hensley, M.L.; Greco, F.A.; Dupont, J.; et al. Phase I Study of the Novel Epothilone Analog Ixabepilone (BMS-247550) in Patients with Advanced Solid Tumors and Lymphomas. *J. Clin. Oncol.* **2007**, *25*, 1082–1088. [CrossRef] [PubMed]
23. Shimizu, T.; Yamamoto, N.; Yamada, Y.; Fujisaka, Y.; Yamada, K.; Fujiwara, Y.; Takayama, K.; Tokudome, T.; Klimovsky, J.; Tamura, T. Phase I clinical and pharmacokinetic study of 3-weekly, 3-h infusion of ixabepilone (BMS-247550), an epothilone B analog, in Japanese patients with refractory solid tumors. *Cancer Chemother. Pharmacol.* **2008**, *61*, 751–758. [CrossRef] [PubMed]
24. Hurwitz, H.I.; Cohen, R.B.; McGovren, J.P.; Hirawat, S.; Petros, W.P.; Natsumeda, Y.; Yoshinari, T. A phase I study of the safety and pharmacokinetics of edotecarin (J-107088), a novel topoisomerase I inhibitor, in patients with advanced solid tumors. *Cancer Chemother. Pharmacol.* **2007**, *59*, 139–147. [CrossRef] [PubMed]
25. Yamada, Y.; Tamura, T.; Yamamoto, N.; Shimoyama, T.; Ueda, Y.; Murakami, H.; Kusaba, H.; Kamiya, Y.; Saka, H.; Tanigawara, Y.; et al. Phase I and pharmacokinetic study of edotecarin, a novel topoisomerase I inhibitor, administered once every 3 weeks in patients with solid tumors. *Cancer Chemother. Pharmacol.* **2006**, *58*, 173–182. [CrossRef] [PubMed]
26. Raymond, E.; ten Bokkel Huinink, W.; Taïeb, J.; Beijnen, J.; Faivre, S.; Wanders, J.; Ravic, M.; Fumoleau, P.; Armand, J.; Schellens, J. Phase I and Pharmacokinetic Study of E7070, a Novel Chloroindolyl Sulfonamide Cell-Cycle Inhibitor, Administered as a One-Hour Infusion Every Three Weeks in Patients with Advanced Cancer. *J. Clin. Oncol.* **2002**, *20*, 3508–3521. [CrossRef] [PubMed]
27. Yamada, Y.; Yamamoto, N.; Shimoyama, T.; Horiike, A.; Fujisaka, Y.; Takayama, K.; Sakamoto, T.; Nishioka, Y.; Yasuda, S.; Tamura, T. Phase I pharmacokinetic and pharmacogenomic study of E7070 administered once every 21 days. *Cancer Sci.* **2005**, *96*, 721–728. [CrossRef]
28. Zohar, S.; Lian, Q.; Levy, V.; Cheung, K.; Ivanova, A.; Chevret, S. Quality assessment of phase I dose-finding cancer trials: Proposal of a checklist. *Clin. Trials* **2008**, *5*, 478–485. [CrossRef]
29. Comets, E.; Zohar, S. A survey of the way pharmacokinetics are reported in published phase I clinical trials, with an emphasis on oncology. *Clin. Pharmacokinet.* **2009**, *48*, 387–395. [CrossRef]
30. Zohar, S.; Katsahian, S.; O'Quigley, J. An approach to meta-analysis of dose-finding studies. *Stat. Med.* **2011**, *30*, 2109–2116. [CrossRef]

31. Ursino, M.; Röver, C.; Zohar, S.; Friede, T. Random-effects meta-analysis of phase I dose-finding studies using stochastic process priors. *arXiv* **2019**, arXiv:1908.06733.
32. Röver, C.; Friede, T. Dynamically borrowing strength from another study through shrinkage estimation. *Stat. Methods Med. Res.* **2019**, *29*, 293–308. [CrossRef]
33. Thall, P.F.; Cook, J.D. Dose-finding based on efficacy–toxicity trade-offs. *Biometrics* **2004**, *60*, 684–693. [CrossRef] [PubMed]

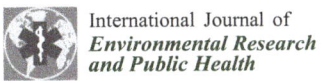

Review

Prior Elicitation for Use in Clinical Trial Design and Analysis: A Literature Review

Danila Azzolina [1,2], Paola Berchialla [3], Dario Gregori [1] and Ileana Baldi [1,*]

1. Unit of Biostatistics, Epidemiology and Public Health, Department of Cardiac Thoracic Vascular Sciences and Public Health, University of Padova, 35128 Padova, Italy; danila.azzolina@uniupo.it (D.A.); dario.gregori@unipd.it (D.G.)
2. Department of Traslational Medicine, University of Eastern Piedmont, 28100 Novara, Italy
3. Department of Clinical and Biological Science, University of Turin, 10124 Turin, Italy; paola.berchialla@unito.it
* Correspondence: ileana.baldi@unipd.it

Abstract: Bayesian inference is increasingly popular in clinical trial design and analysis. The subjective knowledge derived from an expert elicitation procedure may be useful to define a prior probability distribution when no or limited data is available. This work aims to investigate the state-of-the-art Bayesian prior elicitation methods with a focus on clinical trial research. A literature search on the Current Index to Statistics (CIS), PubMed, and Web of Science (WOS) databases, considering "prior elicitation" as a search string, was run on 1 November 2020. Summary statistics and trend of publications over time were reported. Finally, a Latent Dirichlet Allocation (LDA) model was developed to recognise latent topics in the pertinent papers retrieved. A total of 460 documents pertinent to the Bayesian prior elicitation were identified. Of these, 213 (45.4%) were published in the "Probability and Statistics" area. A total of 42 articles pertain to clinical trial and the majority of them (81%) reports parametric techniques as elicitation method. The last decade has seen an increased interest in prior elicitation and the gap between theory and application getting narrower and narrower. Given the promising flexibility of non-parametric approaches to the experts' elicitation, more efforts are needed to ensure their diffusion also in applied settings.

Keywords: prior elicitation; latent dirichlet allocation; clinical trial

1. Introduction

The frequentist inference paradigm has been the main statistical approach to the design and analysis of clinical trials since the 1940s [1].

However, the improvements in statistical computing methods and the introduction of the Markov Chain Monte Carlo (MCMC) algorithm have facilitated the spread of the Bayesian methods, also in the field of clinical trials [2].

The prior distribution is a key element of Bayesian inference and represents the information about a parameter of interest that is combined with the likelihood to yield the posterior distribution. The prior information may be derived from either expert beliefs (subjective prior) or relevant empirical data (objective prior) [3,4].

Especially when few data are available to estimate the likelihood, for example in clinical trials in rare diseases [5] and poor accrual setting [6], an informative inference complemented with an expert elicitation procedure may be useful to translate into prior probability distribution the available expert knowledge about treatment effect [7,8]. The Bayesian priors obtained through the elicitation of expert opinion can be used to augment scarce data about treatment effect, especially in clinical trial design and analysis [9]. Eliciting expert's opinions, in the Bayesian paradigm, may demonstrate the presence of uncertainty in treatment effect belief in a quantifiable and illustrative manner. Moreover, this information can be used to plan a study, for example, the sample size calculations [10] and interim analysis [11]. Elicited prior distributions can be used to augment the information given by scarce therapeutic data [8].

Moreover, it is interesting to consider that, the development of user-friendly interfaces, as SHELF (SHeffield ELicitation Framework) [12] or MATCH (Multidisciplinary Assessment of Technology for Healthcare) [13] software, for prior elicitation, facilitates the application of the method in the clinical research and other applied settings.

The SHELF software carries out elicitation of probability distributions for uncertain quantities from a group of experts. Each expert provides a small number of probability opinions corresponding to points on a cumulative distribution function. The SHELF tool fits a range of parametric distributions displaying them in the form of fitted probabilities and percentiles. For multiple experts, a weighted linear pool of the subjective distributions can be calculated [12].

Another useful tool provided in the literature is MATCH, which provides a web-based interface for the SHELF routine with the aim of being more user-friendly, including also features for the conduction of the elicitation process remotely [13].

The elicitation process is usually performed by asking the experts to report a few summaries of treatment effect, generally medians, modes, and percentiles of the probability distribution.

Some authors assessed that the role of a facilitator is fundamental in the elicitation process. The facilitator translates some percentiles, defined by experts, into a probability distribution. This process is generally based on parametric distributions (Gamma or Beta, Student, Normal or Log-Normal) [14]. This task becomes more complicated when the opinions are asked of several experts. In this case, each expert opinion may be separately translated into distributions, and finally, it is possible to pool them into a unique prior distribution.

The elicitation approach accounts for the subjective expert's uncertainty about the treatment effect under investigation, and the consequences of this uncertainty in final inference can be investigated using sensitivity analysis techniques [8].

Quantiles information about expert beliefs is generally easier to elicit than moments [15]. Probability distributions are in several cases defined by moments, and some authors have investigated procedures to derive the parameters of a distribution using mean and standard deviation [16]. However, instead of considering direct estimates of the mean and standard deviation, it is possible to ask an expert for a specific discrete set of points on the distribution for example quantiles [17]. The mean and standard deviations can be derived from applying specific weights to the quantiles [18], or fitting distributions on the discrete points [19].

Quantiles information are widely adopted, to fit prior probability distributions, not only in a parametric but also in the semiparametric and non-parametric setting; for example, it is possible to ask the expert the quantiles (usually at least two) of the subjective prior distribution. These points may be plotted, and it is possible to smooth a distribution function drawn through them using a semiparametric or non-parametric representation of the expert's opinion [20,21].

In a parametric setting, the elicitation process assumes that experts' opinion may be represented by a good note family of probability distributions identified by hyperparameters. Thus, the elicitation consists of the definition of appropriate values for hyperparameters to represent the experts' belief [7].

It is widely assessed that the main limit of a parametric approach is to constrain expert belief into a pre-specified distribution [22]. Therefore, non-parametric and semi-parametric hybrid approaches have also been proposed in the elicitation process [21].

This work is aimed to investigate the state-of-the-art of Bayesian prior elicitation methods, focusing on the discrepancy between the available methodological approaches in the statistical literature and the elicitation procedures applied within the clinical trial research.

In this general framework, another issue is the identification of the main research topics and the definition of the peculiarities of papers using parametric and non-parametric approaches in a clinical trial concerning identified research themes. A tool that automatically allows classifying the overall elicitation literature could reduce the manual text classification burden and characterise topic patterns over the time.

2. Materials and Methods

2.1. Search Strategy

A search on the Current Index to Statistics (CIS), PubMed, Scopus, Embase, and Web of Science (WOS) electronic databases, finalised to identify all papers dealing with prior elicitation and published from 1 January 1980 to 1 November 2020, was performed. The search string "prior elicitation" was used. This search string is very general to ensure that all relevant results would be included in the final analysis. The pertinent articles were identified after duplicate removal. The overall prior elicitation literature and the articles pertaining to the prior elicitation in the clinical trial have been screened by reading the title and abstract.

2.2. Overall Data Description

Summary statistics were reported to describe the corpus of papers pertinent to the prior elicitation theme.

The prior elicitation-relevant articles have been classified in those published in "Probability and Statistics" journals (here in after referred to as Statistical papers) according to the Journal Citation Reports® [23] classification. The prior elicitation publication trend according to the statistical papers versus other journals has been reported.

As for articles concerning drug clinical trials, the frequencies of published papers have been reported according to publication time and prior elicitation methods, in parametric and in not (or semi) parametric settings.

2.3. State-of-the-Art of Prior Elicitation in Clinical Trials

Methodological approaches to the prior elicitation currently used in clinical trial literature have been described, evaluating the main characteristics of parametric and non-parametric approaches adopted in trial design and analysis distinguishing by type of outcome considered in the study.

For a general comparison purpose, available methods for expert elicitation in the overall pertinent prior elicitation literature have been also reported and described.

2.4. Text Mining Analysis

2.4.1. LDA Algorithm

A text mining (topic model) analysis has been conducted to automatically identify the main topics characterising the overall publications on prior elicitation. The literature on clinical trials could constitute a limited subset of the total literature on prior Elicitation. For this reason, this subset was used as a validation set by classifying the documents manually and comparing the outcome of the manual classification with the automatic one. Topic modelling is an unsupervised machine learning technique that is capable of automatically clustering word groups (topics) and similar expressions that best characterise a set of documents [24].

2.4.2. Data Pre-Processing

The titles and abstracts of prior elicitation pertinent papers have been pre-processed. Punctuation, stop words, white spaces, and numbers were removed. Redundant words (prior, elicitation, expert, Bayesian, analysis) were also removed. All words were converted to lowercase.

Once the text corpus has been cleaned, a Document-Term Matrix (DTM) has been created. A DTM is a matrix, reporting documents (articles) by rows and words by columns; a generic element of DTM is the word counts.

To detect topics, a Latent Dirichlet Allocation (LDA) [24] analysis has been performed on the DTM matrix of pertinent articles. LDA is a technique leading to the automatic discovery of themes in a collection of documents. The method assumes that each document (articles) is a mixture of topics. Documents and words are observed elements instead topics are latent structures discovered by the LDA algorithm.

The method aims to infer the latent topic structure given the words and document. LDA recreates the documents in the corpus by adjusting the relative importance of topics in documents iteratively using a Gibbs sampler algorithm [25].

Gibbs sampling works by performing a random walk. The starting point of the walk is chosen at random; for this reason, it may be useful to discard the first steps (burn-in period). Overall, 10,000 iterations have been considered in the computation, and 100 draws have been discarded as burn-in. A total of five Markov chains with different starting points were generated.

2.4.3. Number of Topics

The number of topics has been chosen following the maximisation criterion of the Deveaud measure [26]. The method is based on the idea of computing distances between pairs of topics over several instances of the model while varying the number of topics. The model iterations are done by varying the number of topics of the LDA model, then estimating again the Dirichlet distributions. The optimal amount of topics is reached when the overall Kullback–Leibler dissimilarity between topics achieves its maximum value [27].

2.4.4. Validation and Convergence Assessment

The algorithm has been validated on the clinical trial pertinent articles. Furthermore, the overall accuracy has been calculated, comparing the manual and automatic classification.

The convergence of the LDA algorithm has been evaluated showing the Log-Likelihood in correspondence of the first 500 iterations. If the Log-Likelihood estimate stabilises after the first iterations, then the convergence is deemed acceptable [25].

2.4.5. Results

Once the algorithm has been validated, the distribution of the publication topics identified by the algorithm on the prior elicitation literature has been characterised according to the year of publication and the field of application (trial versus other pertinent literature).

Computations have been performed using R 3.3.2 [28] System with topicmodels [29] package.

3. Results
3.1. Overall Data Description

A total of 3725 articles have been found performing the literature review. Among them, 470 articles are identified as pertinent to the Bayesian prior elicitation theme (Figure 1). Of these, 213 are published in Statistical Journals according to Journal Citation Reports® classification [23].

As per the temporal pattern of the prior elicitation literature, it is possible to observe that, until 2010, there is a greater number of publications in the statistical literature compared to other research areas; the pattern is reversed starting from 2009 to November 2020 (Figure 2).

Concerning the clinical trial research setting, it is possible to observe that 42 articles out of 470 deal with this research argument. Moreover, according to temporal trends, an increase in the number of publications concerning clinical trials is observed over time; 2 articles between 1992 and 2000, 10 in the period comprised between 2001 and 2008, 15 between 2009 and 2016, and 15 between 2017 and 2020.

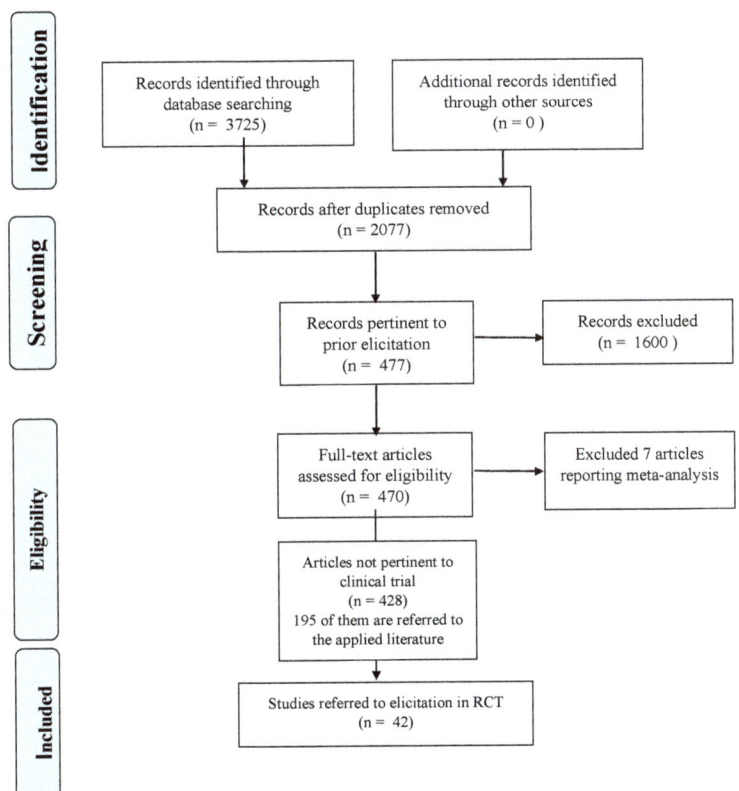

Figure 1. Prisma Flowchart.

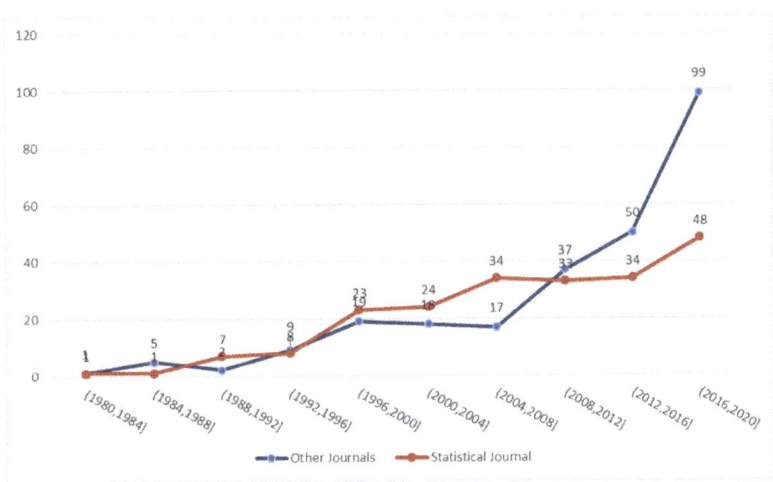

Figure 2. Articles pertinent to Prior Elicitation (n = 470) according to Journal type and year.

3.2. State-of-the-Art Prior Elicitation in the Clinical Trial

Table 1 shows the characteristics of the 42 papers pertinent to clinical trial literature.

Table 1. Articles treating prior elicitation in clinical trial classified according to publication year, first author, title, main approach, the prior distribution, trial phase, prior information, software used for elicitation, manual classification.

Publication Year	Author	Title	Approach	Prior Distribution	Trial Phase	Prior Information	Software	Manual Classification
2020	(Alhussain et al., 2020) [30]	Assurance for clinical trial design with normally distributed outcomes: Eliciting uncertainty about variances	Parametric	Normal	Study design	Sensitivity with different levels of prior variability	SHELF	Applied
2019	(Aupiais et al., 2019) [31]	A Bayesian non-inferiority approach using experts' margin elicitation-application to the monitoring of safety events	Parametric	Beta	Phase III monitoring	Non-informative Beta and informative with parameters defined by expert opinions	Betareg R	Applied
2004	(Bekele & Thall, 2004) [32]	Dose-finding based on multiple toxicities in a soft tissue sarcoma trial	Parametric	Multinormal	Phase I	Sensitivity analysis by randomly perturbing the elicited toxicity weight vector	None	Applied
2019	(Berchialla et al., 2019) [33]	Bayesian sample size determination for phase IIA clinical trials using historical data and semi-parametric prior's Elicitation	Semiparametric	B-Spline	Study design	Uninformative and best fit to the expert opinions	None	Theoretical
2019	(Boulet et al., 2019) [34]	Bayesian variable selection based on clinical relevance weights in small sample studies-Application to colon cancer	Parametric	Mixture of normal	Not applicable	Informative	None	Applied
2017	(Browne et al., 2017) [35]	A Bayesian Analysis of a Randomised Clinical Trial Comparing Antimetabolite Therapies for Non-Infectious Uveitis	Parametric	Normal	Phase II-III	Informative	Matematica and R	Applied

Table 1. *Cont.*

Publication Year	Author	Title	Approach	Prior Distribution	Trial Phase	Prior Information	Software	Manual Classification
1993	(Chaloner et al., 1993) [36]	Graphical Elicitation of a prior distribution for a clinical trial	Non-Parametric	Non-parametric adjustments via copula combinations of the marginal distribution	Phase II-III	Informative	XLISP-STAT software	Theoretical
1999	(Chen et al., 1999) [37]	A new Bayesian model for survival data with a surviving fraction	Parametric	Gamma and Normal	Phase III	Non-informative and Informative prior	None	Theoretical
2002	(Cheung, 2002) [38]	On the use of nonparametric curves in phase I trials with low toxicity tolerance	Parametric	Beta	Phase I	Informative	None	Theoretical
2012	(Cook et al., 2012) [39]	A questionnaire elicitation of surgeons' belief about learning within a surgical trial	Parametric	Learning curve	Phase II	Informative	None	Applied
2008	(Gajewski, Simon, & Carlson, 2008) [40]	Predicting accrual in clinical trials with Bayesian posterior predictive distributions	Parametric	Inverse Gamma	Not applicable	Non-Informative or informative	Accrual R package	Theoretical
2015	(Hampson et al., 2015) [41]	Elicitation of Expert Prior Opinion: Application to the MYPAN Trial in Childhood Polyarteritis Nodosa	Parametric	Beta and Normal	Phase III	Informative	Shiny app created by authors	Applied
2009	(Hiance et al., 2009) [42]	A practical approach for eliciting expert prior beliefs about cancer survival in phase III randomised trial	Parametric	Normal	Phase III	Informative	None	Applied

Table 1. Cont.

Publication Year	Author	Title	Approach	Prior Distribution	Trial Phase	Prior Information	Software	Manual Classification
2011	(Higgins et al., 2011) [43]	A Bayesian approach demonstrating that the incorporation of practitioners' clinical beliefs into research design is crucial for effective knowledge transfer	Parametric	Beta	Not applicable	Informative	SHELF	Applied
2012	(Higgins, Dryden, & Green, 2012) [44]	A Bayesian elicitation of veterinary beliefs regarding systemic dry cow therapy: Variation and importance for the clinical trial design	Parametric	Beta	Not applied	Informative	SHELF	Applied
2020	(Jansen et al., 2011) [45]	Elicitation of prior probability distributions for a proposed Bayesian randomised clinical trial of whole blood for trauma resuscitation	Parametric	Beta	Phase III	Informative	SHELF	Applied
2011	(Johnson et al., 2011) [9]	Effect of warfarin on survival in scleroderma-associated pulmonary arterial hypertension (SSc-PAH) and idiopathic PAH. Belief elicitation for Bayesian priors	Non-parametric	Density histogram	Phase III	Sensitivity analysis to different Informative priors	None	Applied
2013	(Kinnersley, N.; Day, S., 2013) [46]	A structured approach to the Elicitation of expert beliefs for a Bayesian-designed clinical trial: A case study	Parametric	Beta	Phase II	Informative	SHELF	Applied

Table 1. *Cont.*

Publication Year	Author	Title	Approach	Prior Distribution	Trial Phase	Prior Information	Software	Manual Classification
2001	(Legedza & Ibrahim, 2001) [47]	Heterogeneity in phase I clinical trials: prior Elicitation and computation using the continual reassessment method	Non-parametric	Ibrahim Prior (Ibrahim et al., 1998)	Phase I	Informative	S plus	Theoretical
2020	(Lin et al., 2020) [48]	An adaptive trial design to optimise dose-schedule regimes with delayed outcomes	Parametric	Bivariate Normal	Phase I–II clinical trial design	Informative	None	Applied
2013	(Moatti et al., 2013) [49]	Modeling of experts' divergent prior beliefs for a sequential phase III clinical trial	Parametric	Mixture of normal	Phase III	Informative	Mixdist package R	Theoretical
2018	(Muff et al., 2011) [50]	Bias away from the null due to miscounted outcomes? A case study on the TORCH trial	Parametric	Normal Log-Normal	Phase III	Informative	None	Applied
2009	(O'Leary et al., 2009) [51]	Comparison of three expert elicitation methods for logistic regression on predicting the presence of the threatened brush-tailed rock-wall by Petrogale penicillata	Parametric	Normal and Multinormal	Not applicable	Informative and Non-Informative prior	GIS, a map-based software developed by authors	Theoretical
2020	(Ollier et al., 2011) [52]	An adaptive power prior for sequential clinical trials-Application to bridging studies	Non-parametric	Ibrahim power Prior (Ibrahim et al., 1998)	Phase I	Informative	None	Theoretical
2019	(Psioda et al., 2011) [53]	Bayesian clinical trial design using historical data that inform the treatment effect	Non-parametric	Ibrahim adaptive power Prior (Ibrahim et al., 1998)	Study design	Informative	None	Theoretical

Table 1. Cont.

Publication Year	Author	Title	Approach	Prior Distribution	Trial Phase	Prior Information	Software	Manual Classification
2019	(Ramanan et al., 2011) [54]	Defining consensus opinion to develop randomised controlled trials in rare diseases using Bayesian design: An example of a proposed trial of adalimumab versus pamidronate for children with CNO/CRMO	Parametric	Normal	Phase II	Informative	Shiny web app proposed by authors	Applied
2014	(Ren & Oakley, 2014) [55]	Assurance calculations for planning clinical trials with time-to-event outcomes	Parametric	Log-Normal	Study design	Informative	Software implemented by the authors	Theoretical
2011	(Rietbergen et al., 2011) [56]	Incorporation of historical data in the analysis of randomised therapeutic trials	Parametric	Beta	Phase II-III	Informative with power prior	None	Theoretical
2005	(Rosenberger et al., 2005) [57]	Development of interactive software for Bayesian optimal phase 1 clinical trial design	Parametric	Uniform	Phase I	Uninformative by default	IDose software	Applied
2005	(Rovers et al., 2005) [58]	Bayes' theorem: A negative example of an RCT on grommets in children with glue ear	Parametric	Beta	Not applicable	Informative	None	Applied
2012	(See et al., 2012) [59]	Prior Elicitation and Bayesian Analysis of the Steroids for Corneal Ulcers Trial	Parametric	Mixture of normal	Phase 3	Informative	Mathematica	Applied
2002	(Stevens & O'Hagan, 2002) [60]	Incorporation of genuine prior information in cost-effectiveness analysis of clinical trial data	Parametric	Log-Normal	Not applicable	Informative and Non-Informative prior	None	Applied

Table 1. *Cont.*

Publication Year	Author	Title	Approach	Prior Distribution	Trial Phase	Prior Information	Software	Manual Classification
2013	(Sun et al., 2013) [61]	Expert Prior Elicitation and Bayesian Analysis of the Mycotic Ulcer Treatment Trial I	Non-Parametric	Density histogram	Phase III	Informative and Non-Informative prior	Mathematica	Applied
2003	(Tan et al., 2003) [62]	Elicitation of prior distributions for a phase III randomised controlled trial of adjuvant therapy with surgery for hepatocellular carcinoma	Parametric	Normal	Phase III	Sensitivity to informative priors	None	Applied
2017	(Thall et al., 2017) [63]	Bayesian treatment comparison using parametric mixture priors computed from elicited histograms	Parametric	Mixture of Normal	Phase II–III	Informative and Non-Informative prior	None	Theoretical
2009	(Turner et al., 2009) [64]	Bias modeling in evidence synthesis	Parametric	Log-Normal	Not applicable	Informative	None	Applied
2017	(Veen, Stoel, Zondervan-Zwijnenburg, & van de Schoot, 2017) [65]	Proposal for a Five-Step Method to Elicit Expert Judgment	Parametric	Normal	Not applicable	Informative	MATCH	Applied
2003	(Wang & Ghosh, 2003) [66]	Bayesian analysis of bivariate competing risks models with covariates	Parametric	Laplace and Jeffreys Prior	Not applicable	Informative and Non-Informative prior	None	Theoretical
2019	(Wheeler et al., 2011) [67]	Quantal Risk Assessment Database: A Database for Exploring Patterns in Quantal Dose-Response Data in Risk Assessment and its Application to Develop Priors for Bayesian Dose-Response Analysis	Parametric	Beta and Log-Normal	Not applicable	Informative and Non-Informative prior	None	Applied

Table 1. Cont.

Publication Year	Author	Title	Approach	Prior Distribution	Trial Phase	Prior Information	Software	Manual Classification
2005	(White et al., 2005) [68]	Eliciting and using expert opinions about the influence of patient characteristics on treatment effects: a Bayesian analysis of the CHARM trials	Parametric	Normal	Phase III	Informative and Non-Informative prior	None	Applied
2020	(Wiesenfarth et al., 2005) [69]	Quantification of prior impact in terms of effective current sample size	Parametric	Normal and Beta prior	Study design	Informative and Non-Informative prior	None	Applied
2011	(Zohar et al., 2011) [70]	Planning a Bayesian early-phase I/II study for human vaccines in HER2 carcinomas	Non-parametric	Non-parametric expert quantiles distribution	Phase I-II	Informative and Non-Informative prior	None	Applied

3.2.1. Parametric Approaches

Continuous and Time to Event Outcomes

Considering continuous and time to event outcomes, Normal or Log-Normal priors are the preferred distributions for the elicitation procedure in 22 research articles.

The Normal prior distribution is used in several fields of application:

- Survival endpoints

The Gaussian distribution is a used solution to define priors on hyper-parameters for a survival function assuming a Weibull time to event shape relation [37]. The author proposed Bayesian methods for right-censored survival data for populations with a surviving (cure) fraction. A real dataset from a melanoma clinical trial has been considered for the application. The normal random variable has been considered to parametrise the Weibull scale hyperparameter in an uninformative manner with high variance [37]. In fact, according to the Bayes and Laplace postulate, the absence of information concerning the treatment effect may be translated into equal prior probabilities for a discrete event and a flat prior (high variance) for the continuous endpoints [71].

In several cases, log-hazard ratios are also modelled as a normal distribution. Histograms representing the prior beliefs of each investigator were constructed and interpolating the Log Hazard ratio with a Gaussian distribution [49,62]. This approach has been employed also in cancer survival studies by performing a weighted averaging pooling of expert opinions [42].

The poling of the expert opinion may be performed by calculating the average of the height of the prior distributions for each parameter value (average pooling) or computing a geometric mean of the original densities (logarithmic pooling). Both techniques allow for different weights to be given to each opinion depending on the clinician's experience in the area under study [72].

- Models hyperparameters

The normal approximation of experts' opinion is also implemented to model parameters of Bayesian logistic regression. The method models the response as a Bernoulli random variable assuming the regression coefficients as a mixture of three normal distributions reflecting increase, decrease, and no substantive change in the response [51].

Moreover, the Gaussian priors have been considered also to define the hyperparameters for an adjusted hierarchical model for the miscounting count predictions of the Poisson and negative binomial models. The parametrisation has been proposed and applied to a large randomised controlled trial on Chronic Obstructive Pulmonary Disease [50]. The author derived the prior parameters from the historical information by using an adaptive prior weighting approach, accounting for a potential prior-data conflict. The idea is to discounting the prior information whatever the prior-data conflict exists [73].

- Study design

The Normal distribution has been also proposed in multi-stage trials to elicitate a prior for the treatment effect estimation and then calculating the probability that the trial will produce a favourable outcome; the decision to proceed with a larger trial has been translated in a prior probability distribution incorporating the information provided by a smaller trial [30]. The treatment effect has been elicitated via univariate quartile elicitation method: the Gaussian prior parameters have been derived fitting a probability distribution on the expert quantiles via least-squares procedure [13].

The normal prior elicitation is also considered for the Bayesian clinical trial design. Recent research evaluates the prior impact on the observed data model by introducing the effective current sample size (ECSS) prior approach. Special emphasis is put on the robust mixture, power, and commensurate priors defined on a normal and beta parametrisation [69].

The Gaussian random variable is considered in literature also to perform a prior elicitation for a survival function in the context of a Bayesian clinical trial planning [55].

The author proposes an assurance method, which is an alternative to a power calculation analysis based on the probability of a successful trial outcome computation via Elicitation of a prior probability distribution about the study treatment effect. The prior distribution for the difference in the time point-specific survival rate between treatment and control arm has been elicited via univariate quantile elicitation method [13] by using a truncated Gaussian prior ensuring the support of the time-specific survival rate would be comprised between 0 and 1 [55].

- Treatment effect estimation

Another application of this prior parametrisation is used to elicit the mean change score in a rare disease trial once the consensus among the experts has been reached [54]. The study endpoint under consideration was a mean change score measured 100 mm visual analog scale (VAS) assumed to follow a Gaussian distribution. The prior parameters were elicited by averaging individual quantile opinions among experts.

In other cases, continuous outcomes, defined on log scales, are modelled eliciting experts' opinions with normal distributions [59]. Individual responses achieved from the graphical elicitation method were summed and normalised to obtain a unique prior distribution which is the mean of the single expert normal priors [59].

Additionally, cost data, typically highly skewed, are elicited using Log-Normal transformation [60]. The research showed that the use of genuine prior information can provide more realistic conclusions in particular for cost-effectiveness analyses of trial data where sample sizes are relatively small. A genuine prior is represented by an informative distribution which assumes a higher probability to some values than to others within parametric space [60].

- Multivariate distributions and mixture of priors

In several cases, the overall prior distribution is developed by a weighted mixture of the single expert priors [63]. The mixture of expert's Log-Normal priors has been used also to elicit a prior distribution for the sources of bias affecting the final trial estimate which may be reported in a meta-analysis. The elicited opinions are used to develop prior distributions representing the biases in each study useful to perform a bias-adjusted meta-analysis [64].

A Bayesian method has been proposed and applied to a colon cancer trial where the expert information is used to perform a variable selection procedure [34]. A bivariate Normal random variable has been considered to parametrise the covariate effect, instead, a Beta variable is used to define the covariate weight in the feature selection procedure. The expert's opinions have been pooled using a Bayesian Model Average approach [74].

In the CHARM clinical trial, the log-hazard of cardiovascular death has been modelled via Multivariate Normal distribution [68]. The analysis has been performed on a specific group of patients; the group-specific treatment effects have been estimated by using a Bayesian approach with informative Multi-Normal priors obtained eliciting expert's opinions, interpolating the single opinion histogram with a normal random variable, and averaging across opinions.

The bivariate normal parametrisation has been also considered, in a two-stage phase I–II clinical trial design to optimise dose–schedule regimes where a flexible Bayesian hierarchical model has been used to account for the relation among patients subgroups and treatment regimens [48].

Other parametric distributions are considered in the literature for the continuous outcomes, for example, surgical learning curve parameters (first procedure and plateau level) are obtained averaging different experts' opinion, using a power–law function [39].

The inverse gamma distributions served, instead, to model the accrual rate monitoring in a clinical trial. The posterior predictive accrual distribution has been obtained combining prior information on the accrual rate, provided by experts or historical data, with the information known up to the monitoring time point [40].

In another case, Laplace's and Jeffreys's priors are elicited to estimate a competing risks model with covariates [75]. Laplace's prior has been considered for nonidentifiable model parameters, instead, Jeffreys's prior has been considered for identifiable parameters [75].

Laplace's distribution is a continuous probability distribution also note as a double exponential because its density can be seen as the association of two densities of exponential laws. Laplace's law can also be obtained from the difference of two independent exponential variables with the same parameter [76]. This distribution has been used extensively as a sparsity-inducing mechanism to perform feature selection simultaneously within classification or regression. The mechanism is implemented in the LASSO regression. This prior places stronger confidence on zero regression coefficient than does a normal prior centred on zero [77].

The Jeffreys prior instead is a non-informative prior distribution. In agreement with the Jeffreys rule, a prior distribution is uninformative if its density function is proportional to the square root of the determinant of the Fisher information matrix [71,78].

Categorical Outcomes

Generally, prior probability distributions for binary outcomes are elicited in terms of Beta priors [31,45,46,56,58]. Aupiais and colleagues, for example, proposed a non-inferiority approach, in a Bayesian framework, for sequential monitoring of rare dichotomous safety events, incorporating experts' opinions to define the margin. The acceptable difference between adverse event rates across arms, according to the expert opinions, was modelled using a mixture of beta distributions [31].

- SHELF elicitation procedure

The SHELF elicitation procedure is a widely used approach to elicitate Beta event rate in a clinical trial [12] and is the most commonly used software for elicitation (Table 1). Jansen et al. [45], for example, elicited the prior distribution for the 24-h trauma mortality in patients with haemorrhagic complications combining beta distributions using the SHELF elicitation procedure. The single expert distributions were elicited using the roulette method than a linear poling of the distributions has been performed [45].

In the roulette method, the expert provides probabilities of the treatment effect lying in a particular "bin" by allocating "gaming chips" to that bin. The method provides a graphical representation of the provided expert beliefs [14].

Another research underlines the feasibility of a SHELF elicitation procedure for the evaluation of drug safety or efficacy in a hypothetical early-stage trial. A beta prior has been considered for the elicitation of the expert's opinions [46].

A sequential update of the experts' opinion is also reported in veterinary trials by using a SHELF elicitation procedure on the beta event rate. This research has demonstrated the usefulness of probabilistic elicitation for evaluating the diversity and strength of experts' beliefs concerning the efficacy of systemic antibiotics as dry cow therapy [43].

This software is often used for the computer-based elicitation procedure; the distributions are interactively elicited by showing to the experts the priors obtained through the software. Other elicitation procedures are based on (1) informal discussion (2) structured questionnaires (3) Structured interviewing with poling of opinions [72].

- Dose-response curves

In some cases, a normal distribution has been assumed on parameters characterising the dose-toxicity curve in Phase I clinical trial [32]. A phase I clinical trial is generally aimed to find a maximum tolerated dose, which is often a monotonically increasing dose-response curve following a logistic distribution. For example, the definition of a toxicity response may be based on the approach of eliciting a range for the probability of toxicity at the lowest dose level, and the value of the maximum tolerated dose. The prior for both parameters distribution may be considered as a uniform distribution over these ranges [57]. A non-parametric shape function, for a maximum, tolerated dose may also be reported.

Another option, addressed in the literature, is the of the toxicity probability at each dose level considering a Beta prior distribution [38].

The Log-Normal and Normal prior parametrisation has been used also to develop generalised priors for different Bayesian Dose–Response parametric models [67].

A parametric distribution is also adopted in the literature for categorical endpoints by using the log transformation of odds ratios modelling binary data using elicited Normal priors [5]. Opinion on the relative efficacy of treatment was modelled as a normal distribution, the parameters of which were determined by asking experts questions concerning the distribution quantile.

3.2.2. Non-Parametric Approaches

A total of eight articles [9,33,36,47,52,53,61,70] out of 42 treating expert elicitation in clinical trials consider non-parametric methods for the elicitation of the expert opinion. The principal non-parametric approaches applications are classified within:

- Histogram approach

Graphical visualisation of the expert opinion in histogram defined on parameters of a log-hazard function is a possible approach used to perform elicitation of the expert opinion. The method is flexible leading to define hazard regression coefficient with parametric distributions also allowing for non-parametric adjustments using more general copula combinations of marginal distribution [36]. Individual expert histograms representing the prior beliefs about the treatment effect are also used in other cases to derive non-parametric prior averaging individual expert opinion [9,61].

- Study design and power prior approach

The use of historical information to define the prior distribution in a non-parametric context is a method recently used in the literature [53]. Informative prior elicitation is typically a challenging task even in the presence of historical data (objective prior) [79]. Ibrahim and Chen [80] proposed the power prior approach to incorporate the historical data in the analysis of a current study. The method is based on the raising of the likelihood function of the historical data to a power parameter between 0 and 1 (power parameter). This parameter represents the proportion of the historical data incorporated in the prior. Diaconis and Ylvisaker [81] and Morris [13] studied conjugate priors for the exponential families by assuming a fixed power parameter. Ibrahim and Chen [80] considered the uncertainty component on power parameters.

The approach is widely used for the design and analysis of clinical trial data. The method is useful for handling problems related to a lack of exchangeability between the historical and current data, and the risk that prior information overwhelms the clinical trial data information [82].

In a sequential clinical trial, for example, a power prior approach is considered to weight the prior information together with the ESS (Effective Sample Size) approach is used to set the maximum desired amount of information to be shared from historical data at each step of the trial [52]. The ESS method leads to define the prior in terms of the number of hypothetical patients used to develop the prior. The procedure leads to quantify how is informative a prior distribution [83].

Recently, some efforts are evidenced in the literature to incorporate, in the study design phase, the alternative procedure to the prior definition. The method is tailored on a phase IIA trial and represents a Bayesian counterpart of a Simon two-stage design using historical data and semi-parametric prior's elicitation methods [33].

- Dose findings in early phase trials

Non-parametric approaches are also considered to find a maximum tolerated dose in Phase I clinical trials using the Continual Reassessment Method design and proposing a suitable informative prior distribution on the relationship between outcome data and covariates [47,84]. In a dose-finding trial, non-parametric elicitation procedures are used eliciting expert quantiles opinion corresponding to the toxicity probability at each dose level [70].

3.2.3. Field of Application

Phase II-III trial. The prior elicitation has been applied (16 studies) to the trials for an efficacy assessment within phase II or III trials (Table 1). The priors are defined for the drug efficacy assessment, especially in an informative setting (Table 1). However, in several cases, sensitivity analyses to the prior choices have been proposed, including both the results for the non-informative and informative analysis [31,37,61,63,68]. Concerning the prior distribution sensitivity analysis, the robust Bayesian approach has been proposed by Greenhouse and Wasserman and applied to the clinical trial data, especially to help the monitoring committee to decide whether or not early stopping a trial. The method investigates how the inferences might change as the prior varies over a class of distributions [85].

In other cases, different hypotheses are defined on the informative prior parameters [9,62]. Different levels of discounting are also considered on the historical information incorporated in the prior definition by using a power prior approach [56].

Early Phase I-II. Seven studies implemented the prior elicitation in early phases trial for the safety assessment (Table 1); the greater part of them (4) considered informative priors [38,47,48,52].

3.3. Topic Model Analysis

The analysis was performed on textual data of 470 articles. Two topics were selected for analysis because the maximum value of the Deveaud metric is 2.3 and has been reached in correspondence of two topics. Among the most frequent words (Figure S1, Supplementary Material), the redundant words ("result", "assess", "data", "probabl", "approach", "propos", "provid", "base", "knowledge", "approach", "develop", "perform", "also", "present") have been removed from the LDA computation algorithm.

The features pertinent to each topic are shown in Table 2. The most pertinent word on each topic, allow to characterise them by their structure of meaning.

1. The first one, here in after referred to as applied topic, is more related to the empirical application of the prior elicitation methods
2. The second topic, here in after referred to as theoretical topic, seems to be related to the theoretical implications of the prior elicitation procedure

Table 2. Pertinent words according to each LDA topic. In bold are represented the most important words.

	Applied	Theoretical
1	study	model
2	effect	distribut
3	estim	inform
4	opinion	paramet
5	uncertainti	posterior
6	test	sampl
7	process	function
8	risk	paper
9	practic	statist
10	case	predict

Table 1 shows that 28 papers are manually classified as applied works (applied topic), and 14 papers concern a theoretical topic. The articles reporting both theoretical and practical applications have been classified as applied topic papers. The overall accuracy computed on manually screened 42 trial articles is equal to 83% (7 articles have been misclassified by the LDA algorithm).

Observing the predictions of the LDA algorithm according to publication year (Figure 3) it is possible to observe that the prior elicitation procedure is prevalently addressed in Theoretical topic literature until 2010. The pattern is reversed in recent years evidencing an increasing interest on prior elicitations methods also in the generally applied research literature. The number of published papers concerning the prior elicitation increases both in a theoretical and applied framework. This growth continues in parallel with the increase of interest of the scientific literature for the Bayesian approach in general. The pattern of publication of papers containing the word "Bayes" on Pubmed (Figure S2, Supplementary Material), we observe a relevant growth starting from the first half of 2000.

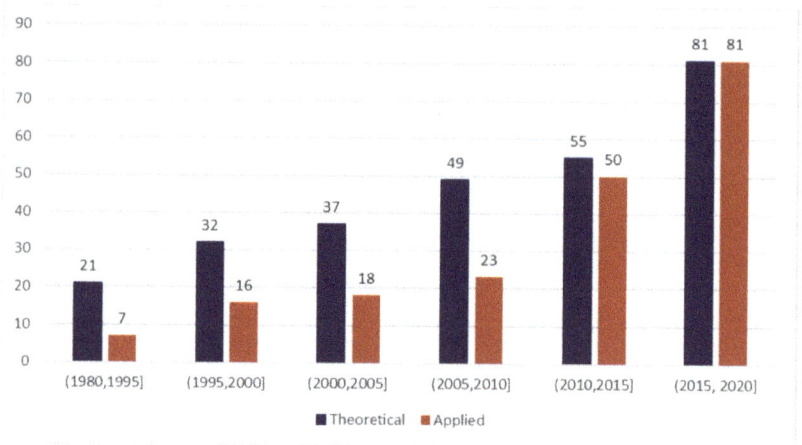

Figure 3. Classification of prior elicitation pertinent articles according to LDA topics and publication years.

Moreover, comparing LDA results about trial articles with the overall pertinent literature on prior elicitation, it is possible to observe a greater proportion of applied papers in trial pertinent literature, and evidence that a consistent part of theoretical literature is allocated in not pertinent articles (Table 3).

Table 3. Classification of articles according to LDA topics and pertinence to the clinical trial literature.

	Applied	Theoretical	Total
Pertinent to clinical trials	16% (31)	4% (11)	42
Not pertinent to clinical trials	84% (164)	96% (264)	428
Total	195	275	470

4. Discussion

Study findings indicate that starting from 2010, it is also possible to observe a spreading of the prior elicitation techniques in research fields different from the theoretical statistics. This aspect may be related to the recent increase in the popularity of the Bayesian methods in a general setting and the clinical trial research [2]. In recent years, Bayesian methods have increasingly being used in the design, monitoring, and analysis of clinical trials due to their flexibility [86].

The increase in popularity of Bayesian methods in a clinical trial involves a need for statisticians to define tools useful for the definition of robust and defensible informative prior distributions [87].

Empirical data may be used to define such priors (objective prior) whenever possible. However, in some cases, the limitations in data availability may preclude the construction of a data-based prior. In this situation, an expert elicitation procedure may be a solution used to define prior distributions [87].

In clinical trial publications, parametric distributions are mostly employed in applied settings. Semi-parametric or non-parametric priors are poorly used within this field, confining them mainly to the theoretical field. This aspect concerns especially less diffused approaches involving non-parametric methods for prior elicitation method. The reason behind the limited application of the non-parametric methods is surely related to the computational effort associated with the definition of a prior distribution which is more flexible and adaptable to the expert opinion but, in several cases, leads to obtaining posterior distributions difficult to be expressed in the closed-form [88].

It is important to consider that, in some research contexts, the translation of the experts' opinions into a pre-specified family distribution may be considered a limitation because many different distributions may be more suitable to the experts' opinions generally expressed in quantiles [14].

In recent years, not only parametric but also non-parametric methods to the elicitation of expert opinion are treated especially in the theoretical literature.

However, in clinical trial research, the conventional parametric methods are the more adopted procedures to the elicitation of expert opinion, leaving non-parametric methods predominantly in a statistical field.

Given the potential of prior elicitation to a better decision on making, more efforts are needed to ensure diffusion of the prior elicitation facilities, not only in theoretical statistical research but also in applied clinical trial settings, both at the design and analysis stage.

5. Conclusions

The prior elicitation methods are recently appealing not only to statistical literature but also in other research settings. It is possible to observe that the methods are increasingly used in general literature and clinical trial research.

However, in this framework, conventional parametric methods are more popular in clinical trial research. The non-parametric approaches are, in several cases, treated specially in the theoretical literature which is mainly focused on a statistical argumentation.

Supplementary Materials: The following are available online at https://www.mdpi.com/1660-4601/18/4/1833/s1, Figure S1: Most frequent word within the Document Term Matrix, Figure S2: PubMed published articles containing the word "Bayes" according to the publication year.

Author Contributions: Conceptualization, I.B. and P.B.; methodology, I.B.; formal analysis, D.A.; writing—original draft preparation, D.A.; writing—review and editing, D.A., D.G., I.B.; supervision, I.B.; All authors have read and agreed to the published version of the manuscript.

Funding: This research received no external funding.

Institutional Review Board Statement: Not applicable.

Informed Consent Statement: Not applicable.

Data Availability Statement: Data sharing not applicable.

Conflicts of Interest: The authors declare no conflict of interest.

References

1. Jack Lee, J.; Chu, C.T. Bayesian Clinical Trials in Action. *Stat. Med.* **2012**, *31*, 2955–2972. [CrossRef]
2. Chevret, S. Bayesian Adaptive Clinical Trials: A Dream for Statisticians Only? *Stat. Med.* **2012**, *31*, 1002–1013. [CrossRef]
3. Chaloner, K.; Rhame, F.S. Quantifying and Documenting Prior Beliefs in Clinical Trials. *Stat. Med.* **2001**, *20*, 581–600. [CrossRef] [PubMed]

4. Dolan, J.G.; Bordley, D.R.; Mushlin, A.I. An Evaluation of Clinicians' Subjective Prior Probability Estimates. *Med. Decis. Mak.* **1986**, *6*, 216–223. [CrossRef]
5. Hampson, L.V.; Whitehead, J.; Eleftheriou, D.; Brogan, P. Bayesian Methods for the Design and Interpretation of Clinical Trials in Very Rare Diseases. *Stat. Med.* **2014**, *33*, 4186–4201. [CrossRef]
6. Quintana, M.; Viele, K.; Lewis, R.J. Bayesian Analysis: Using Prior Information to Interpret the Results of Clinical Trials. *JAMA* **2017**, *318*, 1605–1606. [CrossRef]
7. Garthwaite, P.H.; Kadane, J.B.; O'Hagan, A. Statistical Methods for Eliciting Probability Distributions. *J. Am. Stat. Assoc.* **2005**, *100*, 680–701. [CrossRef]
8. O'Hagan, A. Eliciting Expert Beliefs in Substantial Practical Applications (Disc: P55-68). *J. R. Stat. Soc. Ser. D Stat.* **1998**, *47*, 21–35.
9. Johnson, S.R.; Granton, J.T.; Tomlinson, G.A.; Grosbein, H.A.; Hawker, G.A.; Feldman, B.M. Effect of Warfarin on Survival in Scleroderma-Associated Pulmonary Arterial Hypertension (SSc-PAH) and Idiopathic PAH. Belief Elicitation for Bayesian Priors. *J. Rheumatol.* **2011**, *38*, 462–469. [CrossRef] [PubMed]
10. Spiegelhalter, D.; Freedman, L.S. A Predictive Approach to Selecting the Size of a Clinical Trial, Based on Subjective Clinical Opinion. *Stat. Med.* **1986**, *5*, 1–13. [CrossRef] [PubMed]
11. Spiegelhalter, D. Incorporating Bayesian Ideas into Health-Care Evaluation. *Stat. Sci.* **2004**, *19*, 156–174. [CrossRef]
12. Oakley, J.E.; O'Hagan, A. *SHELF: The Sheffield Elicitation Framework (Version 2.0)*; School of Mathematics and Statistics, University of Sheffield: Sheffield, UK, 2010.
13. Morris, D.E.; Oakley, J.E.; Crowe, J.A. A Web-Based Tool for Eliciting Probability Distributions from Experts. *Environ. Model. Softw.* **2014**, *52*, 1–4. [CrossRef]
14. O'Hagan, A.; Buck, C.E.; Daneshkhah, A.; Eiser, J.R.; Garthwaite, P.H.; Jenkinson, D.J.; Oakley, J.E.; Rakow, T. *Uncertain Judgements: Eliciting Experts' Probabilities*; John Wiley: Chichester, UK, 2006.
15. Kiefer, N.M. Incentive-Compatible Elicitation of Quantiles. *arXiv* **2016**, arXiv:1611.00868.
16. Lau, H.-S.; Lau, A.H.-L. An Improved PERT-Type Formula for Standard Deviation. *IIE Trans.* **1998**, *30*, 273–275. [CrossRef]
17. Zapata-Vazquez, R.E.; O'Hagan, A.; Bastos, L.S. Eliciting Expert Judgements about a Set of Proportions. *J. Appl. Stat.* **2014**, *41*, 1919–1933. [CrossRef]
18. Keefer, D.L. Certainty Equivalents for Three-Point Discrete-Distribution Approximations. *Manag. Sci.* **1994**, *40*, 760–773. [CrossRef]
19. Abbas, A.E.; Budescu, D.V.; Yu, H.-T.; Haggerty, R. A Comparison of Two Probability Encoding Methods: Fixed Probability vs. Fixed Variable Values. *Decis. Anal.* **2008**, *5*, 190–202. [CrossRef]
20. Winkler, R.L. The Assessment of Prior Distributions in Bayesian Analysis. *J. Am. Stat. Assoc.* **1967**, *62*, 776–800. [CrossRef]
21. Bornkamp, B.; Ickstadt, K. A Note on B-Splines for Semiparametric Elicitation. *Am. Stat.* **2009**, *63*, 373–377. [CrossRef]
22. Oakley, J.E.; O'Hagan, A. Uncertainty in Prior Elicitations: A Nonparametric Approach. *Biometrika* **2007**, *94*, 427–441. [CrossRef]
23. Thomson Reuters. *Journal Citation Reports*; Thomson Reuters: Toronto, ON, Canada, 2011.
24. Blei, D.M.; Lafferty, J.D. Topic models. In *Text Mining*; Chapman and Hall/CRC: Boca Raton, FL, USA, 2009; pp. 101–124.
25. Porteous, I.; Newman, D.; Ihler, A.; Asuncion, A.; Smyth, P.; Welling, M. Fast Collapsed Gibbs Sampling for Latent Dirichlet Allocation. In Proceedings of the 14th ACM SIGKDD International Conference on Knowledge Discovery and Data Mining, Las Vegas, NV, USA, 24–27 August 2008; ACM: New York, NY, USA, 2008; pp. 569–577.
26. Deveaud, R.; SanJuan, E.; Bellot, P. Accurate and Effective Latent Concept Modeling for Ad Hoc Information Retrieval. *Doc. Numér.* **2014**, *17*, 61–84. [CrossRef]
27. Blei, D.M.; Ng, A.Y.; Jordan, M.I. Latent Dirichlet Allocation. *J. Mach. Learn. Res.* **2003**, *3*, 993–1022.
28. R Development Core Team. *R: A Language and Environment for Statistical Computing*; R Foundation for Statistical Computing: Vienna, Austria, 2015.
29. Hornik, K.; Grün, B. Topicmodels: An R Package for Fitting Topic Models. *J. Stat. Softw.* **2011**, *40*, 1–30.
30. Alhussain, Z.A.; Oakley, J.E. Assurance for Clinical Trial Design with Normally Distributed Outcomes: Eliciting Uncertainty about Variances. *Pharm. Stat.* **2020**, *19*, 827–839. [CrossRef] [PubMed]
31. Aupiais, C.; Alberti, C.; Schmitz, T.; Baud, O.; Ursino, M.; Zohar, S. A Bayesian Non-Inferiority Approach Using Experts' Margin Elicitation Application to the Monitoring of Safety Events. *BMC Med. Res. Methodol.* **2019**, *19*, 187. [CrossRef] [PubMed]
32. Bekele, B.N.; Thall, P.F. Dose-Finding Based on Multiple Toxicities in a Soft Tissue Sarcoma Trial. *J. Am. Stat. Assoc.* **2004**, *99*, 26–35. [CrossRef]
33. Berchialla, P.; Zohar, S.; Baldi, I. Bayesian Sample Size Determination for Phase IIA Clinical Trials Using Historical Data and Semi-parametric Prior's Elicitation. *Pharm. Stat.* **2019**, *18*, 198–211. [CrossRef]
34. Boulet, S.; Ursino, M.; Thall, P.; Jannot, A.S.; Zohar, S. Bayesian Variable Selection Based on Clinical Relevance Weights in Small Sample Studies-Application to Colon Cancer. *Stat. Med.* **2019**, *38*, 2228–2247. [CrossRef] [PubMed]
35. Browne, E.N.; Rathinam, S.R.; Kanakath, A.; Thundikandy, R.; Babu, M.; Lietman, T.M.; Acharya, N.R. A Bayesian Analysis of a Randomized Clinical Trial Comparing Antimetabolite Therapies for Non-Infectious Uveitis. *Ophthalmic Epidemiol.* **2017**, *24*, 63–70. [CrossRef] [PubMed]
36. Chaloner, K.; Church, T.; Louis, T.A.; Matts, J.P. Graphical Elicitation of a Prior Distribution for a Clinical Trial. *J. R. Stat. Soc. Ser. D Stat.* **1993**, *42*, 341–353. [CrossRef]

37. Chen, M.H.; Ibrahim, J.G.; Sinha, D. A New Bayesian Model for Survival Data with a Surviving Fraction. *J. Am. Stat. Assoc.* **1999**, *94*, 909–919. [CrossRef]
38. Cheung, Y.K. On the Use of Nonparametric Curves in Phase I Trials with Low Toxicity Tolerance. *Biometrics* **2002**, *58*, 237–240. [CrossRef] [PubMed]
39. Cook, J.A.; Ramsay, C.R.; Carr, A.J.; Rees, J.L. A Questionnaire Elicitation of Surgeons' Belief about Learning within a Surgical Trial. *PLoS ONE* **2012**, *7*, e49178. [CrossRef] [PubMed]
40. Gajewski, B.J.; Simon, S.D.; Carlson, S.E. Predicting Accrual in Clinical Trials with Bayesian Posterior Predictive Distributions. *Stat. Med.* **2008**, *27*, 2328–2340. [CrossRef]
41. Hampson, L.V.; Whitehead, J.; Eleftheriou, D.; Tudur-Smith, C.; Jones, R.; Jayne, D.; Hickey, H.; Beresford, M.W.; Bracaglia, C.; Caldas, A.; et al. Elicitation of Expert Prior Opinion: Application to the MYPAN Trial in Childhood Polyarteritis Nodosa. *PLoS ONE* **2015**, *10*, e0120981. [CrossRef] [PubMed]
42. Hiance, A.; Chevret, S.; Levy, V. A Practical Approach for Eliciting Expert Prior Beliefs about Cancer Survival in Phase III Randomized Trial. *J. Clin. Epidemiol.* **2009**, *62*, 431–437. [CrossRef] [PubMed]
43. Higgins, H.M.; Dryden, I.L.; Green, M.J. A Bayesian approach demonstrating that incorporation of practitioners' clinical beliefs into research design is crucial for effective knowledge transfer. In *Udder Health and Communication*; Springer: Berlin/Heidelberg, Germany, 2011; pp. 133–140.
44. Higgins, H.M.; Dryden, I.L.; Green, M.J. A Bayesian Elicitation of Veterinary Beliefs Regarding Systemic Dry Cow Therapy: Variation and Importance for Clinical Trial Design. *Prev. Vet. Med.* **2012**, *106*, 87–96. [CrossRef]
45. Jansen, J.O.; Wang, H.; Holcomb, J.B.; Harvin, J.A.; Richman, J.; Avritscher, E.; Stephens, S.W.; Truon, V.T.T.; Marques, M.B.; DeSantis, S.M.; et al. Elicitation of Prior Probability Distributions for a Proposed Bayesian Randomized Clinical Trial of Whole Blood for Trauma Resuscitation. *Transfusion* **2020**, *60*, 498–506. [CrossRef]
46. Kinnersley, N.; Day, S. Structured Approach to the Elicitation of Expert Beliefs for a Bayesian-Designed Clinicaltrial: A Case Study. *Pharm. Stat.* **2013**, *12*, 104–113. [CrossRef]
47. Legedza, A.T.R.; Ibrahim, J.G. Heterogeneity in Phase I Clinical Trials: Prior Elicitation and Computation Using the Continual Reassessment Method. *Stat. Med.* **2001**, *20*, 867–882. [CrossRef] [PubMed]
48. Lin, R.; Thall, P.F.; Yuan, Y. An Adaptive Trial Design to Optimize Dose-Schedule Regimes with Delayed Outcomes. *Biometrics* **2020**, *76*, 304–315. [CrossRef]
49. Moatti, M.; Zohar, S.; Facon, T.; Moreau, P.; Mary, J.Y.; Chevret, S. Modeling of Experts' Divergent Prior Beliefs for a Sequential Phase III Clinical Trial. *Clin. Trials* **2013**, *10*, 505–514. [CrossRef] [PubMed]
50. Muff, S.; Puhan, M.A.; Held, L. Bias Away from the Null Due to Miscounted Outcomes? A Case Study on the TORCH Trial. *Stat. Methods Med. Res.* **2018**, *27*, 3151–3166. [CrossRef]
51. O'Leary, R.A.; Choy, S.L.; Murray, J.V.; Kynn, M.; Denham, R.; Martin, T.G.; Mengersen, K. Comparison of Three Expert Elicitation Methods for Logistic Regression on Predicting the Presence of the Threatened Brush-Tailed Rock-Wallaby Petrogale Penicillata. *Environmetrics* **2009**, *20*, 379–398. [CrossRef]
52. Ollier, A.; Morita, S.; Ursino, M.; Zohar, S. An Adaptive Power Prior for Sequential Clinical Trials-Application to Bridging Studies. *Stat. Methods Med. Res.* **2020**, *29*, 2282–2294. [CrossRef]
53. Psioda, M.A.; Ibrahim, J.G. Bayesian Clinical Trial Design Using Historical Data That Inform the Treatment Effect. *Biostatistics* **2019**, *20*, 400–415. [CrossRef] [PubMed]
54. Ramanan, A.V.; Hampson, L.V.; Lythgoe, H.; Jones, A.P.; Hardwick, B.; Hind, H.; Jacobs, B.; Vasileiou, D.; Wadsworth, I.; Ambrose, N.; et al. Defining Consensus Opinion to Develop Randomised Controlled Trials in Rare Diseases Using Bayesian Design: An Example of a Proposed Trial of Adalimumab versus Pamidronate for Children with CNO/CRMO. *PLoS ONE* **2019**, *14*, e0215739. [CrossRef]
55. Ren, S.; Oakley, J.E. Assurance Calculations for Planning Clinical Trials with Time-to-Event Outcomes. *Stat. Med.* **2014**, *33*, 31–45. [CrossRef] [PubMed]
56. Rietbergen, C.; Klugkist, I.; Janssen, K.J.; Moons, K.G.; Hoijtink, H.J. Incorporation of Historical Data in the Analysis of Randomized Therapeutic Trials. *Contemp. Clin. Trials* **2011**, *32*, 848–855. [CrossRef]
57. Rosenberger, W.F.; Canfield, G.C.; Perevozskaya, I.; Haines, L.M.; Hausner, P. Development of Interactive Software for Bayesian Optimal Phase 1 Clinical Trial Design. *Drug Inf. J.* **2005**, *39*, 89–98. [CrossRef]
58. Rovers, M.M.; van der Wilt, G.J.; van der Bij, S.; Straatman, H.; Ingels, K.; Zielhuis, G.A. Bayes' Theorem: A Negative Example of a RCT on Grommets in Children with Glue Ear. *Eur. J. Epidemiol.* **2005**, *20*, 23–28. [CrossRef] [PubMed]
59. See, C.W.; Srinivasan, M.; Saravanan, S.; Oldenburg, C.E.; Esterberg, E.J.; Ray, K.J.; Glaser, T.S.; Tu, E.Y.; Zegans, M.E.; McLeod, S.D.; et al. Prior Elicitation and Bayesian Analysis of the Steroids for Corneal Ulcers Trial. *Ophthalmic Epidemiol.* **2012**, *19*, 407–413. [CrossRef]
60. Stevens, J.W.; O'Hagan, A. Incorporation of Genuine Prior Information in Cost-Effectiveness Analysis of Clinical Trial Data. *Int. J. Technol. Assess. Health Care* **2002**, *18*, 782–790. [CrossRef]
61. Sun, C.Q.; Prajna, N.V.; Krishnan, T.; Mascarenhas, J.; Rajaraman, R.; Srinivasan, M.; Raghavan, A.; O'Brien, K.S.; Ray, K.J.; McLeod, S.D.; et al. Expert Prior Elicitation and Bayesian Analysis of the Mycotic Ulcer Treatment Trial I. *Investig. Ophthalmol. Vis. Sci.* **2013**, *54*, 4167–4173. [CrossRef] [PubMed]

62. Tan, S.B.; Chung, Y.F.; Tai, B.C.; Cheung, Y.B.; Machin, D. Elicitation of Prior Distributions for a Phase III Randomized Controlled Trial of Adjuvant Therapy with Surgery for Hepatocellular Carcinoma. *Control. Clin. Trials* **2003**, *24*, 110–121. [CrossRef]
63. Thall, P.F.; Ursino, M.; Baudouin, V.; Alberti, C.; Zohar, S. Bayesian Treatment Comparison Using Parametric Mixture Priors Computed from Elicited Histograms. *Stat. Methods Med. Res.* **2019**, *28*, 404–418. [CrossRef] [PubMed]
64. Turner, R.M.; Spiegelhalter, D.J.; Smith, G.C.S.; Thompson, S.G. Bias Modelling in Evidence Synthesis. *J. R. Stat. Soc. Ser. A Stat. Soc.* **2009**, *172*, 21–47. [CrossRef]
65. Veen, D.; Stoel, D.; Zondervan-Zwijnenburg, M.; van de Schoot, R. Proposal for a Five-Step Method to Elicit Expert Judgment. *Front. Psychol.* **2017**, *8*, 2110. [CrossRef]
66. Wang, C.P.; Ghosh, M. Bayesian Analysis of Bivariate Competing Risks Models with Covariates. *J. Stat. Plan. Inference* **2003**, *115*, 441–459. [CrossRef]
67. Wheeler, M.W.; Piegorsch, W.W.; Bailer, A.J. Quantal Risk Assessment Database: A Database for Exploring Patterns in Quantal Dose-Response Data in Risk Assessment and Its Application to Develop Priors for Bayesian Dose-Response Analysis. *Risk Anal.* **2019**, *39*, 616–629. [CrossRef] [PubMed]
68. White, I.R.; Pocock, S.J.; Wang, D. Eliciting and Using Expert Opinions about Influence of Patient Characteristics on Treatment Effects: A Bayesian Analysis of the CHARM Trials. *Stat. Med.* **2005**, *24*, 3805–3821. [CrossRef]
69. Wiesenfarth, M.; Calderazzo, S. Quantification of Prior Impact in Terms of Effective Current Sample Size. *Biometrics* **2020**, *76*, 326–336. [CrossRef]
70. Zohar, S.; Baldi, I.; Forni, G.; Merletti, F.; Masucci, G.; Gregori, D. Planning a Bayesian Early-Phase Phase I/II Study for Human Vaccines in HER2 Carcinomas. *Pharm. Stat.* **2011**, *10*, 218–226. [CrossRef]
71. Lesaffre, E.; Lawson, A.B. Choosing the Prior Distribution. In *Bayesian Biostatistics*; John Wiley & Sons, Ltd.: Chichester, UK, 2012; pp. 104–138. ISBN 978-1-119-94241-2.
72. Spiegelhalter, D.J.; Abrams, K.R.; Myles, J.P. Prior Distributions. In *Bayesian Approaches to Clinical Trials and Health-Care Evaluation*; John Wiley & Sons, Ltd.: Chichester, UK, 2004; pp. 139–180. ISBN 978-0-470-09260-6.
73. Held, L.; Sauter, R. Adaptive Prior Weighting in Generalized Regression: Adaptive Prior Weighting in Generalized Regression. *Biometrics* **2017**, *73*, 242–251. [CrossRef]
74. Raftery, A.E.; Madigan, D.; Hoeting, J.A. Bayesian Model Averaging for Linear Regression Models. *J. Am. Stat. Assoc.* **1997**, *92*, 179–191. [CrossRef]
75. Coolen, F.P.A.; Mertens, P.R.; Newby, M.J. A Bayes-Competing Risk Model for the Use of Expert Judgment in Reliability Estimation. *Reliab. Eng. Syst. Saf.* **1992**, *35*, 23–30. [CrossRef]
76. Norton, R.M. The Double Exponential Distribution: Using Calculus to Find a Maximum Likelihood Estimator. *Am. Stat.* **1984**, *38*, 135–136. [CrossRef]
77. Kabán, A. On Bayesian Classification with Laplace Priors. *Pattern Recognit. Lett.* **2007**, *28*, 1271–1282. [CrossRef]
78. Zhu, M.; Lu, A.Y. The Counter-Intuitive Non-Informative Prior for the Bernoulli Family. *J. Stat. Educ.* **2004**, *12*. [CrossRef]
79. Ibrahim, J.G.; Chen, M.-H.; Gwon, Y.; Chen, F. The Power Prior: Theory and Applications. *Stat. Med.* **2015**, *34*, 3724–3749. [CrossRef]
80. Ibrahim, J.G.; Chen, M.H. Power Prior Distributions for Regression Models. *Stat. Sci.* **2000**, *15*, 46–60.
81. Diaconis, P.; Ylvisaker, D. Conjugate Priors for Exponential Families. *Ann. Stat.* **1979**, *7*, 269–281. [CrossRef]
82. De Santis, F. Power Priors and Their Use in Clinical Trials. *Am. Stat.* **2006**, *60*, 122–129. [CrossRef]
83. Morita, S.; Thall, P.F.; Müller, P. Evaluating the Impact of Prior Assumptions in Bayesian Biostatistics. *Stat. Biosci.* **2010**, *2*, 1–17. [CrossRef] [PubMed]
84. Ibrahim, J.G.; Ryan, L.M.; Chen, M.-H. Using Historical Controls to Adjust for Covariates in Trend Tests for Binary Data. *J. Am. Stat. Assoc.* **1998**, *93*, 1282–1293. [CrossRef]
85. Greenhouse, J.B.; Waserman, L. Robust Bayesian Methods for Monitoring Clinical Trials. *Stat. Med.* **1995**, *14*, 1379–1391. [CrossRef] [PubMed]
86. Baldi, I.; Gregori, D.; Desideri, A.; Berchialla, P. Accrual Monitoring in Cardiovascular Trials. *Open Heart* **2017**, *4*, e000720. [CrossRef] [PubMed]
87. Dallow, N.; Best, N.; Montague, T.H. Better Decision Making in Drug Development through Adoption of Formal Prior Elicitation. *Pharm. Stat.* **2018**, *17*, 301–316. [CrossRef]
88. Ghahramani, Z. Bayesian Non-Parametrics and the Probabilistic Approach to Modelling. *Phil. Trans. R. Soc. A* **2013**, *371*, 20110553. [CrossRef] [PubMed]

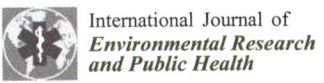

Article

Handling Poor Accrual in Pediatric Trials: A Simulation Study Using a Bayesian Approach

Danila Azzolina [1,2], Giulia Lorenzoni [1], Silvia Bressan [3], Liviana Da Dalt [3], Ileana Baldi [1] and Dario Gregori [1,*]

[1] Unit of Biostatistics, Epidemiology and Public Health, Department of Cardiac Thoracic Vascular Sciences and Public Health, University of Padova, 35128 Padova, Italy; danila.azzolina@uniupo.it (D.A.); giulia.lorenzoni@unipd.it (G.L.); ileana.baldi@unipd.it (I.B.)
[2] Department of Translational Medicine, University of Eastern Piedmont, 28100 Novara, Italy
[3] Department of Women's and Children's Health, University of Padova, 35128 Padova, Italy; silvia.bressan.1@unipd.it (S.B.); liviana.dadalt@unipd.it (L.D.D.)
* Correspondence: dario.gregori@unipd.it

Citation: Azzolina, D.; Lorenzoni, G.; Bressan, S.; Da Dalt, L.; Baldi, I.; Gregori, D. Handling Poor Accrual in Pediatric Trials: A Simulation Study Using a Bayesian Approach. *Int. J. Environ. Res. Public Health* **2021**, *18*, 2095. https://doi.org/10.3390/ijerph18042095

Academic Editor: Paul B. Tchounwou

Received: 7 January 2021
Accepted: 13 February 2021
Published: 21 February 2021

Publisher's Note: MDPI stays neutral with regard to jurisdictional clai-ms in published maps and institutio-nal affiliations.

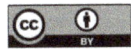

Copyright: © 2021 by the authors. Licensee MDPI, Basel, Switzerland. This article is an open access article distributed under the terms and conditions of the Creative Commons Attribution (CC BY) license (https://creativecommons.org/licenses/by/4.0/).

Abstract: In the conduction of trials, a common situation is related to potential difficulties in recruiting the planned sample size as provided by the study design. A Bayesian analysis of such trials might provide a framework to combine prior evidence with current evidence, and it is an accepted approach by regulatory agencies. However, especially for small trials, the Bayesian inference may be severely conditioned by the prior choices. The Renal Scarring Urinary Infection (RESCUE) trial, a pediatric trial that was a candidate for early termination due to underrecruitment, served as a motivating example to investigate the effects of the prior choices on small trial inference. The trial outcomes were simulated by assuming 50 scenarios combining different sample sizes and true absolute risk reduction (ARR). The simulated data were analyzed via the Bayesian approach using 0%, 50%, and 100% discounting factors on the beta power prior. An informative inference (0% discounting) on small samples could generate data-insensitive results. Instead, the 50% discounting factor ensured that the probability of confirming the trial outcome was higher than 80%, but only for an ARR higher than 0.17. A suitable option to maintain data relevant to the trial inference is to define a discounting factor based on the prior parameters. Nevertheless, a sensitivity analysis of the prior choices is highly recommended.

Keywords: power-prior; poor accrual; Bayesian trial

1. Introduction

Difficulties in the enrolment of the overall trial sample size, as indicated at the design stage, could be caused by several factors (i.e., high costs, regulatory barriers, narrow eligibility criteria, and cultural attitudes toward research in almost all research fields). Effects can be different depending on the population's characteristics and the intervention under evaluation [1].

Prior research evaluating the reasons for termination across a broad range of trials reported that insufficient enrolment is the most common reason, with a frequency ranging from 33.7% to 57%, depending on the definition used [2,3]. The slow or low accrual problem is common in clinical research on adults, primarily in oncology [4–6] and cardiology [7], as well as in pediatric research, in which 37% of clinical trials are terminated early due to inadequate accrual [8]. Pediatrics is a research field that requires particular attention, since accrual issues are associated with methodological and ethical challenges [9]. It is essential to consider that the management and conduct of pediatric trials are more complicated than those of adult trials in terms of practical, ethical, and methodological problems [10].

From a statistical point of view, low accrual results in a reduced sample size, compromising the ability to accurately answer the primary research question due to a reduction in the likelihood of detecting a treatment effect [11]. The scientific community has conveyed that early termination of a trial due to poor accrual leads to inefficiency in clinical research, with consequent increases in costs [12] and a waste of resources, as well as a waste of the efforts of the children involved in the trial [13].

For these reasons, alternative and innovative approaches to pediatric clinical trial design have been a recent topic of debate in the scientific community [9,14]. Alternative methods for pediatric trial design and analysis have been proposed by recent guidelines in the field, i.e., the ICH (International Council for Harmonisation) Topic E11 guidelines [15], the guidance for trial planning and design in the pediatric context [16], and the EMA (European Medicines Agency) guidelines [16–18].

It is noteworthy that data from trials terminated prematurely for poor accrual can provide useful information for reducing the uncertainty about the treatment effect in a Bayesian framework [11].

In recent years, Bayesian methods have increasingly been used in the design, monitoring, and analysis of clinical trials due to their flexibility [19,20]. Considering the research setting described in this work, the Bayesian methods used for accrual monitoring are also interesting [21]. These methods are well suited to designing and analyzing studies conducted with small sample sizes and are particularly appropriate for studies involving children, even in cases of rare disease outcomes [9].

In clinical trials that are candidates for early termination due to poor accrual reasons, a Bayesian approach may be useful for incorporating the available knowledge on the investigated treatment effect, reported in the literature or elicited by experts' opinions [22]. In addition, in a Bayesian setting, prior information combined with data may support the final inference for a trial conducted on a limited number of enrolled patients [23,24].

In pediatric trials, for example, the awareness that a treatment is effective in adults increases the probability of its efficacy in children. This knowledge may be quantitatively translated into a prior probability distribution [9,14].

However, when there is a small sample size, the final inference may be severely conditioned by a misleading prior definition [24]. In this framework, the Food and Drug Administration (FDA) suggests performing a sensitivity analysis on prior definitions [25], especially for very small sample sizes [26]. In this regard, the power prior approach is used to design and analyze small trials to control for the weight of historical information, translated into prior distributions, through prior discounting factors [27,28]. The use of historical information to define the prior distribution in a nonparametric context is a method recently used in the literature [29]. Informative prior elicitation is typically a challenging task even in the presence of historical data (objective prior) [30]. Ibrahim and Chen [28] proposed the power prior approach to incorporate the historical data in the analysis of a current study. The method is based on the raising of the likelihood function of the historical data to a power parameter between 0 and 1 (power parameter). This parameter represents the proportion of the historical data incorporated in the prior.

Hobbs modified the conventional approach, accounting for commensurability of the information in the historical and current data to determine how much the historical information is used in the inference [31]. Other power-prior proposals calibrate the type I error by controlling the degree of similarity between the new and historical data [32,33]. The prior-data conflict has also been addressed and incorporated in the power prior in a commensurability parameter defined by using a measure of distribution distance in a group sequential design clinical trial [34]. A mixture of priors, for the one-parameter exponential family, has been also considered in a sequential trial, to incorporate the historical data accounting for rapid reaction to prior-data conflicts by adding an extra weakly-informative mixture component [35].

In general, the power prior approach is widely used for the design and analysis of clinical trial data. The method is useful for handling problems related to a lack of exchangeability between the historical and current data, and the risk that prior information overwhelms the clinical trial data information [27].

The optimal amount of discounting factors for an informative prior remains to be discussed [14].

This study investigated the effects of the prior choices on the final inference, especially for studies conducted with limited sample sizes, such as pediatric trials. A pediatric trial candidate for early termination due to underrecruitment, the RESCUE trial, served as a motivating example for the simulation study proposed.

A set of possible trial outcomes were simulated. The simulation plan was designed to evaluate the effects of the prior choices on the trial results by evaluating different scenarios depending on the number of patients involved in the study and the magnitude of the true treatment effect.

2. Materials and Methods

2.1. Motivating Example

The RESCUE trial was a randomized controlled double-blind trial. The purpose of the study was to evaluate the effect of adjunctive oral steroids in preventing renal scarring in young children and infants with febrile urinary tract infections. The primary outcome was the renal scar absolute risk reduction (ARR) between the treatment arms. The study was designed expecting an ARR of 0.20 to determine a renal scar reduction from 40% to 20%.

After two years, only 17 recruited patients completed the follow-up for the study outcome (6 in treatment and 11 in control) due to procedural problems and poor compliance with the study therapy and final diagnosis [16–18].

2.2. Simulation Plan

The possible trial outcomes were simulated by assuming several scenarios combining different sample sizes and true ARRs. The simulated data were analyzed via the Bayesian approach using a beta prior distribution whose parameters were derived from trials conducted in research settings similar to the RESCUE trial. The beta-binomial model was considered because it is the most widely used approach among the Bayesian methods to summarize event rates in clinical trials [36]. This parametrization is easily computationally tractable and is very precise [37].

Informative, low-informative, and uninformative priors were selected for the analyses according to the discounting levels placed on the prior parameters.

The classical, non-Bayesian approach was considered a benchmark.

This simulation study is defined by:

1. Data generation hypotheses.
2. Analysis of simulated data.
3. Presentation of the results of simulations.

A flowchart synthesizing the simulation plan is reported in Figure S1, Supplementary Material.

2.3. Data Generation Hypotheses

2.3.1. Simulation Scenarios

The simulation plan consisted of 50 scenarios. Each scenario represents a single combination of the treatment effect (ARR) and the sample size used to generate the data. Fifty scenarios were considered, since they combined ten different sample sizes (ranging from 15 to 240) within five assumed ARRs (Table 1). The ARR ranged from −0.07 to −0.27, with an increment of 0.07, according to the treatment effects suggested by the literature [38,39].

Table 1. Simulation scenarios.

Scenario	1	2	3	4	5	6	7	8	9	10	11	12	13	14	15	16	17	18	19	20	21	22	23	24	25
Sample size	15	40	65	90	115	140	165	190	215	240	15	40	65	90	115	140	165	190	215	240	15	40	65	90	115
True ARR	0.07	0.07	0.07	0.07	0.07	0.07	0.07	0.07	0.07	0.07	0.12	0.12	0.12	0.12	0.12	0.12	0.12	0.12	0.12	0.12	0.17	0.17	0.17	0.17	0.17
Scenario	26	27	28	29	30	31	32	33	34	35	36	37	38	39	40	41	42	43	44	45	46	47	48	49	50
Sample size	140	165	190	215	240	15	40	65	90	115	140	165	190	215	240	15	40	65	90	115	140	165	190	215	240
True ARR	0.17	0.17	0.17	0.17	0.17	0.22	0.22	0.22	0.22	0.22	0.22	0.22	0.22	0.22	0.22	0.27	0.27	0.27	0.27	0.27	0.27	0.27	0.27	0.27	0.27

ARR=Absolute Risk Reduction.

2.3.2. Data Generation within Scenarios

For each scenario, the trial data were randomly generated 5000 times. The data were drawn from a binomial random variable, assuming a true event rate in the control arm of $\pi_{control} = 0.33$. This event rate is in-between the results provided by Huang et al. [38] and Shaikh et al. [39] for the control group.

The treatment arm data were generated using a binomial random variable hypothesizing an ARR, one for each experiment, in compliance with the simulation plan provided in Table 1, where the sample size is showed overall. However, it is assumed that the control arm contains 60% of the sample size to reflect the group imbalance in the motivating example.

2.4. Analysis of the Simulated Data

The 5000 randomly generated data points were analyzed via the Bayesian method by considering: (1) the informative prior, (2) the low-informative prior, and (3) the uninformative prior. A frequentist analysis was performed for comparison purposes.

The data were simulated 5000 times by a binomial random variable in a frequentist approach. For each of the repeated simulations, the ARR was calculated and the binomial confidence interval was estimated.

2.4.1. Prior Definition

A mixture of beta priors was considered for the outcome evaluation, using data provided by the literature [38,39]. The clinical trial results were combined in a mixture of distributions. The beta distributions comprising the mixture of priors for each scar event rate in the treatment and control groups were derived from other trials' historical information [27].

The functional form of the distribution is characterized by the shape α and scale β parameters $\Pi \sim Beta(\alpha, \beta)$ [40], where Π is the parameter that characterizes the event rate on which to make inference. The shape value α is defined by the number of events x observed in other trials, while the β value corresponds to the number of subjects not experiencing the event $(n - x)$ [41].

1. Huang et al. [38] reported probabilities of scarring of $\hat{\pi}_{treat\ (Huang)} = \frac{6}{18} = 0.33$ and $\hat{\pi}_{control\ (Huang)} = \frac{39}{65} = 0.66$ in the treatment and control arms, respectively. Considering this information, the informative beta prior can be derived as:

$$\Pi_{treat\ (Huang)} \sim Beta(6, 12)$$

$$\Pi_{control\ (Huang)} \sim Beta(39, 26)$$

2. Shaikh et al. [39] reported, instead, probabilities of scarring of $\hat{\pi}_{treat\ (Shaikh)} = 0.098$ (12 | 123) and $\hat{\pi}_{control\ (Shaikh)} = 0.168$ (22 | 131) in the treatment and control arms,

respectively. Considering this information, the informative beta prior can be derived as:

$$\Pi_{\text{treat (Shaikh)}} \sim \text{Beta}(12, 111)$$

$$\Pi_{\text{control(Shaikh)}} \sim \text{Beta}(22, 109)$$

The information was combined in a mixture of beta priors:

- For the treatment arm, the beta mixture is defined as:

$$\Pi_{\text{treat}} = \gamma \Pi_{\text{treat (Huang)}} + (1 - \gamma) \Pi_{\text{treat (Shaikh)}}$$

The expected value for the mixture random variable is, for the treatment arm, a weighted mean of the expectations over the mixture components:

$$E\left[\Pi_{\text{treat}}\right] = \gamma E[\Pi_{\text{treat(Huang)}}] + (1 - \gamma) E[\Pi_{\text{treat(Shaikh)}}]$$

If we denote the beta shape $\alpha_{\text{treat(Huang)}}$ and $\alpha_{\text{treat(Shaikh)}}$, respectively for the Huang and Shaikh studies, and $\beta_{\text{treat(Huang)}}$ and $\beta_{\text{treat(Shaikh)}}$ the scales for the considered studies, the mixture expected value may be computed as:

$$E[\Pi_{\text{treat}}] = \gamma E\left[\Pi_{\text{treat(Huang)}}\right] + (1 - \gamma) E\left[\Pi_{\text{treat(Shaikh)}}\right]$$

$$E[\Pi_{\text{treat}}] = \gamma \frac{\alpha_{\text{treat(Huang)}}}{\alpha_{\text{treat(Huang)}} + \beta_{\text{treat(Huang)}}} + (1 - \gamma) \frac{\alpha_{\text{treat(Shaikh)}}}{\alpha_{\text{treat(Shaikh)}} + \beta_{\text{treat(Shaikh)}}}$$

$$= \gamma \frac{6}{6 + 12} + (1 - \gamma) \frac{12}{12 + 111}$$

If we assume an equal weight value $\gamma = 0.5$, $E[\Pi_{\text{treat}}] = 0.215$.

- The mixture variance is given by:

$$\text{Var}[\Pi_{\text{treat}}] = \left[\gamma \left(\text{Var}\left[\Pi_{\text{treat(Huang)}}\right] + E\left[\Pi_{\text{treat(Huang)}}\right] - E[\Pi_{\text{treat}}]\right)\right] +$$
$$+ \left[(1 - \gamma)\left(\text{Var}\left[\Pi_{\text{treat(Shaikh)}}\right] + E\left[\Pi_{\text{treat(Shaikh)}}\right] - E[\Pi_{\text{treat}}]\right)\right]$$

where the variances of the mixture components are:

$$\text{Var}\left[\Pi_{\text{treat(Huang)}}\right] = \frac{\alpha_{\text{treat(Huang)}} \beta_{\text{treat(Huang)}}}{(\alpha_{\text{treat(Huang)}} + \beta_{\text{treat(Huang)}})^2 (\alpha_{\text{treat(Huang)}} + \beta_{\text{treat(Huang)}} + 1)}$$

$$\text{Var}[\Pi_{\text{treat(Shaikh)}}] = \frac{\alpha_{\text{treat(Shaikh)}} \beta_{\text{treat(Shaikh)}}}{(\alpha_{\text{treat(Shaikh)}} + \beta_{\text{treat(Shaikh)}})^2 (\alpha_{\text{treat(Huang)}} + \beta_{\text{treat(Shaikh)}} + 1)}$$

Equal weight was assumed for the components of the mixture, therefore, $\gamma = 0.5$, $E[\Pi_{\text{treat}}] = 0.215$, and $SD[\Pi_{\text{treat}}] = 0.08$.

- For the treatment arm, the mixture is defined as:

$$\Pi_{\text{control}} = \gamma \Pi_{\text{control (Huang)}} + (1 - \gamma) \Pi_{\text{control (Huang)}}$$

with $E[\Pi_{\text{control}}] = 0.38$ and $SD[\Pi_{\text{control}}] = 0.05$ and $\gamma = 0.5$.

2.4.2. Discounting the Priors: The Power Prior Approach

Different levels of penalization (discounting) were provided for the historical information using a power prior approach [28] to perform a sensitivity analysis on the prior choices. The historical information can be included in the final inference using a Beta(α_1, β_1) prior, where:

$$\alpha_1 = 1 + \alpha_0 d_0$$

$$\beta_1 = 1 + \beta_0 d_0$$

The α_0 and β_0 values are the parameters defined by the number of successes and failures derived from the literature and are α_0 and β_0, respectively. The value d_0 defines the amount of historical information to be included in the final inference. The discounting factor is otherwise defined as $(1 - d_0) \times 100$ and represents the level of penalization (discounting) of the historical information derived from other studies.

1. If $d_0 = 0$, the data provided by the literature are not considered, indicating a 100% discount of the historical information. According to this scenario, the prior is an uninformative Beta(1, 1) distribution.
2. If $d_0 = 1$, then all of the information provided by the literature is considered in setting the prior, indicating a 0% discount of the historical data.

Analyses of the simulated trials were conducted using three different priors:

- Power prior without discounting (informative, $d_0 = 1$). A beta informative prior was derived considering the number of successes and failures found in the literature [42], as defined in the method section.
- Power prior 50% discounting (low-informative, $d_0 = 0.5$). The beta prior with a 50% discount, defined in the literature as a substantial-moderate discounting factor [43], was defined based on the beta parameters comprising the mixture of priors specified in the informative scenario.
- Power prior 100% discounting (uninformative, $d_0 = 0$). A mixture of Beta(1, 1) priors was defined.

Effective Sample Size (ESS) Calculation

The ESS was computed on the mixture of beta distribution by using the Morita approach to quantify the prior influence on the final inference using the RBesT package in R (R Foundation for Statistical Computing, Vienna, Austria) [44]. For the mixture of beta prior (equal weight) without power prior discounting ($d_0 = 1$), an ESS of 55 and 98 was achieved for treatment and control arm. However, discounting the beta parameters for $d_0 = 0.5$ (low-informative prior), the ESS is equal to 24 and 48.

The prior distributions are presented in Figure 1.

2.4.3. Posterior Estimation

A beta-binomial model was employed to analyze the difference in event rates between arms [45]. The posterior distribution for the ARR outcome requires the estimation of the posterior distribution of the scar proportion in each arm separately, and was computed with the following Markov chain Monte Carlo (MCMC) resampling procedure [46]:

- A first resampling of the proportion of scarring Π^*_{treat} from $\Pi_{treat}|X_{treat}$, which is the posterior distribution for the treatment group.
- A second resampling of $\Pi^*_{control}$ from $\Pi_{control}|X_2$.
- The posterior distribution for the parameter related to the difference in proportions was obtained by calculating $ARR = \Pi^*_{treat} - \Pi^*_{control}$ from the distributions previously resampled [47].

The resampling procedures were performed using an MCMC estimation algorithm, as indicated in the literature [46], using 3 chains, 6000 iterations, and 1000 adaptations.

An example of the inference results is reported in the Supplementary Material, showing the priors and the posterior distributions calculated on a single database generated by assuming an ARR equal to 0.17.

The computations were performed using OpenBUGS (Free Software Foundation, Boston, MA, USA) [48] and R version 3.3.2 [49]; the simulation R codes are reported in the Supplementary Material.

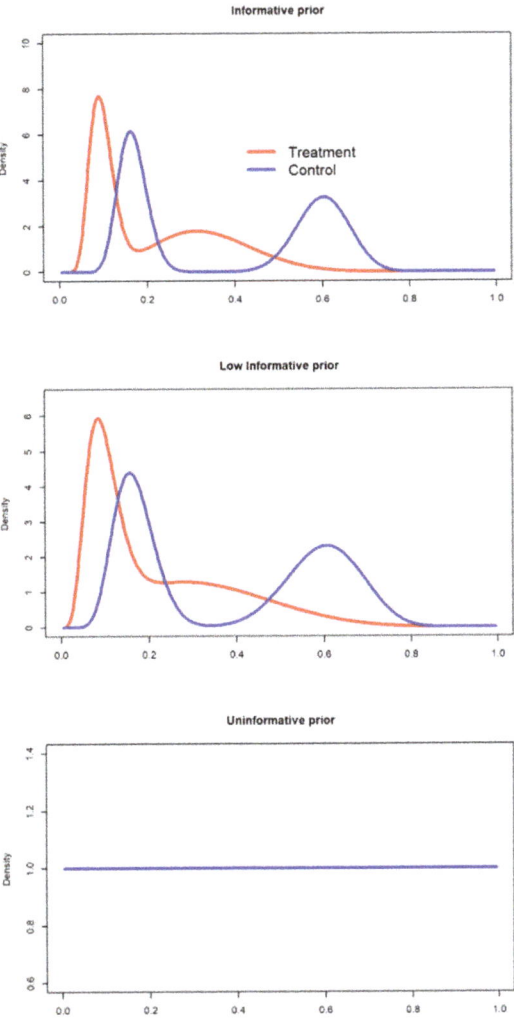

Figure 1. Prior distributions: The prior distributions are defined by an equal-weighted mixture ($\gamma = 0.5$) of beta priors. The components of the mixture prior are, for the treatment arm, $\Pi_{\text{treat (Huang)}} \sim \text{Beta}(6, 12)$ and $\Pi_{\text{treat (Shaikh)}} \sim \text{Beta}(12, 111)$. The mixture of priors ($\gamma = 0.5$) for the control arm is defined by $\Pi_{\text{control (Huang)}} \sim \text{Beta}(39, 26)$ and $\Pi_{\text{control(Shaikh)}} \sim \text{Beta}(22, 109)$. No discounting on the beta priors parameters has been provided ($d_0 = 1$) for the Informative priors. The information has been partially discounted for the low-informative prior scenario ($d_0 = 0.5$). The priors parameters are full discounted for the uninformative prior scenario ($d_0 = 0$), collapsing to a Beta$(1, 1)$ distribution.

2.4.4. Convergence Assessment

The Geweke method [50] was considered to assess the convergence of the MCMC results within iterations. Geweke's statistics test was computed for each analysis conducted on the simulated data. Geweke's Z-score plot was also visually inspected to assess the convergence.

2.5. Results of the Simulations

Four sets of 200 results summarizing 50 scenarios in combination with four methods of analysis were defined as:

1. The proportion of the 5000 simulated trials for which the credibility intervals (CIs), or confidence intervals, for a frequentist analysis do not contain an ARR equal to 0. The proportion of intervals not containing the 0 and containing the data generator ARR was also calculated.
2. The mean length across 5000 simulated trials of the CI.
3. The mean of the posterior median estimate across 5000 simulated trials or the mean of the point-estimated ARR across 5000 simulated trials for the frequentist analysis.
4. The mean absolute percentage error (MAPE):

$$\text{MAPE} = \frac{1}{n} \sum_{t=1}^{n} \left| \frac{\text{ARR}_{\text{true}} - \hat{\text{ARR}}_t}{\text{ARR}_{\text{true}}} \right|$$

ARR_{true} is the true treatment effect considered to generate the data; $\hat{\text{ARR}}_t$ is the estimated treatment effect (posterior median, or point estimate, for the frequentist analysis) achieved for each simulation t within the n = 5000 simulated trials.

3. Results

The proportion of 5000 simulated trials ensuring that the 95% CI does not contain an ARR equal to zero is greater than 90% for all of the informative scenarios, even if the sample size is smaller than 50, except for the 0.07 true ARR. For the 0.07 ARR, this proportion declines as the data used to estimate the likelihood increases (Figure 2, Panel A). This proportion is higher than 80% only for sample sizes greater than 70, and the true ARR is greater than 0.17 for the low-informative priors (Figure 2, Panel B). The pattern of the simulation results is similar, considering the proportion of simulations for which the CI does not include the 0, and includes the true data generator ARR (Figure S3, Supplementary Material).

Similar behavior is observed among the uninformative Bayesian (Figure 2, Panel C) and frequentist (Figure 2, Panel D) estimates, for which this proportion reaches 80% for an ARR greater than 0.22 and sample sizes greater than 120.

The 95% CI length decreases as the sample size increases for all of the Bayesian parametrizations and the frequentist estimates (Table S1, Supplementary Material). The informative (Figure 3, Panel A) and low-informative priors (Figure 3, Panel B) showed more variability in the posterior length of the CIs across different true ARR values. The CI lengths are more similar for different data generation ARR assumptions for the uninformative (Figure 3, Panel C) and frequentist (Figure 3, Panel D) simulations. In general, especially for smaller sample sizes, the estimates are less precise for the frequentist and Bayesian uninformative prior scenarios than for the informative and low-informative prior estimates (Table 1).

The posterior median ARR estimates are influenced by the prior choices, especially for the informative prior. The estimated ARRs are similar to each other for smaller sample sizes across the true treatment effect, while the posterior median ARR estimates converge to the true ARR for larger sample sizes (Figure 4, Panel A). A similar pattern is observed for the low-informative scenarios; however, for smaller sample sizes, greater variability in the posterior median estimates is observed across the different ARRs used to generate the data (Figure 4, Panel B). The ARR is overestimated for small sample sizes in the uninformative prior scenarios (Figure 4, Panel C). Instead, the frequentist estimates across the simulated trial are similar to the true treatment effect for all of the sample sizes (Figure 4, Panel D).

The MAPE estimate decreases as the sample size increases for all the prior parametrizations (Table S1, Supplementary Material). A lower true ARR (i.e., 0.07) ensures a decreasing effect that is more evident than a higher true ARR (Table S1, Supplementary Material).

Also, the MAPE seems to be constant for a higher true ARR in informative (Figure 5, Panel A) and low-informative prior (Figure 5, Panel B) simulations. For the uninformative (Figure 5, Panel C) and frequentist scenarios (Figure 5, Panel D), instead, a reduction in MAPE is also evident for higher true ARR values. The MAPE values are higher for the frequentist scenarios than all of the Bayesian estimates, including those provided via the uninformative prior (Table S1, Supplementary Material).

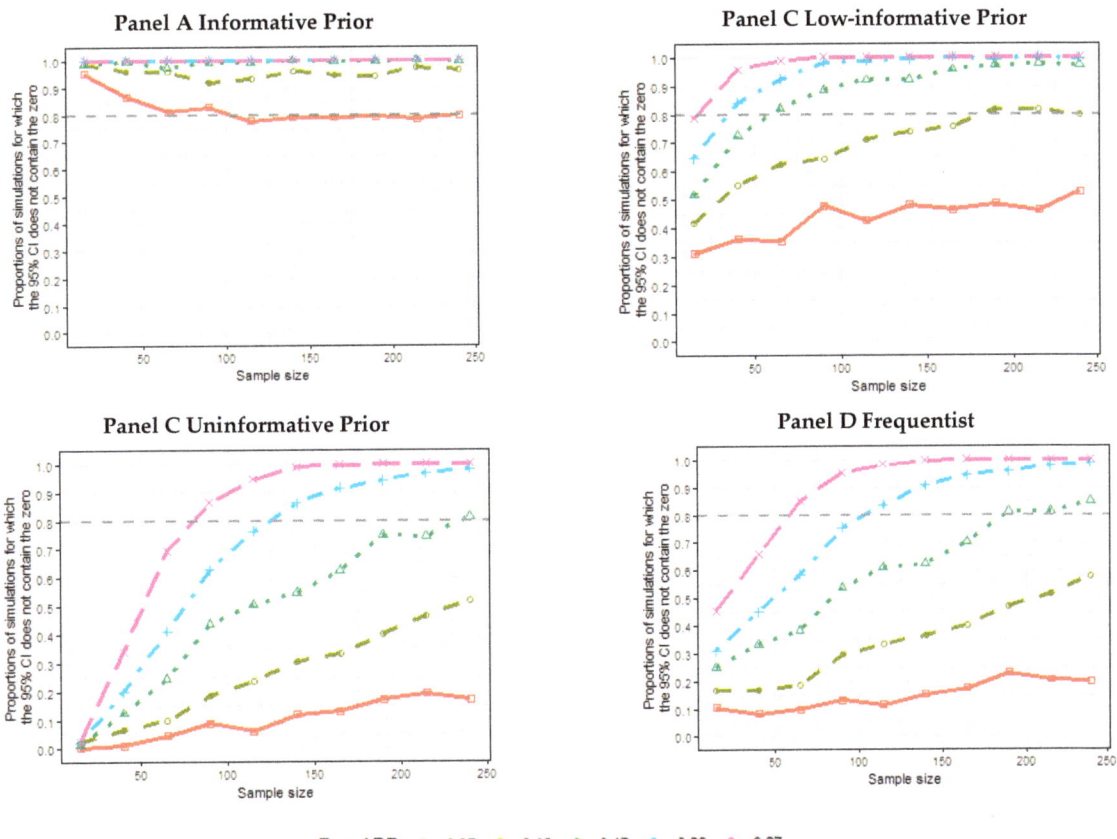

Figure 2. The proportion of CIs within simulated trials not including the zero absolute risk reduction (ARR) according to the sample size, and true ARR for informative prior (Panel A), low-informative prior (Panel B), uninformative prior (Panel C), and frequentist analysis (Panel D).

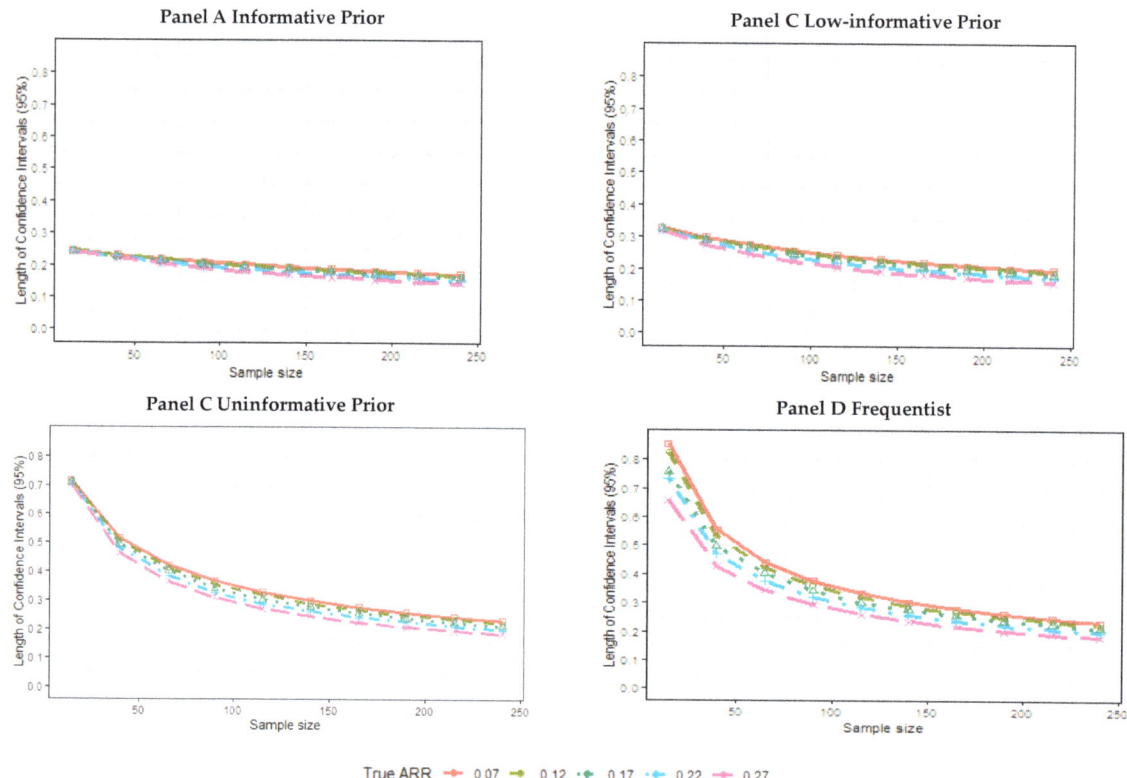

Figure 3. Simulation results for the 95% CI length according to the sample size and true ARR for informative prior (Panel A), low-informative prior (Panel B), uninformative prior (Panel C), and frequentist analyses (Panel D).

The hypothesis of the stationarity of the chain was not rejected according to Geweke's statistic for all of the analyses conducted on the simulated data and for all of the prior parametrizations. The Z-scores within iterations was also visually inspected. An example within simulations (ARR = 0.07 and sample size = 65) is reported in the Figure S2, Supplementary Material. The Z-score lies within the acceptance stationarity region (±2) or all chains and all the prior parametrizations; the pattern is very similar for all the considered scenarios.

An example of a possible inference result is shown in the Supplementary Material. The posteriors were calculated for a generated trial data reporting 8 events over 56 in the treatment arm ($\hat{\pi}_{treat}$ = 0.14) and 30 events over 84 in the control arm ($\hat{\pi}_{control}$ = 0.36). The data generator ARR is 0.17, while the observed ARR is 0.22. Considering the different priors, the inference results are located in mean on the same event rate; however, the uncertainty in the posterior distribution increases, considering the uninformative prior assumption (Figure S4, Supplementary Material).

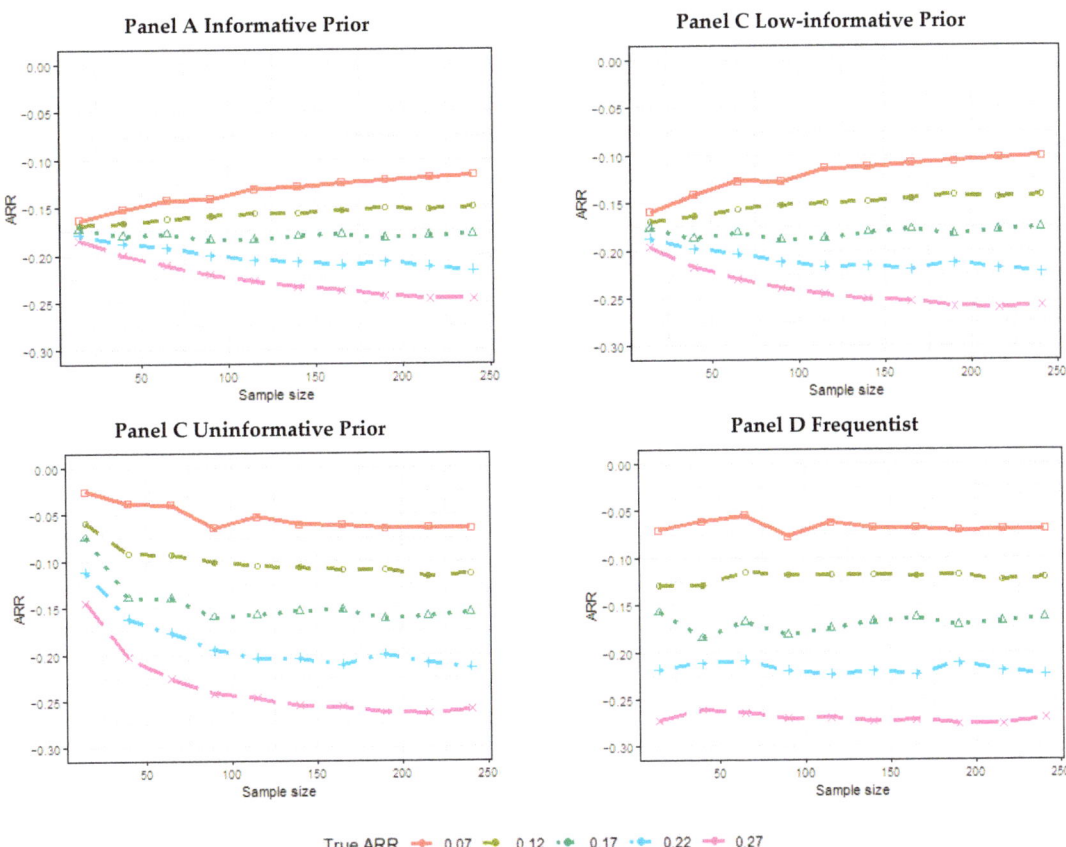

Figure 4. Simulation results for the estimated ARR (posterior median, or point estimate, for frequentist analysis) according to the sample size and true ARR for informative prior (Panel A), low-informative prior (Panel B), uninformative prior (Panel C), and frequentist analyses (Panel D).

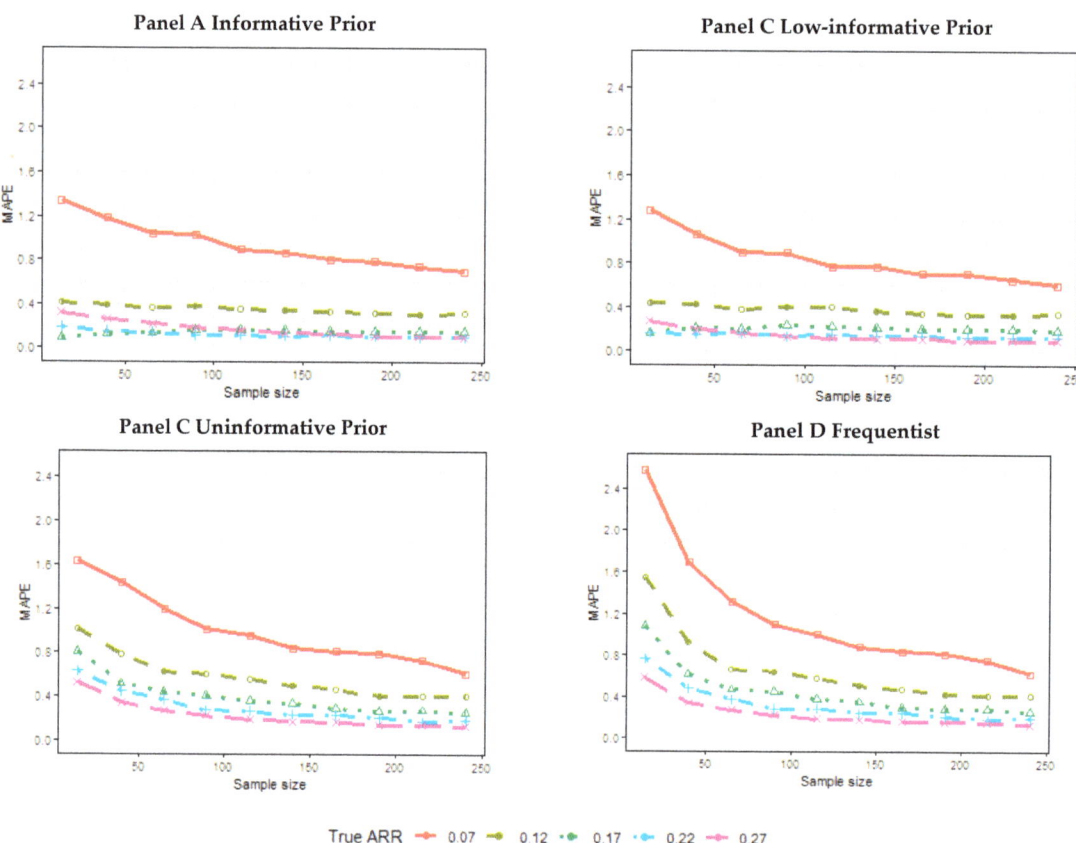

Figure 5. Simulation results for the mean absolute percentage error (MAPE) estimate according to the sample size and true ARR for informative prior (Panel A), low-informative prior (Panel B), uninformative prior (Panel C), and frequentist analyses (Panel D).

4. Discussion

Regulatory agencies advocate an increase in pediatric research, which is motivated by the need for more information on treatment labeling to guide pediatricians and to offer more suitable and safe treatments for children [14]. However, in various cases, pediatric trials have demonstrated difficulties in enrolling participants [51]. The RESCUE trial represents a typical example of a complex trial in pediatric research affected by poor accrual. The difficulties encountered in the enrolment and retention of participants are related to procedural problems related to the study protocol [51,52] and poor adherence to the therapy.

Bayesian data analysis may overcome challenges in the conduct of trials similar to the RESCUE study, allowing investigators to combine information provided by current trial data with evidence provided by the literature, as recommended by regulatory agencies to deal with small sample sizes [15].

The present findings show that Bayesian inference can detect a small treatment effect for small sample sizes (lower than 50), even if the prior is fully uninformative compared to a maximum likelihood approach. This result confirms the potential benefits of using a Bayesian method on small sample sizes. However, the literature suggests paying attention to the use of uninformative prior distributions for small clinical trials, because there is the possibility of including in the final inference extreme treatment effects that are potentially unexpected from a clinical point of view. For this reason, it is suggested to use evidence from previous trials to inform these prior distributions [53].

For this reason, a key issue in Bayesian analysis is the choice of prior. This simulation study demonstrated that, especially for small studies, the trial results could be influenced by the prior choices and weakly influenced by the data when using fully informative priors. In particular, a prior distribution incorporating favorable treatment effect information on small sample sizes is likely to conditionate the inference in favor of the treatment, even if, in truth, the effect is null or minimal. All of this implies that the prior in these contexts should be defined by using validated empirical evidence [27]. Conversely, this study suggests that the full informative prior elicited by considering large effect size tends to direct the inference towards the existence of a treatment effect for all the sample size scenarios. For this reason, we recommend, especially when the treatment effect hypothesized for the study design is large and the sample size is small, the use of a low-informative prior for achieving more data-driven results.

The situation is different if a discounting factor is placed on the prior parameters. Looking at the estimated values of ESS, the historical information retained in the prior in the low-informative scenario is halved, compared to the informative parameterization. This implies that the inference is more data-oriented, assuming a discounting of 0.5. The probability of confirming the trial results is demonstrated to be more data-dependent and, for sample sizes less than 50, is higher than 80% only for ARRs higher than 0.17.

As the power prior parameter increases, the prior becomes more informative, and the estimated precision (length of CI) increases. Looking at the differences between observed and estimated ARR, the inferential results, comparing the various parameterizations of the prior discounting factor, tend to converge toward the same conclusions in the direction of the generating data effect size starting from a sample size of 150 subjects. All this implies that, for studies conducted on a considerable number of patients, it is possible to tune the prior toward a more informative solution ($d_0 > 0.5$), obtaining results representing a suitable compromise between the available historical information and what is suggested by the data.

In the literature, some reasons are addressed for a suitable discounting of historical prior information. First, the historical data and the current trial evidence may be heterogeneous concerning the study design and conduct [28]. Moreover, as also demonstrated by this simulation analysis, especially for small trials, an informative historical prior may overwhelm the current trial evidence [27].

Another issue outlined in this paper is the potentially misleading information on the treatment effect provided by the posterior median effect for a sample size smaller than 50 patients. This source of bias is evident not only for informative inference but also for low-informative and uninformative analyses. Conversely, the frequentist point estimate is unbiased in terms of the mean because of the proportion estimator's asymptotical unbiasedness over repeated resamples. However, in the frequentist approach, the variability of results across sample replications is very high for small samples, even though the effect, on average, is unbiased [54]. Bayesian estimates, on the other hand, return scenarios of inferential results that are less variable, especially if a minimum amount of historical information is incorporated into the prior.

The frequentist approach considers all the parameters to be fixed; the data are a realization of a random variable. Instead, Bayesian methods assume that all the parameters are random and the data are fixed [54]. This point of view leads to incorporating the available knowledge on the prior parameters into a probability distribution. For this reason, it is important to ensure that the information on which informative priors are based is accurate; otherwise, the resulting estimates and posterior standard deviations could be biased if misleading informative priors are utilized [55].

In this regard, the Bayesian approach leads to thinking about inference in terms of a probability distribution on the treatment effect, rather than a point estimate or confidence interval. Therefore, a Bayesian approach is oriented toward a progressive uncertainty reduction (on a posterior probability distribution) in treatment effect estimation. Historical information contributes sequentially to the reduction of this uncertainty [56]. The uncertainty can be measured in terms of the CI width. The simulation results demonstrate a narrower CI for small sample sizes (similarly across different true ARRs) for Bayesian analyses compared to the frequentist approach. This effect has also been reported in the literature [57].

The present results show that Bayesian methods can outperform frequentist methods with small samples by providing increased efficiency and an increased ability to determine non-null effects. However, the appropriate prior distribution choice, especially on small datasets, plays a fundamental role. Researchers might need to consult experts, meta-analyses, or review studies in the area of interest to obtain informative, accurate priors that can meaningfully contribute to posterior distributions. Furthermore, a sensitivity analysis on priors (i.e., defining the robustness of conclusions that may be affected by decisions made on the priors) is highly recommended for pediatric trials [14], which is in line with the literature [24] and FDA recommendations [25].

Study Limitations

This study was conducted considering only the conjugate prior beta setting. It may be interesting to explore the impact of inference in the posterior case obtained in a nonclosed form. For example, instead of directly placing a parameter derived on the beta prior, it may be advisable to consider expert elicitation about treatment effects to define the specific prior distribution. Moreover, future research development is needed to investigate the effect of an eventual prior-data conflict on the trial results according to different study size.

5. Conclusions

Bayesian inference is a flexible tool compared to frequentist inference, especially for trials conducted in a poor accrual setting. A full informative Bayesian inference, conducted on small samples, can generate data-insensitive results. On the other hand, the use of an uninformative prior distribution may include, in the final inference, clinically unproven extreme treatment effect hypotheses. A power prior approach on sample sizes smaller than 50 patients seems to be a good compromise between these two methods. However, the choice of parameters and discounting factors should be negotiated with expert pediatricians and should be guided by an appropriate consultation of the scientific literature. In agreement with the FDA recommendations, a sensitivity analysis of priors is highly recommended.

Supplementary Materials: The following are available online at https://www.mdpi.com/1660-4601/18/4/2095/s1, Figure S1: Simulation Plan, Figure S2: Geweke's Z-statistics for Informative, Figure S3: The proportion of CIs within simulated trials, Figure S4. Prior and posterior density estimates, Table S1: Simulation results according to the prior choices, and Simulation Codes.

Author Contributions: Conceptualization: D.G. and D.A.; methodology: I.B.; formal analysis: D.A.; writing—original draft preparation: D.A. and D.G.; writing—review and editing: D.A., D.G., G.L., I.B., S.B., and L.D.D.; supervision: D.G. All authors have read and agreed to the published version of the manuscript.

Funding: This research received no external funding.

Institutional Review Board Statement: Not applicable.

Informed Consent Statement: Not applicable.

Data Availability Statement: Data sharing not applicable.

Conflicts of Interest: The authors declare no conflict of interest.

References

1. Kadam, R.A.; Borde, S.U.; Madas, S.A.; Salvi, S.S.; Limaye, S.S. Challenges in Recruitment and Retention of Clinical Trial Subjects. *Perspect. Clin. Res.* **2016**, *7*, 137–143. [CrossRef]
2. Pak, T.R.; Rodriguez, M.; Roth, F.P. Why Clinical Trials Are Terminated. *bioRxiv* **2015**, bioRxiv:021543. [CrossRef]
3. Williams, R.J.; Tse, T.; DiPiazza, K.; Zarin, D.A. Terminated Trials in the ClinicalTrials.gov Results Database: Evaluation of Availability of Primary Outcome Data and Reasons for Termination. *PLoS ONE* **2015**, *10*, e0127242. [CrossRef]
4. Rimel, B. Clinical Trial Accrual: Obstacles and Opportunities. *Front. Oncol.* **2016**, *6*, 103. [CrossRef]
5. Mannel, R.S.; Moore, K. Research: An Event or an Environment? *Gynecol. Oncol.* **2014**, *134*, 441–442. [CrossRef]
6. Stensland, K.D.; McBride, R.B.; Latif, A.; Wisnivesky, J.; Hendricks, R.; Roper, N.; Boffetta, P.; Hall, S.J.; Oh, W.K.; Galsky, M.D. Adult Cancer Clinical Trials That Fail to Complete: An Epidemic? *J. Natl. Cancer Inst.* **2014**, *106*, dju229. [CrossRef] [PubMed]
7. Baldi, I.; Lanera, C.; Berchialla, P.; Gregori, D. Early Termination of Cardiovascular Trials as a Consequence of Poor Accrual: Analysis of ClinicalTrials.gov 2006–2015. *BMJ Open* **2017**, *7*, e013482. [CrossRef] [PubMed]
8. Pica, N.; Bourgeois, F. Discontinuation and Nonpublication of Randomized Clinical Trials Conducted in Children. *Pediatrics* **2016**, e20160223. [CrossRef]
9. Baiardi, P.; Giaquinto, C.; Girotto, S.; Manfredi, C.; Ceci, A. Innovative Study Design for Paediatric Clinical Trials. *Eur. J. Clin. Pharmacol.* **2011**, *67*, 109–115. [CrossRef]
10. Greenberg, R.G.; Gamel, B.; Bloom, D.; Bradley, J.; Jafri, H.S.; Hinton, D.; Nambiar, S.; Wheeler, C.; Tiernan, R.; Smith, P.B.; et al. Parents' Perceived Obstacles to Pediatric Clinical Trial Participation: Findings from the Clinical Trials Transformation Initiative. *Contemp. Clin. Trials Commun.* **2018**, *9*, 33–39. [CrossRef]
11. Billingham, L.; Malottki, K.; Steven, N. Small Sample Sizes in Clinical Trials: A Statistician's Perspective. *Clin. Investig.* **2012**, *2*, 655–657. [CrossRef]
12. Kitterman, D.R.; Cheng, S.K.; Dilts, D.M.; Orwoll, E.S. The Prevalence and Economic Impact of Low-Enrolling Clinical Studies at an Academic Medical Center. *Acad. Med. J. Assoc. Am. Med Coll.* **2011**, *86*, 1360–1366. [CrossRef]
13. Joseph, P.D.; Craig, J.C.; Caldwell, P.H. Clinical Trials in Children. *Br. J. Clin. Pharmacol.* **2015**, *79*, 357–369. [CrossRef]
14. Huff, R.A.; Maca, J.D.; Puri, M.; Seltzer, E.W. Enhancing Pediatric Clinical Trial Feasibility through the Use of Bayesian Statistics. *Pediatric Res.* **2017**, *82*, 814. [CrossRef] [PubMed]
15. ICH Topic E 11. Clinical Investigation of Medicinal Products in the Paediatric Population. In *Note for Guidance on Clinical Investigation of Medicinal Products in the Paediatric Population (CPMP/ICH/2711/99)*; European Medicines Agency: London, UK, 2001.
16. European Medicines Agency. *Guideline on the Requirements for Clinical Documentation for Orally Inhaled Products (OIP) Including the Requirements for Demonstration of Therapeutic Equivalence between Two Inhaled Products for Use in the Treatment of Asthma and Chronic Obstructive Pulmonary Disease (COPD) in Adults and for Use in the Treatment of Asthma in Children and Adolescents*; European Medicines Agency: London, UK, 2009.
17. Committee for Medicinal Products for Human Use. *Guideline on the Clinical Development of Medicinal Products for the Treatment of Cystic Fibrosis*; European Medicines Agency: London, UK, 2009.
18. Committee for Medicinal Products for Human Use. *Note for Guidance on Evaluation of Anticancer Medicinal Products in Man*; The European Agency for the Evaluation of Medical Products: London, UK, 1996.
19. O'Hagan, A. Chapter 6: Bayesian Statistics: Principles and Benefits. In *Handbook of Probability: Theory and Applications*; Rudas, T., Ed.; Sage: Thousand Oaks, CA, USA, 2008; pp. 31–45.
20. Azzolina, D.; Berchialla, P.; Gregori, D.; Baldi, I. Prior Elicitation for Use in Clinical Trial Design and Analysis: A Literature Review. *Int. J. Environ. Res. Public Health* **2021**, *18*, 1833. [CrossRef]
21. Gajewski, B.J.; Simon, S.D.; Carlson, S.E. Predicting Accrual in Clinical Trials with Bayesian Posterior Predictive Distributions. *Stat. Med.* **2008**, *27*, 2328–2340. [CrossRef] [PubMed]
22. O'Hagan, A. Eliciting Expert Beliefs in Substantial Practical Applications. *J. R. Stat. Soc. Ser. D Stat.* [CD-ROM P55-68]. **1998**, *47*, 21–35.
23. Lilford, R.J.; Thornton, J.; Braunholtz, D. Clinical Trials and Rare Diseases: A Way out of a Conundrum. *BMJ* **1995**, *311*, 1621–1625. [CrossRef]
24. Quintana, M.; Viele, K.; Lewis, R.J. Bayesian Analysis: Using Prior Information to Interpret the Results of Clinical Trials. *Jama* **2017**, *318*, 1605–1606. [CrossRef]
25. Office of the Commissioner; Office of Clinical Policy and Programs. *Guidance for the Use of Bayesian Statistics in Medical Device Clinical Trials*; CDRH: Rockville, MD, USA; CBER: Silver Spring, MD, USA, 2010. Available online: https://www.fda.gov/regulatory-information/search-fda-guidance-documents/guidance-use-bayesian-statistics-medical-device-clinical-trials (accessed on 2 February 2021).
26. Gelman, A. Prior Distribution. Chapter 4: Statistical Theory and Methods. In *Encyclopedia of Environmetrics*; Wiley: Hoboken, NJ, USA, 2006.
27. De Santis, F. Power Priors and Their Use in Clinical Trials. *Am. Stat.* **2006**, *60*, 122–129. [CrossRef]
28. Ibrahim, J.G.; Chen, M.-H. Power Prior Distributions for Regression Models. *Stat. Sci.* **2000**, *15*, 46–60.
29. Psioda, M.A.; Ibrahim, J.G. Bayesian Clinical Trial Design Using Historical Data That Inform the Treatment Effect. *Biostat* **2019**, *20*, 400–415. [CrossRef] [PubMed]

30. Ibrahim, J.G.; Chen, M.-H.; Gwon, Y.; Chen, F. The Power Prior: Theory and Applications. *Stat. Med.* **2015**, *34*, 3724–3749. [CrossRef] [PubMed]
31. Hobbs, B.P.; Carlin, B.P.; Mandrekar, S.J.; Sargent, D.J. Hierarchical Commensurate and Power Prior Models for Adaptive Incorporation of Historical Information in Clinical Trials. *Biometrics* **2011**, *67*, 1047–1056. [CrossRef] [PubMed]
32. Liu, G.F. A Dynamic Power Prior for Borrowing Historical Data in Noninferiority Trials with Binary Endpoint. *Pharm. Stat.* **2018**, *17*, 61–73. [CrossRef]
33. Nikolakopoulos, S.; van der Tweel, I.; Roes, K.C.B. Dynamic Borrowing through Empirical Power Priors That Control Type I Error: Dynamic Borrowing with Type I Error Control. *Biom* **2018**, *74*, 874–880. [CrossRef]
34. Ollier, A.; Morita, S.; Ursino, M.; Zohar, S. An Adaptive Power Prior for Sequential Clinical Trials—Application to Bridging Studies. *Stat. Methods Med. Res.* **2020**, *29*, 2282–2294. [CrossRef] [PubMed]
35. Schmidli, H.; Gsteiger, S.; Roychoudhury, S.; O'Hagan, A.; Spiegelhalter, D.; Neuenschwander, B. Robust Meta-Analytic-Predictive Priors in Clinical Trials with Historical Control Information: Robust Meta-Analytic-Predictive Priors. *Biom* **2014**, *70*, 1023–1032. [CrossRef]
36. Chuang-Stein, C. An Application of the Beta-Binomial Model to Combine and Monitor Medical Event Rates in Clinical Trials. *Drug Inf. J.* **1993**, *27*, 515–523. [CrossRef]
37. Zaslavsky, B.G. Bayes Models of Clinical Trials with Dichotomous Outcomes and Sample Size Determination. *Stat. Biopharm. Res.* **2009**, *1*, 149–158. [CrossRef]
38. Huang, Y.C.; Lin, Y.C.; Wei, C.F.; Deng, W.L.; Huang, H.C. The Pathogenicity Factor HrpF Interacts with HrpA and HrpG to Modulate Type III Secretion System (T3SS) Function and T3ss Expression in *Pseudomonas Syringae* Pv. *Averrhoi. Mol. Plant Pathol.* **2016**, *17*, 1080–1094. [CrossRef]
39. Shaikh, N.; Shope, T.R.; Hoberman, A.; Muniz, G.B.; Bhatnagar, S.; Nowalk, A.; Hickey, R.W.; Michaels, M.G.; Kearney, D.; Rockette, H.E.; et al. Corticosteroids to Prevent Kidney Scarring in Children with a Febrile Urinary Tract Infection: A Randomized Trial. *Pediatr. Nephrol.* **2020**, *35*, 2113–2120. [CrossRef]
40. Lehoczky, J.P. Distributions, Statistical: Special and Continuous. In *International Encyclopedia of the Social & Behavioral Sciences*; Elsevier: Amsterdam, The Netherlands, 2001; pp. 3787–3793. ISBN 978-0-08-043076-8.
41. Wilcox, R.R. A Review of the Beta-Binomial Model and Its Extensions. *J. Educ. Stat.* **1981**, *6*, 3. [CrossRef]
42. Huang, Y.-Y.; Chen, M.-J.; Chiu, N.-T.; Chou, H.-H.; Lin, K.-Y.; Chiou, Y.-Y. Adjunctive Oral Methylprednisolone in Pediatric Acute Pyelonephritis Alleviates Renal Scarring. *Pediatrics* **2011**, peds-2010. [CrossRef]
43. De Santis, F. Using Historical Data for Bayesian Sample Size Determination. *J. R. Stat. Soc. Ser. A* **2007**, *170*, 95–113. [CrossRef]
44. Weber, S. *RBesT: R Bayesian Evidence Synthesis Tools*, Version 1.6-1. Available online: https://cran.r-project.org/web/packages/RBesT/index.html (accessed on 2 February 2020).
45. Albert, J. *Bayesian Computation with R*; Springer Science & Business Media: Berlin/Heidelberg, Germany, 2009; ISBN 0-387-92298-9.
46. Kawasaki, Y.; Shimokawa, A.; Miyaoka, E. Comparison of Three Calculation Methods for a Bayesian Inference of $P(\Pi_1 > \Pi_2)$. *J. Mod. Appl. Stat. Methods* **2013**, *12*, 256–268. [CrossRef]
47. Barry, J. Doing Bayesian Data Analysis: A Tutorial with R and BUGS. *Eur. J. Psychol.* **2011**, *7*, 778–779. [CrossRef]
48. Lunn, D.; Spiegelhalter, D.; Thomas, A.; Best, N. The BUGS Project: Evolution, Critique and Future Directions. *Stat. Med.* **2009**, *28*, 3049–3067. [CrossRef] [PubMed]
49. R Core Team. *R: A Language and Environment for Statistical Computing*; R Foundation for Statistical Computing: Vienna, Austria, 2015.
50. Geweke, J. *Evaluating the Accuracy of Sampling-Based Approaches to the Calculation of Posterior Moments*; Federal Reserve Bank of Minneapolis, Research Department: Minneapolis, MN, USA, 1991; Volume 196.
51. Bavdekar, S.B. Pediatric Clinical Trials. *Perspect. Clin. Res.* **2013**, *4*, 89–99. [CrossRef] [PubMed]
52. Gill, D.; Kurz, R. Practical and Ethical Issues in Pediatric Clinical Trials. *Appl. Clin. Trials* **2003**, *12*, 41–45.
53. Pedroza, C.; Han, W.; Thanh Truong, V.T.; Green, C.; Tyson, J.E. Performance of Informative Priors Skeptical of Large Treatment Effects in Clinical Trials: A Simulation Study. *Stat. Methods Med. Res.* **2018**, *27*, 79–96. [CrossRef] [PubMed]
54. McNeish, D. On Using Bayesian Methods to Address Small Sample Problems. *Struct. Equ. Modeling Multidiscip. J.* **2016**, *23*, 750–773. [CrossRef]
55. Depaoli, S. Mixture Class Recovery in GMM under Varying Degrees of Class Separation: Frequentist versus Bayesian Estimation. *Psychol. Methods* **2013**, *18*, 186–219. [CrossRef] [PubMed]
56. Spiegelhalter, D.J.; Freedman, L.S.; Parmar, M.K.B. Bayesian Approaches to Randomized Trials. *J. R. Stat. Soc. Ser. A* **1994**, *157*, 357. [CrossRef]
57. Albers, C.J.; Kiers, H.A.L.; van Ravenzwaaij, D. Credible Confidence: A Pragmatic View on the Frequentist vs. Bayesian Debate. *Collabra Psychol.* **2018**, *4*, 31. [CrossRef]

Article

Study Protocol: Phase I Dose Escalation Study of Oxaliplatin, Cisplatin and Doxorubicin Applied as PIPAC in Patients with Peritoneal Metastases

Manuela Robella [1,*], Paola Berchialla [2], Alice Borsano [1], Armando Cinquegrana [1], Alba Ilari Civit [1], Michele De Simone [1] and Marco Vaira [1]

1. Unit of Surgical Oncology, Candiolo Cancer Institute, Fondazione del Piemonte per l'Oncologia—IRCCS, 10060 Candiolo, Italy; alice.borsano@ircc.it (A.B.); armando.cinquegrana@ircc.it (A.C.); alba.ilari@ircc.it (A.I.C.); michele.desimone@ircc.it (M.D.S.); marco.vaira@ircc.it (M.V.)
2. Department of Clinical and Biological Sciences, University of Turin, 10124 Turin, Italy; paola.berchialla@unito.it
* Correspondence: manuela.robella@ircc.it

Abstract: Pressurized Intra-Peritoneal Aerosol Chemotherapy (PIPAC) is a novel laparoscopic intraperitoneal chemotherapy approach offered in selected patients affected by non-resectable peritoneal carcinomatosis. Drugs doses currently established for nebulization are very low: oxaliplatin (OXA) 120 mg/sm, cisplatin (CDDP) 10.5 mg/sm and doxorubicin (DXR) 2.1 mg/sm. A model-based approach for dose-escalation design in a single PIPAC procedure and subsequent dose escalation steps is planned. The starting dose of oxaliplatin is 100 mg/sm with a maximum estimated dose of 300 mg/sm; an escalation with overdose and under-dose control (for probability of toxicity less than 16% in case of under-dosing and probability of toxicity greater than 33% in case of overdosing) will be further applied. Cisplatin is used in association with doxorubicin: A two-dimensional dose-finding design is applied on the basis of the estimated dose limiting toxicity (DLT) at all combinations. The starting doses are 15 mg/sm for cisplatin and 3 mg/sm for doxorubicin. Safety is assessed according to Common Terminology Criteria for Adverse Events (CTCAE version 4.03). Secondary endpoints include radiological response according to Response Evaluation Criteria in Solid Tumor (version 1.1) and pharmacokinetic analyses. This phase I study can provide the scientific basis to maximize the optimal dose of cisplatin, doxorubicin and oxaliplatin applied as PIPAC.

Keywords: cisplatin; doxorubicin; oxaliplatin; dose escalation; phase I; PIPAC; peritoneal carcinomatosis

1. Introduction

Peritoneal carcinomatosis (PC) is both a consequence of different primary tumors, synchronous or metachronous, and the clinical presentation of primitive peritoneal neoplasms. Despite significant recent advances in the management of peritoneal carcinomatosis, this diagnosis still is linked frequently to a poor prognosis. The unfavorable outcome is often accompanied by clinical symptoms that dramatically impact on quality of life and represent a real challenge for the managing health care provider.

Curative approach is, unluckily, reserved to a small minority of patients amenable to combined procedures based on cytoreductive surgery and locoregional treatments. The majority of patients is still nowadays treated by palliative approach.

1.1. The Failure of Systemic Treatment

The treatment of PC by palliative systemic chemotherapy (sCT) is still, nowadays, often the standard of care. Some cheering improvement in survival are recorded in PC from colonic cancer in which median survival for non-surgical amenable patients raised from six to 24 months by novel drugs agents, as FolfOX/FolfIRI ± bevacizumab [1]. In other PC, such as from gastric cancer, results are not so encouraging: literature reported median overall survival ranging from 4 to 13 months [2,3]. In ovarian cancer, intravenous chemotherapy with platinum compounds, taxanes, anthracyclines, gemcitabine, topotecan and trabectedin in various combinations and sequences are the mainstay of recurrence treatment. These regimens achieve median overall survival rates after the first, second, third, fourth and fifth relapse of 17.6 (95% CI 16.4–18.6), 11.3 (10.4–12.9), 8.9 (7.8–9.9), 6.2 (5.1–7.7) and 5.0 (3.8–10.4) months, respectively [4]. It is remarkable that the intraperitoneal availability of drugs by sCT is low; consequentially, the systemic treatment is often inefficient in bulky disease. Furthermore, the cumulative toxicity of intravenous repeated chemotherapeutic regimens is responsible for progressive decrease of patients' compliance to therapy.

1.2. The Failure of the Intraperitoneal Chemotherapy

Intraperitoneal chemotherapy (IPC) has the potential to improve drug delivery to the tumor with generally accepted systemic side effects [5]. The rationale of this approach is represented by the possibility to consider the peritoneal cavity as a "pharmacologic sanctuary", due to the presence of the peritoneal-plasma barrier that allows a high drug concentration in the abdominal cavity associated to minimal leakage towards systemic circulation. IPC is reported to be effective but is still burdened by pharmacological limitation, such as low homogeneity in drug distribution in the abdominal cavity [6] and technical problems like the high complication rate related to the intraperitoneal catheter (infections, obstruction, bleeding, dislocation): only 40% of patients are able to complete the expected chemotherapy cycles [7,8]. Furthermore, the poor drug penetration into peritoneal bulky disease (and adhesions-entrapped tumor nodules) in intraperitoneal administration is responsible for mediocre results if IPC is not preceded by optimal cytoreductive surgery [9].

1.3. PIPAC as a Promising Intraperitoneal Chemotherapy Delivery Technique

PIPAC takes advantage of the physical properties of gas and pressure avoiding the pharmacokinetic limitations of IPC [10]: under-pressure application and drug micronization enhance drugs uptake, peritoneal distribution and penetration depth [11–13].

Based on animal experimental data, PIPAC has been tested in patients with recurrent peritoneal carcinomatosis: It has been administered alone or after systemic fluorouracil [13–15]. Concomitant systemic treatment is possible with most used regimens, considering no systemic chemotherapy for two weeks before and one week after PIPAC procedure.

Two intraperitoneal regimens are used for PIPAC procedures: cisplatin in combination with doxorubicin and oxaliplatin as monotherapy. At least three PIPAC procedures are done at six- to eight-week intervals, but treatment can be pursued depending on disease response and patient tolerance.

So far, the dosages of these drugs have been set at approximately 20% of the dose used in HIPEC. Only one phase 1 study increased the doses of cisplatin and doxorubicin applied as PIPAC, setting them to a dosage still too low—10.5 mg/sm and 2.1 mg/sm, respectively [16]. Similarly, the oxaliplatin dose used for PIPAC has recently been the subject of a dose escalation study reporting that the recommended phase 2 dose should be 120 mg/sm [17].

The feasibility, safety and tolerance of repeated PIPAC treatment are confirmed by retrospective and prospective studies. Limited hepatic and renal toxicity are reported, associated to acceptable local toxicity: nausea and diffuse abdominal pain are the most complained complications. No acute or cumulative renal, gastrointestinal and hepatic toxicity are described [18–20]. Furthermore, surgical complications are rare. Whereas no mortality is observed in prospective trials, the mortality in retrospective studies is 2.7% [21].

At least, PIPAC has been shown to be safe regarding occupational health aspects such as operation theatre air contamination with aerosol chemotherapy particles [22].

Considering the efficacy of the procedure, not only retrospective studies, but also phase 2 trials described PIPAC as treatment able to induce regression of peritoneal nodules. Clinical response is reported in 62–88% of patients with ovarian cancer, in 50–91% of patients with gastric cancer, in 71–86% of colorectal cancer and 67–75% of peritoneal mesothelioma [21]. Moreover, in patients with advanced peritoneal carcinomatosis, PIPAC has been able to improve quality of life by up to 89% [23].

On the basis of the cited literature, this phase 1 study aims to determine the dose-related safety profile and tolerability of PIPAC with cisplatin, doxorubicin and oxaliplatin by assessment of dose-limiting toxicities and adverse events.

2. Materials and Methods

This is a prospective, single center, open-label, non-randomized, two-arm study.

The trial was originally designed in 2015 as a single arm study with repeated dose targeting patients not amenable to standard systemic chemotherapy. This approach significantly compromised the progress of the study since the majority of patients presented general clinical conditions suitable for a systemic treatment. The protocol was, therefore, modified, through an amendment, by creating two study arms:

- Cohort A: patients receiving standard systemic chemotherapy cycles in association with PIPAC.
- Cohort B: patients ineligible to receive standard systemic chemotherapy who will be treated using the PIPAC procedure alone. A dose escalation design was planned for this arm.

Ethics approval was obtained according to the guidelines of the Declaration of Helsinki and approved by the Ethics Committee of Candiolo Cancer Institute, FPO—IRCCS (EudraCT number 2015–000866-72 version 3.0—4 February 2018) and by the Italian drug agency (AIFA—Agenzia Italiana del FArmaco—5 April 2018); the trial is registered on ClinicalTrials.gov, number NCT02604784.

2.1. PIPAC Administration

PIPAC procedure is performed as previously described [24]. Briefly, an open access with a midline 5–6 cm incision is performed and a single-port platform (QuadPort+ Olympus) is positioned according to our original technique (Figure 1). A 12 mmHg CO_2 pneumoperitoneum is inflated. Ascites is removed if present and the amount documented. Video documentation is started; PC extent is evaluated according to the Peritoneal Cancer Index (PCI) and multiple peritoneal biopsies are taken for histological examination and baseline tissue drug concentration detection. A nebulizer (Capnopen®, Capnomed, Villingendorf, Germany) is connected to a high-pressure injector and inserted into the peritoneal cavity; the tightness of the abdomen is documented with a CO_2 zero-flow. The camera and the nebulizer are maintained in position by a self-retaining retractor (Thompson). The pressurized aerosol containing cisplatin and doxorubicin or oxaliplatin at the respective dose according to the dose escalating design is applied through the nebulizer. The flow rate is set at 30 mL/min and the maximal upstream pressure is 200 PSI. The injection is remote-controlled in order to avoid occupational exposure. The capnoperitoneum is then maintained for 30 min at 37 °C. At the end, the aerosol is exsufflated through two sequential micro-particle filters into the air-waste system of the hospital. Single-port platform is removed; no abdominal drain tube is applied. Nasogastric tube and urinary catheter are removed at the end of the operation.

2.2. Study Population

Eligible patients should present peritoneal mesothelioma, primary peritoneal tumor or unresectable peritoneal metastasis from ovarian, gastric, intestinal and appendiceal cancer. Suitability and eligibility of the patient have to be validated by a multidisciplinary team.

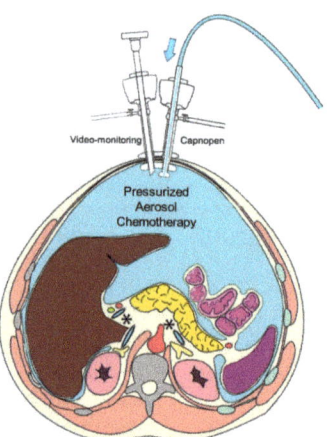

Figure 1. Schematic of single-port PIPAC set-up. The nebulizer connected to a standard injector and a laparoscope are inserted through a Quadport+ platform.

2.3. Inclusion Criteria

Patients eligible for recruitment must meet all of the following criteria:

- Unresectable peritoneal metastasis on peritoneal cytology/histology;
- Age between 18 and 80 years;
- Eastern Cooperative Oncology Group (ECOG) performance status ≤ 2;
- Adequate liver function [AST/SGOT and/or ALT/SGPT $\leq 2.5 \times$ ULN (upper limit of the normal range) or $\leq 5 \times$ ULN if liver metastases are present, serum bilirubin $\leq 1.5 \times$ ULN];
- Adequate renal function (serum creatinine $\leq 1.5 \times$ ULN or creatinine clearance >50 mL/min);
- Cardiac and pulmonary function preserved;
- Adequate bone marrow function [absolute neutrophil count (ANC) $\geq 1.5 \times 10^9$/L, hemoglobin (Hb) ≥ 9 g/dL, platelets (PLT) $\geq 100 \times 10^9$/L];
- Total recovery or a CTCAE grade ≤ 1 from all adverse clinical events of previous chemotherapy, including surgery and radiotherapy, except for alopecia;
- No chemotherapy/major surgery in the last four weeks prior to the PIPAC procedure;
- Written informed consent signed.

2.4. Exclusion Criteria

Any of the following is considered an exclusion criterion:

- Extra abdominal metastatic disease (with the exception of isolated pleural carcinomatosis);
- Bowel obstruction;
- History of allergic reactions to cisplatin/doxorubicin/oxaliplatin or their derivatives;
- Severe renal failure, myelosuppression, severe hepatic failure, severe heart failure, recent myocardial infarction, severe arrhythmia;
- Immunosuppressed patients, undergoing immunosuppressive therapy;
- Previous treatment with reaching the maximum cumulative dose of doxorubicin, daunorubicin, epirubicin, idarubicin and/or other anthracyclines and anthracenedions;
- Pregnancy;
- Patients of both sexes with reproductive potential who refuse to use an adequate method of contraception;
- Major surgery or systemic chemotherapy less than four weeks prior to PIPAC procedure.

2.5. Study Objective

The primary endpoint of the study is to determine the incidence of dose-limiting toxicity of PIPAC with cisplatin, doxorubicin or oxaliplatin (according to the primary pathology) performed once in patients with peritoneal carcinomatosis. Toxicity will be graded using the National Cancer Institute (NCI) Common Terminology Criteria for Adverse Events (CTCAE) version 4.03.

Secondary endpoints will be: pharmacokinetics of cisplatin, doxorubicin and oxaliplatin as pressurized aerosol by the intraperitoneal route; evaluation of the clinical tumor response based on RECIST criteria (version 1.1) after PIPAC.

2.6. Statistical Design

Cisplatin and doxorubicin will be used in patients with peritoneal carcinomatosis of ovarian and gastric origin and in primary tumors of the peritoneum. A dose escalation model based on a two-agents combination design published by Riviere is adopted [25]. It is an extension of the Continual Reassessment Method in case of two-dimensional dose-escalation, which identifies the MTD of the combination of cisplatin and doxorubicin based on the probability of dose limit toxicity (DLT) of each combination of the two agents.

An empirical logistic model in a Bayesian framework is adopted. The model of the probability of toxicity at a given dose combination is defined as following:

$$logit(\pi(d_{1j}, d_{2k} \alpha, \beta_1, \beta_2, \beta_3)) = \alpha + \beta_1 d_{1,j} + \beta_2 d_{2,k} + \beta_3 d_{1,j} d_{2,k} \quad (1)$$

where β_1 represents the toxicity effect of agent 1 (cisplatin), β_2 of agent 2 (doxorubicin), and β_3 is the interaction effect potentially due to the combination of the agents.

For parameters α and β_3, a vague normal prior distribution centered at 0 to indicate that a priori either positive or negative values are favored, letting the observed number of patients with toxicity driving the posteriori distribution. For parameters (β_1, β_2), an exponential distribution with mean 1 is chosen, based on the consideration that (β_1, β_2) should numerically be in a neighborhood of 1.

The working model is defined by dose levels $d_{1,j}$ for cisplatin and $d_{2,k}$ for doxorubicin, which have been identified on the basis of a modified Fibonacci series.

The first cohort of participants will be treated with cisplatin 15 mg/sm body surface in 150 mL NaCl 0.9% and doxorubicin 3 mg/sm (cohort 1); the following cohort will receive CDDP 30 mg/sm and DXR 6 mg/sm (cohort 2) and the third cohort CDDP 50 mg/sm and DXR 10 mg/sm (cohort 3). Dose escalation will be continued by the protocol according to the probability model up to a maximum of CDDP 100 mg/sm (that is the dose currently used in HIPEC procedure) and DXR 30 mg/sm.

The different dose increases will be adopted as reported in Table 1.

Table 1. Cisplatin and doxorubicin dose escalation design.

Level	Cisplatin (CDDP)	Doxorubicin (DXR)
1	15 mg/sm	3 mg/sm
2	30 mg/sm	6 mg/sm
3	50 mg/sm	10 mg/sm
4	67 mg/sm	13 mg/sm
5	88 mg/sm	18 mg/sm
6	93 mg/sm	23 mg/sm
7	100 mg/sm	30 mg/sm

The recommended doses of both agents are those of the dose level combination associated with a probability of DLT closes to the DLT probability target at 25%. An escalation with overdose and under-dose control (for probability of toxicity less than 16% in case of under-dosing; and probability of toxicity greater than 33% in case of overdosing) is further applied. No skipping dose is allowed, nor intra-patient dose escalation.

As a stopping rule, the maximum number of 42 patients is considered.

Oxaliplatin will be used in patients presenting peritoneal carcinomatosis of intestinal origin.

An extension of the Continual Reassessment Method based on a two-parameter probability model proposed by Neuenschwander will be used to identify the recommended dose of oxaliplatin [26].

The first cohort of patients will be treated with oxaliplatin 100 mg/sm body surface in 150 dextrose solution 5% (cohort 1); the following cohort will receive oxaliplatin 135 mg/sm (cohort 2) and 155 mg/sm for the third one (cohort 3).

After each cohort is assessed, a probability of toxicity, given the data observed (i.e., the number of patients who experienced toxicity), is computed on the basis of the following 2-parameters logistic regression model

$$logit(\pi(d^*_j;\alpha,\beta) = log\alpha + \beta \times d^*_j, \alpha,\beta > 0 \qquad (2)$$

where the parameters (α, β), which are positive valued, ensure a monotonically increasing dose-toxicity relationship; d^*_j is a dose standardized to a reference dose, so that log α can be interpreted as the log-odds of toxicity when d^*_i is the reference dose.

Parameters (α, β) will be calibrated to reflect information about toxicities, corresponding to assuming a toxicity probability of oxaliplatin at the maximum dose of 460 mg equal to 25% and a toxicity probability at the starting dose of 120 mg equal to 10. Calibration of the parameters will be carried out according to the approach proposed in Thall [27], assuming a zero a priori correlation.

An escalation with overdose and under-dose control (for probability of toxicity less than 16% in case of under-dosing; and probability of toxicity greater than 33% in case of overdosing) is further applied. No skipping dose is allowed, nor intra-patient dose escalation.

The dose escalation design of oxaliplatin is presented in Table 2.

Table 2. Oxaliplatin dose escalation design.

Level	Oxaliplatin (OXA)
1	100 mg/sm
2	135 mg/sm
3	155 mg/sm
4	180 mg/sm
5	200 mg/sm
6	235 mg/sm
7	270 mg/sm
8	300 mg/sm

2.7. Outcome Measures

Patient demographics, clinical features, surgical treatment details, AEs, clinical laboratory evaluations and safety data of cisplatin, doxorubicin and oxaliplatin administered as PIPAC will be collected.

Toxicity will be graded using CTCAE version 4.03. DLT is defined as any severe chemotherapy-related grade ≥ 3 toxicity. Patients will be assessed on day 0, 1, 2 (until the date of discharge), 15, 28 for toxicities, adverse events, hematology and chemistries.

Clinical response will be assessed with contrast enhanced computed tomography according Response Evaluation Criteria in Solid Tumor (RECIST v. 1.1).

Doxorubicin, cisplatin and oxaliplatin plasma levels will be assayed with blood samples drawn prior to and 30, 60, 120 min and 6, 12, 24 h after PIPAC procedure at each dose level.

3. Discussion

Peritoneal carcinomatosis is still nowadays one of the toughest oncological challenge, with a poor prognosis due to a weak response to systemic treatments.

The intraperitoneal chemotherapy administration was found to be effective [5], but still burdened by complications related to the infusion catheter which have always limited its repeatability. Moreover, its effectiveness is restricted by drug intraperitoneal distribution and tumor penetration [28].

PIPAC seems to have achieved a better distribution and penetration taking advantage of the pressurized drug micronization and aerosolization, while maintaining the virtues of the standard intraperitoneal administration (lower systemic toxicity and higher tissue penetration as compared to systemic chemotherapy).

Not only retrospective studies, but also phase II trials demonstrated promising results in terms of efficacy. A German phase II study reported a histological tumor regression and PC Index improvement in 26/34 (76%) and in 26/34 (76%) patients with advanced ovarian cancer submitted to three PIPAC procedures [18]. Another Italian study with sixty-three patients with peritoneal carcinomatosis of different origins reported an objective response in 14 patients (35%). In this study, PIPAC was often associated to systemic chemotherapy: the combined treatment did not induce significant hepatic and renal toxicity and the author suggested it as valid therapeutic option in patients with advanced peritoneal disease [19]. A further phase 2 study in patients with peritoneal disease from gastric cancer reported a radiological complete, partial response or stable disease in 40% of patients [29].

To date, the promising early results demonstrated encouraging response rates to PIPAC approach, which came along with expected benefit survival and a reduction of symptoms related to the disease diffusion. Higher drugs doses could improve efficacy and make PIPAC a promising treatment for advanced peritoneal diseases or refractory ascites.

This is one of the very few phase 1 studies about PIPAC born from the hypothesis that higher drug doses could be safely administered as pressurized intraperitoneal aerosol [30,31].

High dose of platinum-based chemotherapy given by intraperitoneal route are reported to be well tolerated [32]; moreover, the doses of cisplatin, oxaliplatin and doxorubicin used in HIPEC procedure are usually higher [33–35].

Local drug administration limits systemic toxicities thanks to the possibility to consider the peritoneum as a sanctuary in which the peritoneal layer acts as barrier; with cisplatin 100 mg/sm administered via HIPEC, the maximum drug concentration detected in plasma is 1.71 µg/mL [35].

Platinum based intraperitoneal chemotherapy have dose-dependent efficacy [36]: higher intraperitoneal doses result in higher intratumoral concentrations with a consequent higher efficacy. Moreover, the combination of CDDP and DXR appears to be one of the most effective available regimens with acceptable local-regional toxicity [37]. A dose escalation study is, therefore, essential to evaluate cisplatin, doxorubicin and oxaliplatin pharmacokinetics and relative tissue concentrations.

4. Conclusions

This phase I study aims to identify the recommended doses of oxaliplatin, cisplatin and doxorubicin applied as PIPAC through an evidence-based approach. The results of this study could be the starting point of subsequent phase 2 studies aimed to evaluate and maximize the effectiveness of this promising technique.

Author Contributions: Conceptualization, M.R. and P.B.; validation, M.D.S. and M.V.; formal analysis, P.B.; data curation, A.B., A.C. and A.I.C.; writing—original draft preparation, M.R.; writing—review and editing, M.R. All authors have read and agreed to the published version of the manuscript.

Funding: This research received no external funding.

Institutional Review Board Statement: The study was conducted according to the guidelines of the Declaration of Helsinki, and approved by the Ethics Committee of Candiolo Cancer Institute, FPO—IRCCS (EudraCT number 2015–000866-72 version 3.0, date of approval: 4 February 2018) and by the Italian drug agency (AIFA—Agenzia Italiana del FArmaco, date of approval: 5 April 2018); the trial is registered on ClinicalTrials.gov, number NCT02604784.

Informed Consent Statement: Informed consent will be obtained from all subjects involved in the study.

Data Availability Statement: Not applicable.

Conflicts of Interest: The authors declare no conflict of interest.

References

1. Elias, D.; Lefevre, J.H.; Chevalier, J.; Brouquet, A.; Marchal, F.; Classe, J.-M.; Ferron, G.; Guilloit, J.-M.; Meeus, P.; Goéré, D.; et al. Complete Cytoreductive Surgery Plus Intraperitoneal Chemohyperthermia With Oxaliplatin for Peritoneal Carcinomatosis of Colorectal Origin. *J. Clin. Oncol.* **2009**, *27*, 681–685. [CrossRef] [PubMed]
2. Shirao, K.; Boku, N.; Yamada, Y.; Yamaguchi, K.; Doi, T.; Goto, M.; Nasu, J.; Denda, T.; Hamamoto, Y.; Takashima, A.; et al. Randomized Phase III Study of 5-Fluorouracil Continuous Infusion vs. Sequential Methotrexate and 5-Fluorouracil Therapy in Far Advanced Gastric Cancer with Peritoneal Metastasis (JCOG0106). *Jpn. J. Clin. Oncol.* **2013**, *43*, 972–980. [CrossRef] [PubMed]
3. Thomassen, I.; Van Gestel, Y.R.; Van Ramshorst, B.; Luyer, M.D.; Bosscha, K.; Nienhuijs, S.W.; Lemmens, V.E.; De Hingh, I.H. Peritoneal carcinomatosis of gastric origin: A population-based study on incidence, survival and risk factors. *Int. J. Cancer* **2014**, *134*, 622–628. [CrossRef]
4. Hanker, L.C.; Loibl, S.; Burchardi, N.; Pfisterer, J.; Meier, W.; Pujade-Lauraine, E.; Ray-Coquard, I.; Sehouli, J.; Harter, P.; du Bois, A. The impact of second to sixth line therapy on survival of relapsed ovarian cancer after primary taxane/platinum-based therapy. *Ann. Oncol.* **2012**, *23*, 2605–2612. [CrossRef] [PubMed]
5. Ceelen, W.P.; Flessner, M.F. Intraperitoneal therapy for peritoneal tumors: Biophysics and clinical evidence. *Nat. Rev. Clin. Oncol.* **2009**, *7*, 108–115. [CrossRef]
6. Dedrick, R.L.; Flessner, M.F. Pharmacokinetic Problems in Peritoneal Drug Administration: Tissue Penetration and Surface Exposure. *J. Natl. Cancer Inst.* **1997**, *89*, 480–487. [CrossRef]
7. Yamaguchi, H.; Kitayama, J.; Ishigami, H.; Kazama, S.; Nozawa, H.; Kawai, K.; Hata, K.; Kiyomatsu, T.; Tanaka, T.; Tanaka, J.; et al. Breakthrough therapy for peritoneal carcinomatosis of gastric cancer: Intraperitoneal chemotherapy with taxanes. *World J. Gastrointest. Oncol.* **2015**, *7*, 285–291. [CrossRef] [PubMed]
8. Wright, A.A.; Cronin, A.M.; Milne, D.E.; Bookman, M.A.; Burger, R.A.; Cohn, D.E.; Cristea, M.C.; Griggs, J.J.; Keating, N.L.; Levenback, C.F.; et al. Use and Effectiveness of Intraperitoneal Chemotherapy for Treatment of Ovarian Cancer. *J. Clin. Oncol.* **2015**, *33*, 2841–2847. [CrossRef]
9. Hirose, K.; Katayama, K.; Iida, A.; Yamaguchi, A.; Nakagawara, G.; Umeda, S.-I.; Kusaka, Y. Efficacy of Continuous Hyperthermic Peritoneal Perfusion for the Prophylaxis and Treatment of Peritoneal Metastasis of Advanced Gastric Cancer: Evaluation by Multivariate Regression Analysis. *Oncology* **1999**, *57*, 106–114. [CrossRef]
10. Alkhamesi, N.A.; Ridgway, P.F.; Ramwell, A.; McCullough, P.W.; Peck, D.H.; Darzi, A.W. Peritoneal nebulizer: A novel technique for delivering intraperitoneal therapeutics in laparoscopic surgery to prevent locoregional recurrence. *Surg. Endosc.* **2005**, *19*, 1142–1146. [CrossRef]
11. Jacquet, P.; Stuart, O.A.; Chang, D.; Sugarbaker, P.H. Effects of intra-abdominal pressure on pharmacokinetics and tissue distribution of doxorubicin after intraperitoneal administration. *Anti-Cancer Drugs* **1996**, *7*, 596–603. [CrossRef] [PubMed]
12. Esquis, P.; Consolo, D.; Magnin, G.; Pointaire, P.; Moretto, P.; Ynsa, M.D.; Beltramo, J.-L.; Drogoul, C.; Simonet, M.; Benoit, L.; et al. High Intra-abdominal Pressure Enhances the Penetration and Antitumor Effect of Intraperitoneal Cisplatin on Experimental Peritoneal Carcinomatosis. *Ann. Surg.* **2006**, *244*, 106–112. [CrossRef] [PubMed]
13. Robella, M.; Vaira, M.; De Simone, M. Safety and feasibility of pressurized intraperitoneal aerosol chemotherapy (PIPAC) associated with systemic chemotherapy: An innovative approach to treat peritoneal carcinomatosis. *World J. Surg. Oncol.* **2016**, *14*, 128. [CrossRef]
14. Alyami, M.; Gagniere, J.; Sgarbura, O.; Cabelguenne, D.; Villeneuve, L.; Pezet, D.; Quenet, F.; Glehen, O.; Bakrin, N.; Passot, G. Multicentric initial experience with the use of the pressurized intraperitoneal aerosol chemotherapy (PIPAC) in the management of unresectable peritoneal carcinomatosis. *Eur. J. Surg. Oncol. (EJSO)* **2017**, *43*, 2178–2183. [CrossRef] [PubMed]
15. Giger-Pabst, U.; Demtröder, C.; Falkenstein, T.A.; Ouaissi, M.; Götze, T.O.; Rezniczek, G.A.; Tempfer, C.B. Pressurized IntraPeritoneal Aerosol Chemotherapy (PIPAC) for the treatment of malignant mesothelioma. *BMC Cancer* **2018**, *18*, 442. [CrossRef] [PubMed]
16. Tempfer, C.B.; Giger-Pabst, U.; Seebacher, V.; Petersen, M.; Dogan, A.; Rezniczek, G.A. A phase I, single-arm, open-label, dose escalation study of intraperitoneal cisplatin and doxorubicin in patients with recurrent ovarian cancer and peritoneal carcinomatosis. *Gynecol. Oncol.* **2018**, *150*, 23–30. [CrossRef]
17. Kim, G.; Tan, H.L.; Sundar, R.; Lieske, B.; Chee, C.E.; Ho, J.; Shabbir, A.; Babak, M.V.; Ang, W.H.; Goh, B.C.; et al. PIPAC-OX: A Phase I Study of Oxaliplatin-Based Pressurized Intraperitoneal Aerosol Chemotherapy in Patients with Peritoneal Metastases. *Clin. Cancer Res.* **2021**, *27*, 1875–1881. [CrossRef] [PubMed]
18. Tempfer, C.B.; Winnekendonk, G.; Solass, W.; Horvat, R.; Giger-Pabst, U.; Zieren, J.; Rezniczek, G.A.; Reymond, M.-A. Pressurized intraperitoneal aerosol chemotherapy in women with recurrent ovarian cancer: A phase 2 study. *Gynecol. Oncol.* **2015**, *137*, 223–228. [CrossRef]

19. De Simone, M.; Vaira, M.; Argenziano, M.; Berchialla, P.; Pisacane, A.; Cinquegrana, A.; Cavalli, R.; Borsano, A.; Robella, M. Pressurized Intraperitoneal Aerosol Chemotherapy (PIPAC) with Oxaliplatin, Cisplatin, and Doxorubicin in Patients with Peritoneal Carcinomatosis: An Open-Label, Single-Arm, Phase II Clinical Trial. *Biomedicines* **2020**, *8*, 102. [CrossRef] [PubMed]
20. Nadiradze, G.; Giger-Pabst, U.; Zieren, J.; Strumberg, D.; Solass, W.; Reymond, M.-A. Pressurized Intraperitoneal Aerosol Chemotherapy (PIPAC) with Low-Dose Cisplatin and Doxorubicin in Gastric Peritoneal Metastasis. *J. Gastrointest. Surg.* **2016**, *20*, 367–373. [CrossRef]
21. Alyami, M.; Hübner, M.; Grass, F.; Bakrin, N.; Villeneuve, L.; Laplace, N.; Passot, G.; Glehen, O.; Kepenekian, V. Pressurised intraperitoneal aerosol chemotherapy: Rationale, evidence, and potential indications. *Lancet Oncol.* **2019**, *20*, e368–e377. [CrossRef]
22. Oyais, A.; Solass, W.; Zieren, J.; Reymond, M.; Giger-Pabst, U. Occupational Health Aspects of Pressurised Intraperitoneal Aerosol Chemotherapy (PIPAC): Confirmation of Harmlessness. *Zentralbl. Chir.* **2014**, *141*, 421–424. [CrossRef]
23. Odendahl, K.; Solass, W.; Demtröder, C.; Giger-Pabst, U.; Zieren, J.; Tempfer, C.; Reymond, M. Quality of life of patients with end-stage peritoneal metastasis treated with Pressurized IntraPeritoneal Aerosol Chemotherapy (PIPAC). *Eur. J. Surg. Oncol. (EJSO)* **2015**, *41*, 1379–1385. [CrossRef]
24. Vaira, M.; Robella, M.; Borsano, A.; De Simone, M. Single-port access for Pressurized IntraPeritoneal Aerosol Chemotherapy (PIPAC): Technique, feasibility and safety. *Pleura Peritoneum* **2016**, *1*, 217–222. [CrossRef] [PubMed]
25. Riviere, M.-K.; Yuan, Y.; Dubois, F.; Zohar, S. A Bayesian dose-finding design for drug combination clinical trials based on the logistic model. *Pharm. Stat.* **2014**, *13*, 247–257. [CrossRef] [PubMed]
26. Neuenschwander, B.; Branson, M.; Gsponer, T. Critical aspects of the Bayesian approach to phase I cancer trials. *Stat. Med.* **2008**, *27*, 2420–2439. [CrossRef] [PubMed]
27. Thall, P.F.; Lee, S.-J. Practical model-based dose-finding in phase I clinical trials: Methods based on toxicity. *Int. J. Gynecol. Cancer* **2003**, *13*, 251–261. [CrossRef]
28. Prada-Villaverde, A.; Esquivel, J.; Lowy, A.M.; Markman, M.; Chua, T.; Pelz, J.; Baratti, D.; Baumgartner, J.M.; Berri, R.; Bretcha-Boix, P.; et al. The American Society of Peritoneal Surface Malignancies evaluation of HIPEC with Mitomycin C versus Oxaliplatin in 539 patients with colon cancer undergoing a complete cytoreductive surgery. *J. Surg. Oncol.* **2014**, *110*, 779–785. [CrossRef] [PubMed]
29. Struller, F.; Horvath, P.; Solass, W.; Weinreich, F.-J.; Strumberg, D.; Kokkalis, M.K.; Fischer, I.; Meisner, C.; Königsrainer, A.; Reymond, M.A. Pressurized intraperitoneal aerosol chemotherapy with low-dose cisplatin and doxorubicin (PIPAC C/D) in patients with gastric cancer and peritoneal metastasis: A phase II study. *Ther. Adv. Med Oncol.* **2019**, *11*, 1758835919846402. [CrossRef]
30. Kim, G.; Tan, H.L.; Chen, E.; Teo, S.C.; Jang, C.J.M.; Ho, J.; Ang, Y.; Ngoi, N.Y.L.; Chee, C.E.; Lieske, B.; et al. Study protocol: Phase 1 dose escalating study of Pressurized Intra-Peritoneal Aerosol Chemotherapy (PIPAC) with oxaliplatin in peritoneal metastasis. *Pleura Peritoneum* **2018**, *3*, 20180118. [CrossRef] [PubMed]
31. Dumont, F.; Senellart, H.; Pein, F.; Campion, L.; Glehen, O.; Goere, D.; Pocard, M.; Thibaudeau, E. Phase I/II study of oxaliplatin dose escalation via a laparoscopic approach using pressurized aerosol intraperitoneal chemotherapy (PIPOX trial) for nonresecable peritoneal metastases of digestive cancers (stomach, small bowel and colorectal): Rationale and design. *Pleura Peritoneum* **2018**, *3*, 20180120. [CrossRef] [PubMed]
32. Armstrong, D.K.; Bundy, B.; Wenzel, L.; Huang, H.Q.; Baergen, R.; Lele, S.; Copeland, L.J.; Walker, J.L.; Burger, R.A. Intraperitoneal Cisplatin and Paclitaxel in Ovarian Cancer. *N. Engl. J. Med.* **2006**, *354*, 34–43. [CrossRef]
33. Sugarbaker, P.; Van Der Speeten, K.; Stuart, O.A.; Chang, D. Impact of surgical and clinical factors on the pharmacology of intraperitoneal doxorubicin in 145 patients with peritoneal carcinomatosis. *Eur. J. Surg. Oncol. (EJSO)* **2011**, *37*, 719–726. [CrossRef]
34. Van Der Speeten, K.; Stuart, O.A.; Mahteme, H.; Sugarbaker, P.H. A pharmacologic analysis of intraoperative intracavitary cancer chemotherapy with doxorubicin. *Cancer Chemother. Pharmacol.* **2009**, *63*, 799–805. [CrossRef] [PubMed]
35. Zivanovic, O.; Abramian, A.; Kullmann, M.; Fuhrmann, C.; Coch, C.; Hoeller, T.; Ruehs, H.; Keyver-Paik, M.D.; Rudlowski, C.; Weber, S.; et al. HIPEC ROC I: A phase i study of cisplatin administered as hyperthermic intraoperative intraperitoneal chemoperfusion followed by postoperative intravenous platinum-based chemotherapy in patients with platinum-sensitive recurrent epithelial ovarian cancer. *Int. J. Cancer* **2014**, *136*, 699–708. [CrossRef] [PubMed]
36. Maindrault-Goebel, F.; De Gramont, A.; Louvet, C.; André, T.; Carola, E.; Gilles, V.; Lotz, J.-P.; Tournigand, C.; Mabro, M.; Molitor, J.-L.; et al. Evaluation of oxaliplatin dose intensity in bimonthly leucovorin and 48-hour 5-fluorouracil continuous infusion regimens (FOLFOX) in pretreated metastatic colorectal cancer. *Ann. Oncol.* **2000**, *11*, 1477–1483. [CrossRef] [PubMed]
37. Rossi, C.R.; Mocellin, S.; Pilati, P.; Foletto, M.; Quintieri, L.; Palatini, P.; Lise, M. Pharmacokinetics of intraperitoneal cisplatin and doxorubicin. *Surg. Oncol. Clin. N. Am.* **2003**, *12*, 781–794. [CrossRef]

Article

Adjustment for Baseline Covariates to Increase Efficiency in RCTs with Binary Endpoint: A Comparison of Bayesian and Frequentist Approaches

Paola Berchialla [1,*], Veronica Sciannameo [2], Sara Urru [1], Corrado Lanera [2], Danila Azzolina [3], Dario Gregori [2] and Ileana Baldi [2]

1. Department of Clinical and Biological Sciences, University of Torino, 10100 Torino, Italy; sara.urru@unito.it
2. Unit of Biostatistics, Epidemiology and Public Health, Department of Cardiac, Thoracic, Vascular Sciences and Public Health, University of Padova, 35121 Padova, Italy; veronica.sciannameo@unito.it (V.S.); corrado.lanera@unipd.it (C.L.); dario.gregori@unipd.it (D.G.); ileana.baldi@unipd.it (I.B.)
3. Department of Medical Sciences, University of Ferrara, 44121 Ferrara, Italy; danila.azzolina@unife.it
* Correspondence: paola.berchialla@unito.it

Abstract: Background: In a randomized controlled trial (RCT) with binary outcome the estimate of the marginal treatment effect can be biased by prognostic baseline covariates adjustment. Methods that target the marginal odds ratio, allowing for improved precision and power, have been developed. Methods: The performance of different estimators for the treatment effect in the frequentist (targeted maximum likelihood estimator, inverse-probability-of-treatment weighting, parametric G-computation, and the semiparametric locally efficient estimator) and Bayesian (model averaging), adjustment for confounding, and generalized Bayesian causal effect estimation frameworks are assessed and compared in a simulation study under different scenarios. The use of these estimators is illustrated on an RCT in type II diabetes. Results: Model mis-specification does not increase the bias. The approaches that are not doubly robust have increased standard error (SE) under the scenario of mis-specification of the treatment model. The Bayesian estimators showed a higher type II error than frequentist estimators if noisy covariates are included in the treatment model. Conclusions: Adjusting for prognostic baseline covariates in the analysis of RCTs can have more power than intention-to-treat based tests. However, for some classes of model, when the regression model is mis-specified, inflated type I error and potential bias on treatment effect estimate may arise.

Keywords: randomized controlled trial; causal inference; doubly robust estimation; propensity score

1. Introduction

Baseline covariates impact the outcome in many randomized controlled trials, and a recent systematic review reported that 84% of the trials present adjusted analysis. Among them, 91% pre-specified in the protocol such adjusted analysis [1]. It has been shown that models that adjust for baseline covariates can substantially improve the statistical power of the analysis when the covariates are moderately to strongly prognostic.

While this is justified for continuous outcomes, for binary outcomes, which require non-linear models, covariate adjustment may change the magnitude of the treatment effect, and thus the situation is subtler [2]. Due to the non-collapsibility of odds ratios, the non-adjusted and adjusted analyses estimate the marginal and the conditional treatment effect, respectively. However, the overall effect of adjusting for baseline covariates in logistic regression is still an increase in power. This is because the marginal estimate is always closer to the null effect than the conditional one, and the impact of the loss of precision on the power of the conditional estimate is offset by the larger effect size, leading to a net increase in power for the adjusted analyses [2,3].

The large amount of baseline covariates collected in an RCT opens the possibility to select the combination of covariates that results in the most favorable treatment effect estimate and/or the lowest *p*-value [4].

This is well-recognized in the "Guideline on adjustment for baseline covariates in clinical trials", issued by the European Medicines Agency (EMA) in 2015, which requires pre-specification in the protocol of the variables to be included in the primary analysis for preventing the potential selection of the combination of covariates that may influence the treatment effect, especially in non-linear models [5].

However, pre-specification of the variables to be adjusted for is not always feasible as all prognostic variables may be not known in advance.

Under the frequentist approach, doubly robust and semi-parametric efficient estimators allow for the separation of treatment effect estimation from baseline covariate adjustment [6–8]. This is achieved by the inverse-probability-of-treatment weighting (IPTW) estimator, the parametric G-computation, the semiparametric locally efficient (SLE) estimator and the more recent targeted maximum likelihood estimator (TMLE). Under the Bayesian framework, model averaging is an alternative to the more common approach of model selection [9], which relies on estimation from a single model. While Bayesian model averaging (BMA) successfully accounts for model uncertainty in making a prediction, its advantages are less straightforward when used within the causal inference framework. In the context of causal treatment effect estimation, BMA tends to assign large posterior probabilities to models that may not accurately adjust for confounding. To overcome this drawback, the Bayesian adjustment for confounding (BAC) algorithm has been proposed as an alternative approach based on the specification of both an outcome and a treatment model, as in the propensity score framework [10].

However, since BMA and BAC are based on models that likely contain noisy prognostic covariates, they lose precision in estimating the treatment effect. To overcome this limitation, the generalized Bayesian causal effect estimation (GBCEE) has been proposed as a further unbiased and efficient estimator [11].

This study investigates which methods of adjusting for baseline covariate in the analysis of RCTs with binary endpoint maximize the statistical power while retaining the type I error rate and unbiased estimate of treatment effect. Such comparison is justified because type I error and power are still the study operating characteristics of concern healthcare regulators require when appraising the results of confirmatory clinical trials [12].

In the following, in Section 2.1, the motivation example is introduced. Then in Section 2.2, the simulation study is explained, and the frequentists and Bayesian estimators are briefly presented. Results of both simulation and the illustrative study will be reported in Section 3 and finally discussed in Section 4.

2. Materials and Methods
2.1. Illustrative Study and Simulated Data

Our simulation study was based on the motivating example of re-analyzing the PROLOGUE RCT [13]. The PROLOGUE study is among the largest trials investigating whether DPP-4 inhibitors provide cardiovascular protective effects to patients with type 2 diabetes by slowing carotid stiffness progression associated with conventional diabetes treatment.

The study participants were either allocated to add-on DPP-4 inhibitor (sitagliptin) treatment or to continue therapy with conventional anti-diabetic agents. The primary endpoint was the arterial stiffness of annual changes, which resulted in being not significantly different between the two groups. However, the study showed that the decrease in glycated haemoglobin (HbA1c) in patients treated with sitagliptin was superior to conventional therapy, proving a better glycemic control. As a re-analysis of the PROLOGUE study, we then investigated a potential sitagliptin effect on the improvement of HbA1c.

2.2. Simulation Study

The simulation study was carried out to compare the performance of several estimators applied to obtain a marginal treatment effect estimate in the case of a binomial outcome and was based on the same scheme adopted in Zhang et al. [14].

There was a 50% chance of being assigned to either the treatment or the control group. The treatment assignment variable (Z) was generated as Bernoulli with $P(Z = 1) = P(Z = 0) = 0.5$. The assignment $Z = 1$ corresponds to the treatment group. The baseline covariates were generated as follows:

- X_1, X_3, X_8 follow a Normal (0,1) distribution;
- X_4 follows a Bernoulli (0.3) distribution;
- X_6 follows a Bernoulli (0.5) distribution;
- X_2 was generated as $0.2 \times X_1 + 0.98\, U_1$
- X_5 was generated as $0.1 \times X_1 + 0.2 \times X_2 + 0.97\, U_2$
- X_7 was generated as $0.1 \times X_3 + 0.99\, U_3$

where U_1, U_2, U_3 are Normal (0,1) variables.

Finally, Y was generated as $Y = \text{logit}(P(Y = 1 | Z, X)) = \alpha + \beta Z + \gamma X$, where $X = (X_1, \ldots, X_8)$ is the matrix of covariates, $\alpha = 0.9$, $\beta = 1.3$, $\gamma = (0.5, 1.3, 0.5, 1.5, 0, 0, 0, 0)$. The parameter β is the conditional treatment effect; α is the intercept and γ is the vector of the coefficients of covariates $X_1, \ldots, X_8$. Thus, $X_1, \ldots, X_4$ variables represent prognostic patient features for treatment effect.

To find the marginal treatment effect, one million individuals were simulated, and 30 repetitions were performed. The marginal treatment effect was then calculated as the mean of the treatment effects as the log odds ratios using unadjusted logistic regression. The true marginal treatment effect resulted in being equal to -0.871 ± 0.004.

For the simulation study, 5000 datasets of sample size $n = 200$ were generated. For the frequentist estimators, several scenarios were defined to evaluate the effects of model selection and are reported in Table 1.

Table 1. Scenarios under which the estimators were compared. The model for outcome generation is $Y = \text{logit } P(Y|Z, X) = 0.9 + 1.3Z + 0.5X_1 + 1.3X_2 + 0.5X_3 + 1.5X_4$.

Scenario	Outcome Model Estimated	Prognostic Variables in the Outcome Model Estimated	Non-Prognostic Variables in the Outcome Model Estimated
Correct	$E(Y\|Z, X) = \alpha + \beta Z + \gamma_1 X_1 + \gamma_2 X_2 + \gamma_3 X_3 + \gamma_4 X_4$	X_1, X_2, X_3, X_4	none
Misspecification	$E(Y\|Z, X) = \alpha + \beta Z + \gamma_3 X_3 + \gamma_5 X_5$	X_3	X_8
All-variables	$E(Y\|Z, X) = \alpha + \beta Z + \gamma_1 X_1 + \gamma_2 X_2 + \gamma_3 X_3 + \gamma_4 X_4 + \gamma_5 X_5 + \gamma_6 X_6 + \gamma_7 X_7 + \gamma_8 X_8$	X_1, X_2, X_3, X_4	X_5, X_6, X_7, X_8

Frequentist estimators were compared on all the three scenarios. Bayesian estimators were compared on all-variables scenario, only.

The model estimated under the correct scenario is the same used to generate the outcome data when all prognostic variables are known. The model estimated under the mis-specification scenario includes only one prognostic variable and an additional noisy variable. Finally, the model estimated under the all-variables scenario includes all the prognostic variables as well as non-prognostic variables and mimics the situation of using all patient features for the treatment effect estimation in the case of uncertainty about knowledge on prognostic variables.

2.2.1. Frequentist Estimators

The frequentist estimators employed for the estimation of the treatment effect are briefly presented. In describing the estimators, we will refer to the treatment model as the conditional probability (likelihood) of being treated given the covariates, i.e., $P(Z|X)$, and to the outcome model as the probability, i.e., likelihood, of the outcome given the treatment and the prognostic covariates, i.e., P(Y | Z, X).

G-computation. To address confounding, G-computation relies on the estimation of the outcome model, i.e., the conditional expectation of the outcome given the treatment and the prognostic covariates. Contrary to the propensity score methods, it does not require estimating the exposure mechanism or treatment model, i.e., the conditional probability of being treated given the observed confounders [15].

Doubly Robust Estimation. Doubly robust (DR) estimation combines the outcome model and treatment model. Both the models are unbiased only if they are correctly specified. The DR estimation ensures that when combining the two models for the treatment effect estimation, only one of them must be correctly specified to obtain an unbiased estimate. The estimates of the parameters of interest of the outcome model and the treatment model are used to predict patients' responses under the treatment condition and the treatment assignment (propensity score), respectively. Inversely weighting the expected response under treatment condition by the propensity score allows us to represent the estimator of the quantity of interest as an unbiased estimate plus a second term. This term reduces to 0 if either the treatment model or the outcome model are correctly specified and if, and only if, the possibly incorrect conditional density has the same support as the true conditional density [6].

Semi-Parametric Locally Efficient Estimator. It uses a semi-parametric model for the outcome model, which is used to generate predicted values separately from the treatment model. Finally, it computes the average treatment effect as the mean difference in predicted outcome pair across individuals [16].

Targeted Maximum Likelihood Estimator. TMLE is a doubly robust, maximum-likelihood–based estimation method that includes a secondary targeting step that optimizes the bias-variance tradeoff for the estimation of the parameter of interest. TMLE is particularly attractive for causal effect estimation in RCT analysis. First, it is a doubly robust method, which yields unbiased estimates if the treatment model is correctly specified, which is the case of RCT setup [17].

Augmented Inverse Probability Weighting. Propensity scores are estimated and used to create inverse probability weights; all observations are weighted. Finally, it computes the average treatment effect as the mean difference between weighted outcomes among exposed and unexposed [18].

2.2.2. Bayesian Estimators

Bayesian Model Averaging. BMA is an extension of the Bayesian inference methods. In addition to the usual modelling of parameter uncertainty through the prior distribution, it models the uncertainty of the model selection process, obtaining a posterior parameter and posterior probability model through Bayes' theorem. In the present work, we considered Zellner's g distribution as a-priori distribution on coefficients for the variable selection [19] and the Bayesian adaptive sampling algorithm for the model selection [9].

Bayesian Adjustment for Confounding. As in the propensity score framework, BAC requires the definition of the outcome model, which is a function of the treatment and potential confounders, and the treatment model, which is a function of the potential confounders to treatment assignment. Then it applies a Bayesian variable selection process in both models to select covariates and introduces a dependence parameter between the outcome and treatment model, ω, which denotes the prior odds of including a confounder in the outcome model, given that the same confounder is in the exposure model. In the special case of dependence parameter $\omega = 1$, BAC reduces to BMA [10].

Generalized Bayesian Causal Effect Estimation. The generalized Bayesian causal effect estimation (GBCEE) algorithm performs variable selection and delivers doubly robust estimates. It employs a prior distribution that targets the selection of true confounders and predictors of the outcome. It thus takes advantage of the Bayesian framework to account for uncertainty in the model selection process. It is different from BMA in building the prior distribution. It uses a prior distribution tailored to identify the potential confounders, which uses information from the data and thus relies on the empirical Bayes approach. Finally, it adds a doubly robust estimation, employing the posterior distribution of the parameters and adopting the TMLE framework to estimate the causal effect that protects against model mis-specification [11].

3. Results

3.1. Simulation Study

For each method, we computed the bias as the difference between the average of the estimates and the true effect. The standard error (SE) of the estimates, the Monte Carlo standard error for the standard deviation (MC SD) and the coverage probability (CP), i.e., the proportion of simulation replicates in which the 95% confidence intervals included the true effect. For the frequentist estimators, 95% confidence intervals were computed. For the Bayesian estimator GBCEE, 95% confidence intervals were computed as well, using 50 non-parametric bootstrap replicates with the percentile method. For the BAC and BMA approach, the 95% credible intervals were computed.

Type I error and power were also calculated. For both frequentist and Bayesian estimators, type I error was computed simulating 5000 datasets under the null hypothesis that the treatment is not effective. For BAC and BMA, type I error was estimated by the proportion of the simulations incorrectly declared the treatment effective, based on the posterior probability $P(\beta < 0|Y, X_1, \ldots, X_8) \geq 0.95$.

Similarly, the power was calculated as the proportion of simulations that declare the trial successful based on the given decision criteria when the target treatment effect is assumed to be the true value. This approach has been recommended by the FDA [20].

The performance of the frequentist estimators was assessed under three scenarios: the ideal case of the correct model specification (correct scenario); the case of important prognostic variable not identified in the model specification (mis-specification scenario); finally, the case when noisy prognostic variables are introduced in the model (all-variables scenario). In the all-variables scenario, for SLE estimator, a model selection process was foreseen based on backward and forward stepwise techniques.

Bayesian estimators' performance was assessed on the all-variables scenario only since they do not require selecting a final model but allow for averaging over the space of potential models that could have generated the data.

Results of the simulation study are reported in Table 2. The bias is similar across all methods, while more variation is observed in the power of the estimators, ranging between 84.6% and 94.9%. For Bayesian estimators, the power is given by the posterior probability of observing a treatment marginal effect greater than zero. A slight inflation of type I error is observed, except for BMA, however, it is not greater than 6.5%.

3.2. Illustrative Study

To illustrate the effect of baseline adjustment on the treatment effect estimation, we applied the introduced methods to re-analyze the PROLOGUE RCT [13].

The PROLOGUE RCT aimed to investigate whether DPP-4 inhibitors provide cardiovascular protective effects to patients with type 2 diabetes.

The study participants were either allocated to add-on DPP-4 inhibitor (sitagliptin) treatment or to continue therapy with conventional anti-diabetic agents. The study showed that the decrease in glycated haemoglobin (HbA1c) in patients treated with sitagliptin was superior to conventional therapy, proving a better glycemic control.

We set as outcome an improvement of at least 1% in HbA1c, obtaining a dichotomised outcome. This choice is motivated by the observation that two large-scale studies—the UK Prospective Diabetes Study (UKPDS) and the Diabetes Control and Complications Trial (DCCT)—demonstrated that improving HbA1c by 1% (or 11 mmol/mol) for people with type 1 diabetes or type 2 diabetes cuts the risk of microvascular complications by 25%.

Table 2. Results of the simulation study. In semiparametric locally efficient (SLE)/all-variables scenario, a model selection process based on backward (SLE backward) and forward (SLE forward) stepwise techniques were foreseen.

Method	Scenario	BIAS	SE	MC SD	Power	Type II Error	CP	Type I Error
SLE	All variables	−0.010	0.246	0.015	0.947	0.053	0.941	0.061
SLE Backward	All variables	−0.011	0.247	0.015	0.947	0.053	0.941	0.061
SLE Forward	All variables	−0.010	0.246	0.015	0.947	0.053	0.941	0.061
TMLE	All variables	−0.011	0.248	0.015	0.947	0.053	0.939	0.065
G-Comp	All variables	−0.011	0.248	0.015	0.943	0.057	0.944	0.060
AIPTW	All variables	−0.011	0.248	0.015	0.942	0.058	0.942	0.058
DR	All variables	−0.013	0.298	0.010	0.943	0.057	0.940	0.059
SLE	Mis-specification	−0.010	0.246	0.015	0.856	0.144	0.951	0.051
TMLE	Mis-specification	−0.011	0.248	0.016	0.852	0.148	0.947	0.056
G-Comp	Mis-specification	−0.011	0.248	0.016	0.846	0.154	0.949	0.054
AIPTW	Mis-specification	−0.008	0.244	0.015	0.847	0.153	0.948	0.053
DR	Mis-specification	−0.008	0.244	0.015	0.847	0.153	0.948	0.052
SLE	Correct	−0.008	0.244	0.015	0.949	0.051	0.946	0.056
TMLE	Correct	−0.012	0.296	0.010	0.949	0.051	0.946	0.054
G-Comp	Correct	−0.012	0.296	0.010	0.949	0.051	0.947	0.052
AIPTW	Correct	−0.012	0.298	0.011	0.949	0.051	0.948	0.052
DR	Correct	−0.013	0.295	0.011	0.949	0.051	0.947	0.053
GBCEE	All variables	−0.014	0.147	0.022	0.916	0.084	0.952	0.063
BAC	All variables	−0.015	0.299 [1]	0.046	0.902	0.098	0.945	0.045
BMA	All variables	−0.051	0.451 [1]	0.090	0.922	0.078	0.942	0.02

[1] The value is the standard deviation of the posterior distribution. Semi-parametric Locally Efficient (SLE) Estimator: Targeted Maximum Likelihood Estimator (TMLE); G-Computation (G-Comp); Augmented Inverse Probability Weighting (AIPTW); Doubly Robust (DR); Generalized Bayesian Causal Effect Estimation (GBCEE); Bayesian Adjustment for Confounding (BAC); Bayesian Model Average (BMA).

As prognostic covariates, we used age (years), gender (female, male), body mass index (BMI, kg/cm^2), systolic blood pressure (SBP, mmHg), low-density lipoprotein (LDL, mg/dL), high-density lipoprotein (HDL, mg/dL), HbA1c (%), fasting plasma glucose (FPG, mmol/L), dyslipidemia (LDL $\geq$ 130 mg/dL odds ratio (OR) HDL < 35 mg/dL OR triglyceride $\geq$ 150 mg/dL OR total cholesterol (=LDL + HDL + (Triglyceride/5)) $\geq$ 200 mg/dL).

In Figure 1, the unadjusted OR of improving HbA1c by 1% is reported along with 95% confidence interval. Frequentist estimates are reported with 95% confidence intervals, and finally, Bayesian estimates with 95% credible intervals are listed.

Odds Ratio 1% change in Hba1c at 24 months

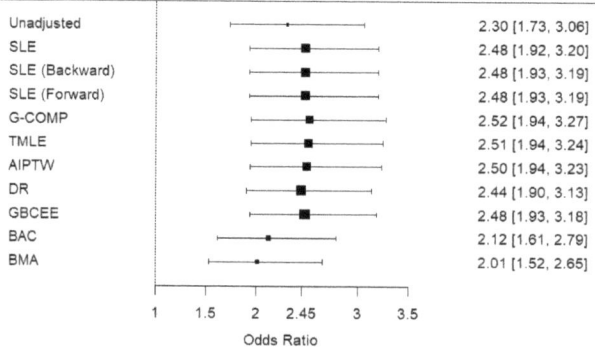

Figure 1. Odds ratio 1% change in Hba1c at 24 months.

4. Discussion

We have presented a study to compare different approaches to address covariate adjustment to estimate treatment effect in RCTs.

Baseline covariates adjustment impacts the outcome in many RCTs in terms of power, type I error and bias of the marginal effect estimation.

In fact, variable selection methods based on *p*-values, and large observed differences between arms and stepwise approaches, have increased type I error rates [4]. The guideline on adjustment for baseline covariates in clinical trials issued by the EMA in 2015 strongly recommends pre-specifying the variables to be included in the primary analysis in the protocol to avoid bias and potential selection of the combination of covariates that may favour the treatment [4]. Moreover, the Consolidated Standards of Reporting Trials (CONSORT) [21] and the International Conference on Harmonization [22] recommend to pre-specify the potential prognostic variables to employ in adjusted analysis. However, there is still debate on how to identify prognostic covariates correctly.

Several approaches have been proposed to estimate a marginal causal effect, which is the standard measure of treatment effect reported when analyzing RCTs [23]. Although it is known from the literature that adjustment for prognostic covariates can increase the efficiency of the analysis, there is still a lack of attempts to assess comparatively the performance of all the methods under real scenarios of analysis, including adjustment for non-prognostic variables and model mis-specification.

We compared several frequentist and Bayesian estimators under different scenarios. The selected estimators were: SLE estimation, TMLE, G-computation, AIPTW, DR estimator, GBCEE, BMA and the Bayesian adjustment for confounding algorithm. We assessed their performance under three scenarios: the ideal case of the correct model specification; the case of important prognostic variable not identified in the model specification (model mis-specification); finally, the case when noisy prognostic variables are introduced in the model (all variables selected in the adjusted analysis). Since the Bayesian estimators can handle the uncertainty of the model selection process assigning a posterior probability to each set of covariates [24], they were assessed only under the scenario of all variables included in the adjusted analysis.

Our results from the simulation study showed that model mis-specification does not increase the bias. This holds also for the G-computation estimator, which is not theoretically guaranteed to be a consistent estimator under model mis-specification.

The approaches that are not doubly robust have increased MC SD. They also showed increased SE under the scenario of mis-specification.

Across different scenarios, frequentist estimators showed a similar precision (SE ranges between 0.244 and 0.298). This observation is particularly interesting since the correct specification of a parametric model with many covariates is nearly impossible [17]. Bayesian estimators behave differently, showing a high precision for GBCEE (SE = 0.147). The uncertainty of BMA is not directly comparable with SE, since it is the standard deviation computed on the posterior distribution. Thus it showed a larger uncertainty (0.451), which is expected since it embeds the uncertainty of estimates in the posterior probability function.

Covariate adjustment reduced type II error but under the scenario of mis-specification of the outcome model. The Bayesian estimators showed a higher type II error than frequentist estimators under the scenario, including all prognostic variables and noisy covariates in the model specification. On the other hand, BMA showed the largest bias, even if offset by the smallest type I error, which is not surprising since it has been shown that the bias can be relevant when covariates are only slightly associated with the outcome [11].

In the re-analysis of PROLOGUE RCT, we estimated the odds ratio of improving HbA1c using the frequentist and the Bayesian estimators introduced for avoiding confounding. Among the Bayesian estimators, GBCEE resulted similar to other frequentist estimators due to its doubly robust property. In contrast, BMA and BAC showed a smaller treatment effect, compared to the unadjusted estimate.

Adjusting for prognostic covariates leads to an increase in power, as seen by observing that the adjusted estimate is farther from the null value of 1 than the unadjusted estimate (odds ratio equal to 1 indicates no treatment effect). Compared to the unadjusted analysis, we did not observe a dramatic increase of SE, thus a loss of precision, except for BMA and BAC. However, the GBCEE Bayesian estimators showed performances comparable to other frequentist estimators.

5. Conclusions

Adjusting for baseline covariates predictive of outcome in the analysis of RCTs can have more power than intention-to-treat based tests. However, for some classes of model, when the regression model is mis-specified, inflated type I error and potential bias on treatment effect estimate may arise. Estimators that allow for separating the baseline covariate adjustment from the treatment effect estimation can avoid potential bias for covariates' post hoc selection retaining the focus on objective inference on treatment effect. Among Bayesian estimators, BMA presents the largest bias.

Our simulations were carried out in the context of a binary outcome. Similar conclusions are likely to be applied to the hazard ratio since odds-ratio and hazard ratio showed the same non-collapsibility issue.

Limitations of this study rely on the assumption of independent, identical distribution of data, which is not necessarily the case in RCTs. Patients in RCTs often have wide variability in their response to treatment resulting in heterogeneity of treatment effect. Further research should include realistic synthetic datasets, which capture the relationships across clinical features among patients. Probabilistic models, classification-based imputation models, and generative adversarial neural networks are an example of data-driven approaches of synthetic data generation methods [25].

Author Contributions: Conceptualization, P.B. and I.B.; formal analysis, P.B.; data curation, C.L.; writing—original draft preparation, P.B.; writing—review and editing, S.U., V.S., D.A. and D.G. All authors have read and agreed to the published version of the manuscript.

Funding: This research was funded by the University of Torino, grant number BERP_RILO_17_01.

Institutional Review Board Statement: Not applicable.

Informed Consent Statement: Not applicable. This study used secondary data already collected and publicly available online.

Data Availability Statement: The data and code for the analysis are available upon request to the authors.

Conflicts of Interest: The authors declare no conflict of interest.

References

1. Ciolino, J.D.; Palac, H.L.; Yang, A.; Vaca, M.; Belli, H.M. Ideal vs. Real: A Systematic Review on Handling Covariates in Randomized Controlled Trials. *BMC Med. Res. Methodol.* **2019**, *19*, 136. [CrossRef] [PubMed]
2. Robinson, L.D.; Jewell, N.P. Some Surprising Results about Covariate Adjustment in Logistic Regression Models. *Int. Stat. Rev. Rev. Int. Stat.* **1991**, *59*, 227. [CrossRef]
3. Kahan, B.C.; Jairath, V.; Doré, C.J.; Morris, T.P. The Risks and Rewards of Covariate Adjustment in Randomized Trials: An Assessment of 12 Outcomes from 8 Studies. *Trials* **2014**, *15*, 139. [CrossRef] [PubMed]
4. Raab, G.M.; Day, S.; Sales, J. How to Select Covariates to Include in the Analysis of a Clinical Trial. *Control. Clin. Trials* **2000**, *21*, 330–342. [CrossRef]
5. Committee for Medicinal Products for Human Use (CHMP) Guideline on Adjustment for Baseline Covariates in Clinical Trials. 2015. Available online: www.Ema.Europa.Eu/Contact (accessed on 20 May 2021).
6. Tsiatis, A.A. Locally Efficient Semiparametric Estimators for Functional Measurement Error Models. *Biometrika* **2004**, *91*, 835–848. [CrossRef]
7. Funk, M.J.; Westreich, D.; Wiesen, C.; Stürmer, T.; Brookhart, M.A.; Davidian, M. Doubly Robust Estimation of Causal Effects. *Am. J. Epidemiol.* **2011**, *173*, 761–767. [CrossRef] [PubMed]
8. Zhang, M.; Gilbert, P.B. Increasing the Efficiency of Prevention Trials by Incorporating Baseline Covariates. *Stat. Commun. Infect. Dis.* **2010**, *2*. [CrossRef]

9. Clyde, M.A.; Ghosh, J.; Littman, M.L. Bayesian Adaptive Sampling for Variable Selection and Model Averaging. *J. Comput. Graph. Stat.* **2011**, *20*, 80–101. [CrossRef]
10. Wang, C.; Parmigiani, G.; Dominici, F. Bayesian Effect Estimation Accounting for Adjustment Uncertainty. *Biometrics* **2012**, *68*, 661–671. [CrossRef]
11. Talbot, D.; Lefebvre, G.; Atherton, J. The Bayesian Causal Effect Estimation Algorithm. *J. Causal Inference* **2015**, *3*, 207–236. [CrossRef]
12. Ryan, E.G.; Brock, K.; Gates, S.; Slade, D. Do We Need to Adjust for Interim Analyses in a Bayesian Adaptive Trial Design? *BMC Med. Res. Methodol.* **2020**, *20*, 150. [CrossRef]
13. Oyama, J.; Murohara, T.; Kitakaze, M.; Ishizu, T.; Sato, Y.; Kitagawa, K.; Kamiya, H.; Ajioka, M.; Ishihara, M.; Dai, K.; et al. The Effect of Sitagliptin on Carotid Artery Atherosclerosis in Type 2 Diabetes: The PROLOGUE Randomized Controlled Trial. *PLoS Med.* **2016**, *13*, e1002051. [CrossRef] [PubMed]
14. Zhang, M.; Tsiatis, A.A.; Davidian, M. Improving Efficiency of Inferences in Randomized Clinical Trials Using Auxiliary Covariates. *Biometrics* **2008**, *64*, 707–715. [CrossRef] [PubMed]
15. Wang, A.; Nianogo, R.A.; Arah, O.A. G-Computation of Average Treatment Effects on the Treated and the Untreated. *BMC Med. Res. Methodol.* **2017**, *17*, 3. [CrossRef] [PubMed]
16. Robins, J.M.; Rotnitzky, A.; Zhao, L.P. Estimation of Regression Coefficients When Some Regressors Are Not Always Observed. *J. Am. Stat. Assoc.* **1994**, *89*, 846–866. [CrossRef]
17. Laan, M.V.D.; Rose, S. *Targeted Learning: Causal Inference for Observational and Experimental Data*; Series in Statistics; Springer: New York, NY, USA, 2011.
18. Glynn, A.N.; Quinn, K.M. An Introduction to the Augmented Inverse Propensity Weighted Estimator. *Polit. Anal.* **2010**, *18*, 36–56. [CrossRef]
19. Liang, F.; Paulo, R.; Molina, G.; Clyde, M.A.; Berger, J.O. Mixtures of g Priors for Bayesian Variable Selection. *J. Am. Stat. Assoc.* **2008**, *103*, 410–423. [CrossRef]
20. U.S. Food and Drug Administration Adaptive Designs for Clinical Trials of Drugs and Biologics: Guidance for Industry. 2019. Available online: https://www.fda.gov/regulatory-information/search-fda-guidance-documents/adaptive-design-clinical-trials-drugs-and-biologics-guidance-industry (accessed on 18 July 2021).
21. Moher, D.; Hopewell, S.; Schulz, K.F.; Montori, V.; Gøtzsche, P.C.; Devereaux, P.J.; Elbourne, D.; Egger, M.; Altman, D.G. CONSORT 2010 Explanation and Elaboration: Updated Guidelines for Reporting Parallel Group Randomised Trials. *J. Clin. Epidemiol.* **2010**, *63*, e1–e37. [CrossRef]
22. ICH Official Web Site: ICH. Available online: https://www.ich.org/ (accessed on 9 July 2021).
23. Martens, E.P.; Pestman, W.R.; Klungel, O.H. Conditioning on the Propensity Score Can Result in Biased Estimation of Common Measures of Treatment Effect: A Monte Carlo Study (p n/a) by Peter C. Austin, Paul Grootendorst, Sharon-Lise T. Normand, Geoffrey M. Anderson, Statistics in Medicine. *Stat. Med.* **2007**, *26*, 3208–3210, author reply 3210–3212. [CrossRef]
24. Volinsky, C.T.; Madigan, D.; Raftery, A.E.; Kronmal, R.A. Bayesian Model Averaging in Proportional Hazard Models: Assessing the Risk of a Stroke. *J. R. Stat. Soc. Ser. C* **1997**, *46*, 433–448. [CrossRef]
25. Goncalves, A.; Ray, P.; Soper, B.; Stevens, J.; Coyle, L.; Sales, A.P. Generation and Evaluation of Synthetic Patient Data. *BMC Med. Res. Methodol.* **2020**, *20*, 108. [CrossRef] [PubMed]

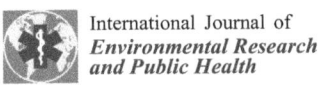

Article

Bayesian Sequential Monitoring of Single-Arm Trials: A Comparison of Futility Rules Based on Binary Data

Valeria Sambucini

Dipartimento di Scienze Statistiche, Sapienza University of Rome, Piazzale Aldo Moro 5, 00185 Rome, Italy; valeria.sambucini@uniroma1.it

Abstract: In clinical trials, futility rules are widely used to monitor the study while it is in progress, with the aim of ensuring early termination if the experimental treatment is unlikely to provide the desired level of efficacy. In this paper, we focus on Bayesian strategies to perform interim analyses in single-arm trials based on a binary response variable. Designs that exploit both posterior and predictive probabilities are described and a slight modification of the futility rules is introduced when a fixed historical response rate is used, in order to add uncertainty in the efficacy probability of the standard treatment through the use of prior distributions. The stopping boundaries of the designs are compared under the same trial settings and simulation studies are performed to evaluate the operating characteristics when analogous procedures are used to calibrate the probability cut-offs of the different decision rules.

Keywords: Bayesian monitoring; futility rules; interim analysis; posterior and predictive probabilities; stopping boundaries

Citation: Sambucini, V. Bayesian Sequential Monitoring of Single-Arm Trials: A Comparison of Futility Rules Based on Binary Data. *Int. J. Environ. Res. Public Health* **2021**, *18*, 8816. https://doi.org/10.3390/ijerph18168816

Academic Editor: Paul B. Tchounwou

Received: 29 May 2021
Accepted: 31 July 2021
Published: 20 August 2021

Publisher's Note: MDPI stays neutral with regard to jurisdictional clai-ms in published maps and institutio-nal affiliations.

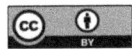

Copyright: © 2021 by the author. Licensee MDPI, Basel, Switzerland. This article is an open access article distributed under the terms and conditions of the Creative Commons Attribution (CC BY) license (https://creativecommons.org/licenses/by/4.0/).

1. Introduction

In clinical trials, the implementation of data monitoring for early termination represents a frequently used strategy. In many trials, participants are followed for a relatively long period and, therefore, it may be desirable to conduct interim analyses during the course of the trial with the aim of early stopping the study if there is convincing evidence of benefit or harm. The Bayesian approach is particularly suited to this experimental context, since it naturally entails sequential updating of the interim decision rules as data accumulate.

Let us focus on single-arm designs that are typically used in phase II trials, whose primary goal is not to provide definitive evidence of drug efficacy, but to avoid further investigations for unpromising drugs. In this early phase, ethical concerns make it especially important to establish convincing futility stopping rules to reduce the number of patients who receive ineffective treatments. A binary efficacy variable is typically considered and the response rate of the experimental treatment is usually compared with a constant target value that should ideally represent the response rate for the standard of care therapy. Generally, this target value is fixed by exploiting historical information about the efficacy of the standard treatment that is typically available.

Under a Bayesian framework, monitoring strategies of single-arm phase II trials are typically based on either posterior probabilities or predictive probabilities [1]. Thall and Simon [2] proposed a Bayesian procedure that continually evaluates, as data accumulate, the posterior probability that the experimental treatment is superior to the standard one, until reaching a maximum planned sample size N. At any interim stage, given the current data, the futility rule determines the termination of the trial if the posterior probability of interest is lower than a fixed threshold. An important feature of the design is that it avoids the specification of a fixed target to evaluate the efficacy of the experimental drug, while accounting for the uncertainty in the response rate of the standard agent by the use of prior distributions. This makes it possible to incorporate in a more realistic way pre-experimental knowledge about the standard treatment [3]. The design proposed by Thall and Simon [2] has been extended to accommodate the monitoring of both efficacy and safety endpoints [4–6]. Zhou et al. [7] presented a unified approach to construct a Bayesian optimal design for phase II trials (BOP2) based on posterior probabilities, that can handle binary and more complicated endpoints through the use of a Dirichlet-multinomial model. Differently from the proposal of Thall and Simon [2], the BOP2 design does not exploit prior distributions to introduce uncertainty in the historical response rate. However, a merit of the design is that its futility rule compares the posterior probability that the response rate of the experimental treatment exceeds the target level with a threshold that varies as a function of n/N, where n is the current sample size. This allows to have a more relaxed stopping rule at the initial stages of the trial, when the accumulated information is limited, in order to avoid early stopping of the study on the basis of fortuitously negative results. More recently, simulation tools have been exploited to compare the use of alternative probability boundaries with different shapes as functions of the interim sample size [8].

For interim monitoring, Bayesian methods based on predictive probabilities are also widely used in practice [9]. The idea is to evaluate the chance of having a desired outcome at the scheduled end of the trial conditional on the observed interim data [10]. Lee and Liu [11] described how to implement predictive decision rules in single-arm phase II trials based on a binary endpoint. The condition to establish if the experimental treatment can be declared successful at the conclusion of the trial is based on the posterior probability that its response rate exceeds a fixed target level. At any interim stage, it is possible to obtain the predictive probability that this condition is attained by enumerating all possible future outcomes. According to the futility rule, the trial is stopped for lack of efficacy if this predictive probability is below a threshold of interest. The predictive probability monitoring is considered conceptually appealing because it takes into account the uncertainty in future data [12]: it mimics the decision-making process of claiming the drug promising or non-promising by projecting the result to the end of the trial [13]. This very flexible approach has been also applied to more complex trial settings, such as randomized phase II trials [14], platform studies [15], trials that simultaneously monitor efficacy and safety [16], and studies based on time-to-event endpoints [17] or longitudinal outcomes [18].

In this paper, we focus on Bayesian single-arm designs based on both posterior and predictive probabilities. More specifically, we aim at comparing the phase II design of Thall and Simon [2] with slightly modified versions of the designs due to Zhou et al. [7] and Lee and Liu [11] that account for the uncertainty in the response rate of the standard treatment. All three designs allow to enumerate the stopping boundaries of the futility rules before the trial starts. For each current sample size of interest, these boundaries are provided in terms of the maximum number of responses that, if observed, leads to the termination of the study for lack of efficacy. This common characteristic makes the designs particularly easy to implement in practice, because it avoids the need to implement Bayesian computation at interim analyses during the trial. We compare the stopping boundaries of the three designs under the same trial settings and using analogous procedures to calibrate the probability cut-offs of the different decision rules. The frequentist performance of the designs have been also evaluated through simulations.

The outline of the paper is as follows. Section 2 provides some preliminaries on the Bayesian problem setting when the focus is on of a single-arm trial based on a binary endpoint. In Sections 3 and 4, we review the futility monitoring rules based on posterior and predictive probabilities, respectively. We also introduce modified versions of the designs due to Zhou et al. [7] and Lee and Liu [11], that exploit prior distributions of the probability efficacy of the standard treatment. The calibration of the probability thresholds is also discussed. In Section 5 we present the results of simulation studies that evaluate and compare the operating characteristics of the Bayesian designs. Finally, Section 6 contains a conclusive discussion.

2. Bayesian Problem Settings

Let us consider a single-arm phase II trial based on a binary endpoint that represents the efficacy of an experimental treatment, E, and assume that a standard treatment, S, exists for the disease under study. The parameter of interest of the trial is the response rate of E, denoted by p_E. Due to the non-comparative nature of the study, p_E is typically compared with a fixed target value p_S^*, usually obtained by exploiting historical data on the efficacy probability of S. In practice, p_S^* is typically set equal to the historical estimate of the response rate of the standard therapy or equal to the estimate plus a minimum clinically meaningful improvement. Then, the new treatment is considered sufficiently promising if p_E exceeds p_S^*.

Let N be the maximum sample size planned for the entire study. We assume that the number of responses in the current n ($n \leq N$) patients at a certain interim time, X, follows a binomial distribution with parameters n and p_E. We denote by $\text{beta}(\cdot; \alpha, \beta)$, and $\text{Beta}(\cdot; \alpha, \beta)$ the probability density function and the cumulative distribution function of a beta distribution with parameters α and β, respectively. By introducing a beta prior distribution for p_E, $\pi(p_E) = \text{beta}(p_E; \alpha_E, \beta_E)$, from standard Bayesian conjugate analysis it follows that the corresponding posterior distribution is still a beta density,

$$\pi(p_E | x, n) = \text{beta}(p_E; \alpha_E + x, \beta_E + n - x). \tag{1}$$

Therefore, the posterior probability that p_E exceeds the target p_S^* can be easily computed as

$$1 - \text{Beta}(p_S^*; \alpha_E + x, \beta_E + n - x). \tag{2}$$

Aside from computational convenience, the beta prior distribution is typically employed because of its capability of assuming a wide variety of shapes reflecting various degrees of prior belief. In general terms, in order to elicit different kinds of available information or to represent reasonable skeptical or enthusiastic opinions regarding a success probability p, the hyperparameters α and β of a beta prior are often expressed in terms of (i) a *measure of central location* and (ii) a parameter representing the *prior sample size*. For instance, by setting

$$\alpha = n^{prior} p^{prior} + 1 \quad \text{and} \quad \beta = n^{prior}(1 - p^{prior}) + 1,$$

we obtain a prior density with mode at p^{prior} and prior sample size n^{prior}, that reflects the dispersion of the distribution around its mode. The larger the value of n^{prior}, the more concentrated is the beta prior [19]. A similar and alternative way of proceeding is to choose the prior mean as the measure of centrality of interest, p^{prior}. In this latter case, the hyperparameters are fixed as $\alpha = n^{prior} p^{prior}$ and $\beta = n^{prior}(1 - p^{prior})$.

3. Futility Rules Based on Posterior Probabilities

3.1. The Design of Thall and Simon

Thall and Simon [2] proposed a Bayesian single arm design for phase II trials, where at each interim look the futility rule is based on the posterior probability that the experimental treatment is more effective than the standard one. In the original proposal, data are monitored continuously until the maximum planned sample size is reached, but actually the design can be implemented by using cohorts of different sizes.

Let us denote by p_S the unknown response rate of the standard treatment. Instead of using a pre-specified target value p_S^* in order to establish if the treatment E can be considered sufficiently promising, the authors fully exploit the Bayesian approach and treat both p_E and p_S as random variables. Thus, we consider two independent prior distributions,

$$\pi(p_E) = \text{beta}(p_E; \alpha_E, \beta_E) \quad \text{and} \quad \pi(p_S) = \text{beta}(p_S; \alpha_S, \beta_S).$$

The prior $\pi(p_S)$ is constructed as an informative distribution based on historical data about S, whose weight can be discounted by using suitable procedures that allow to enlarge the prior variance [20,21]. Alternative strategies to build informative prior distributions for a response rate in phase II trials are provided in the literature [22–24]. For p_E, instead, it could be reasonable to elicit a non-informative or a very diffuse prior density, since little pre-experimental information is generally available about the novel therapy. Many authors suggest to center this prior density at a value p_E^{prior} considered the most likely, while fixing the prior sample size equal to one [8,19,25,26]. As stated by Tan and Machin [26] "such a prior distribution is sufficiently vague to allow for the possibility that p_E may take any value in the range $(0,1)$, although its most likely value is p_E^{prior}".

Then, given x responses observed out of n current patients treated with the experimental agent, the joint posterior distribution of (p_E, p_S) is

$$\pi(p_E, p_S | x, n) \propto \text{beta}(p_E; \alpha_E + x, \beta_E + n - x)\text{beta}(p_S; \alpha_S, \beta_S). \quad (3)$$

The experimental drug is considered sufficiently promising if $p_E > p_S + \delta$, where δ denotes the minimally acceptable increment in the efficacy rate for E compared with S. Therefore, the posterior probability that the experimental treatment is worthy of further evaluation can be computed as

$$\Pi_{E,S}(p_E > p_S + \delta | x, n) = \int_0^{1-\delta} \Big[1 - \text{Beta}(p_S + \delta; \alpha_E + x, \beta_E + n - x) \Big] \text{beta}(p_S; \alpha_S, \beta_S) \mathrm{d}p_S, \quad (4)$$

where $\Pi_{E,S}$ indicates the probability measure corresponding to the posterior distribution in (3). The integral in (4) can be evaluated numerically. The use of a prior distribution for p_S allows to incorporate uncertainty in the historical response rate of the standard agent and, if no uncertainty is introduced by setting $\pi(p_S)$ equal to a degenerate density at the target p_S^*, the posterior quantity in (4) is simply reduced to (2) for $\delta = 0$.

The futility stopping rule consists in terminating the trial and declaring the experimental drug not sufficiently promising if

$$\Pi_{E,S}(p_E > p_S + \delta | x, n) \leq C, \quad (5)$$

where C is a pre-specified probability threshold. Thall and Simon [2] suggest to set C as a small value, so that the criterion in (5) allows to terminate the study if, given the current data, it is very unlikely that the experimental treatment has superior efficacy over the standard one. However, regulators currently require the attainment of targeted frequentist operating characteristics to approve Bayesian designs, and simulations are commonly used to adjust tuning parameters to satisfy pre-specified constraints on the type I error probability [27].

In our setting, and under the hypothesis testing framework, an appropriate null hypothesis H_0 specifies values of the parameters under which the novel treatment is considered not worthy of further evaluation, while the alternative H_1 specifies values of the parameters under which the treatment is considered sufficiently promising. Therefore, we have that $H_0 : p_E \leq p_S + \delta$ and $H_1 : p_E > p_S + \delta$. Of course, the rejection of H_0 corresponds to the continuation of the trial. As C increases, it becomes harder to reject the null hypothesis and the type I error rate decreases. Therefore, assuming a suitable scenario under H_0, C is typically calibrated through simulation techniques as the smallest value that controls the type I error probability at a desired level. For instance, let us consider a trial with $N = 40$, $\delta = 0.1$ and interim analyses conducted continuously after the first $N_{min} = 10$ patients have been treated. Suppose that historical data indicate 0.4 as the estimate of the response rate of the standard treatment and suggest that is highly feasible that p_S lies in the range $[0.3, 0.5]$. To take into account this prior knowledge when eliciting the beta prior distribution for p_S, we express the hyperparameters in terms of the prior mode and a suitable value for the prior sample size, as described in Section 2. Specifically, we set the mode equal to 0.4 and fix the prior sample size so that it is approximatively equal to 0.99 the prior probability assigned to the interval [0.3, 0.5]. This way of proceeding leads to the prior $\pi(p_S) = \text{beta}(p_S; 63, 94)$, based on a prior sample size equal to 155. The beta prior density for p_E is assumed to be $\pi(p_E) = \text{beta}(p_E; 1.4, 1.6)$, which also has its mode at 0.4, but is much more diffuse being based on a prior sample size equal to 1. Then, for each element in a set of possible thresholds C, we simulate 100000 clinical trials assuming that the true p_E is equal to 0.4 (scenario under H_0) and compute the type I error rate as the frequency of simulated trials that reach the maximum sample size and conclude rejecting the null hypothesis. The calibrated value of the threshold is the smallest element in the set that controls the error probability at the level 0.1. In the specific case considered we obtain the value 0.278.

Furthermore, since $\Pi_{E,S}(p_E > p_S + \delta | x, n)$ is a monotonic function of the number of current responses, it is possible to obtain the rejection regions of the design prior to the onset of the trial. Under the setup described above, the stopping boundaries are provided in Table 1.

Table 1. Stopping boundaries of the design by Thall and Simon [2], when $N = 40$, $N_{min} = 10$, $\delta = 0.1$, $\pi(p_S) = \text{beta}(p_S; 63, 94)$, $\pi(p_E) = \text{beta}(p_E; 1.4, 1.6)$ and the nominal level for the type I error rate is 0.1.

n	10	13	15	17	19	21	23	26	28	30	32	34	36	38	40
r_n	4	5	6	7	8	9	10	11	12	13	14	15	16	17	18

In practice, the trial terminates for low efficacy if the number of responses after treating n patients is less than or equal to the corresponding boundary r_n.

3.2. The BOP2 Design

Zhou et al. [7] proposed a Bayesian optimal phase II (BOP2) design that is based on posterior probabilities and accommodates various types of endpoints. In the case of a binary efficacy endpoint, two essential differences from the design of Thall and Simon [2] are:

1. the experimental treatment is considered sufficiently promising if p_E exceeds a constant target p_S^*;
2. the posterior probability of interest is compared with a threshold that varies with the interim sample size.

In other words, in line with the majority of phase II Bayesian designs, the BOP2 design does not introduce uncertainty on the efficacy rate of the standard therapy. Moreover, the design takes into account the weight of the current information in relation to the amount of future data. Let us recall that the decision rule in (5) depends on the constant cut-off C: the larger the cut-off is chosen, the more stringent is the criterion for going on with the trial. Instead of considering a fixed probability threshold, Zhou et al. [7] allow it to monotonically increase with the fraction of accumulated information, n/N. The idea is that, when n is small, a more relaxed stopping rule, based on smaller values of the probability threshold, is preferred to avoid terminating the trial for fortuitously negative results. As the trial proceeds and more data are accumulated, it is desirable to have a more stringent condition, based on larger values of the cut-off, in order to correctly identify ineffective treatments.

At a certain stage of the trial, when x responses have been observed out of n current patients, the futility rule of the BOP2 design consists in stopping the trial if

$$\Pi_E(p_E > p_S^* | x, n) \leq C(n),$$

where Π_E indicates the probability measure corresponding to the posterior distribution in (1) and

$$C(n) = \lambda \left(\frac{n}{N}\right)^\gamma. \tag{6}$$

The strictly positive tuning parameters, λ and γ, are selected by maximizing the power of the design while controlling the type I error rate at a certain level under suitable scenarios. As an alternative strategy, Zhou et al. [7] suggest to choose λ, γ and the maximum sample size N that yield the minimum expected sample size under H_0, while ensuring desirable levels for the type I and type II error rates. In this latter case, N is not fixed, but represents a design parameter to be optimized.

3.2.1. Accounting for Uncertainty on p_S in the BOP2 Design

In line with Thall and Simon [2], we modify the decision rule of the BOP2 design by introducing a prior distribution on p_S that accounts for the uncertainty in the response rate of the standard treatment. The trial, therefore, terminates at the interim look if

$$\Pi_{E,S}(p_E > p_S + \delta | x, n) \leq C(n), \tag{7}$$

where $C(n)$ is the threshold in (6) whose tuning parameters can be calibrated by using the strategies described above. From now on, we will refer to the design based on the modified futility rule in (7) by using the acronym BOP2m, while the design of Thall and Simon [2] will be indicated as the TS design.

Let us consider again the trial continuously monitored with $N = 40$, $N_{min} = 10$, $\delta = 0.1$, $\pi(p_S) = \text{beta}(p_S; 63, 94)$, and $\pi(p_E) = \text{beta}(p_E; 1.4, 1.6)$. We calibrate the tuning parameters λ and γ through simulations by maximizing the statistical power when p_E is equal to 0.6 (scenario under H_1), while ensuring that the type I error rate is smaller than or equal to the nominal level 0.1 when the true p_E is 0.4 (scenario under H_0). More details about the grid search algorithm used to adjust the parameters will be provided in Section 5. The resulting calibrated values are $\lambda = 0.38$ and $\gamma = 0.95$ and we provide the corresponding stopping boundaries in Table 2.

Table 2. Stopping boundaries of the modified version of the design by Zhou et al. [7], when $N = 40$, $N_{min} = 10$, $\delta = 0.1$, $\pi(p_S) = \text{beta}(p_S; 63, 94)$, $\pi(p_E) = \text{beta}(p_E; 1.4, 1.6)$ and the nominal level for the type I error rate is 0.1.

n	10	11	13	15	17	19	21	22	24	26	28	30	32	33	35	37	39	40
r_n	2	3	4	5	6	7	8	9	10	11	12	13	14	15	16	17	18	19

In the left panel of Figure 1 we show the behavior of the calibrated thresholds C and $C(n)$ as a function of the current sample size n. Differently from the threshold used in the TS design, that remains constant, the threshold of the BOP2m design increases as data accumulate: it is smaller than C for very low values of n and exceeds C when n approaches the maximum planned sample size. As a consequence, the BOP2m design makes it harder to terminate the trial at early stages of the study, while it is easier to stop at later stages, as it is evident looking at the right panel of Figure 1 where the stopping boundaries of both the designs are represented.

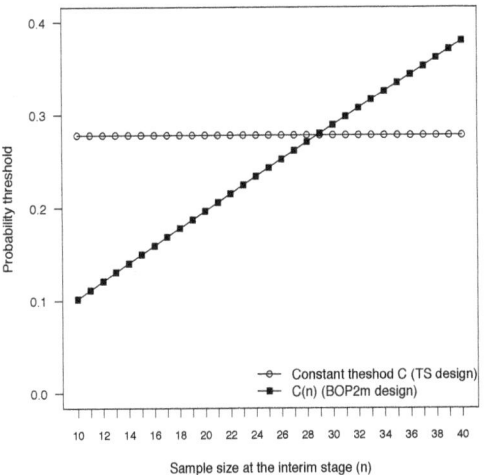 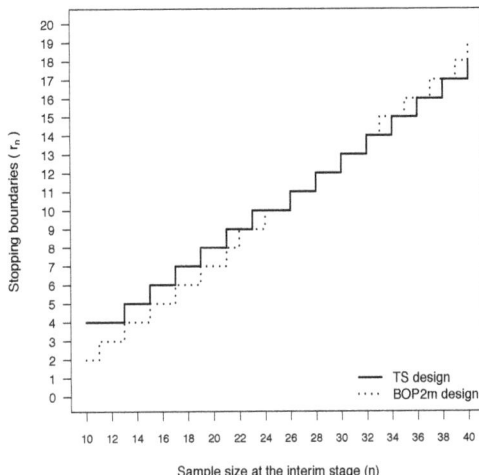

Figure 1. Behavior of the calibrated thresholds C and $C(n)$ as a function of n (**left panel**) and stopping boundaries of the TS and BOP2m designs (**right panel**), when $\lambda = 0.38$, $\gamma = 0.95$, $N = 40$, $N_{min} = 10$, $\delta = 0.1$, $\pi(p_S) = \text{beta}(p_S; 63, 94)$, $\pi(p_E) = \text{beta}(p_E; 1.4, 1.6)$ and the nominal level for the type I error rate is 0.1.

4. Futility Rules Based on Predictive Probabilities

4.1. The Design of Lee and Liu

In the Bayesian phase II design proposed by Lee and Liu [11], at any interim analysis, the futility rule is based on the evaluation of the predictive probability that the trial will show a conclusive result at the planned end of the study, given the observed data.

Given x responses observed in the current n patients, let Y be the random variable representing the number of responses out of the potential future $N - n$ patients. It is well known that the posterior predictive distribution of Y is

$$m_N(y|x,n) = \text{beta-binom}(y; N - n, \alpha_E + x, \beta_E + n - x), \tag{8}$$

for $y = 0, 1, \cdots, N - n$. At the conclusion of the study, when the result $Y = y$ will be available, the experimental treatment will be declared sufficiently promising if the following condition will be satisfied

$$\Pi_E(p_E > p_S^* | x + y, N) > \theta_T,$$

where θ_T is a pre-specified probability cut-off. However, at the interim look Y has not yet been observed and it is possible to exploit the posterior predictive distribution in (8) to calculate the probability of a positive conclusion should the trial be conducted to the maximum planned sample size, that is

$$PP = \sum_{y=0}^{N-n} m_N(y|x,n) I\{\Pi_E(p_E > p_S^* | x + y, N) > \theta_T\}, \tag{9}$$

where $I\{\cdot\}$ denotes the indicator function. In practice, PP is obtained by summing the predictive probabilities of all the possible future outcomes that, given the accumulated information, will allow to declare that the experimental treatment is sufficiently promising at the end of the trial. The futility rule of the design is, therefore, to stop the trial and consider the experimental treatment not sufficiently good if PP is below a suitable fixed threshold θ_L. A low value of PP in fact indicates that the new drug is likely to be declared ineffective by the end of the study. The thresholds θ_T and θ_L can be specified in order to optimize frequentist operating characteristics of the design.

Let us notice that this predictive design has two similarities with the BOP2: it does not account for uncertainty in the response rate of the standard treatment and it makes a compromise between the current information and the amount of future data. In fact, no prior distribution on p_S is considered. Moreover, the decision rule based on predictive probability in (9) focuses on the expected results at the scheduled end of the trial and is affected by the number of remaining patients. More specifically, while in the BOP2 design the posterior quantity of interest is compared with a threshold that varies as a function of n, in the design of Lee and Liu the probability threshold θ_L is fixed, but the predictive probability PP varies as a function of the number of future patients and the futility rule generally results to be less stringent at the initial stages of the trial, when there is still a large number of patients to enrol.

4.1.1. Accounting for Uncertainty on p_S in the Design of Lee and Liu

Similarly to the BOP2 design, the predictive design of Lee and Liu [11] can also be modified to account for the uncertainty in the response rate of the standard therapy by introducing a beta prior distribution on p_S. Then, the decision rule stops accrual for futility if

$$PPm = \sum_{y=0}^{N-n} m_N(y|x,n) I\left\{\Pi_{E,S}(p_E > p_S + \delta | x+y, N) > \theta_T\right\} < \theta_L. \tag{10}$$

Let us notice that PPm is reduced to PP if p_S has a point mass distribution at p_S^* and $\delta = 0$. From now on, the abbreviation LLm will be used to indicate the design based on the futility rule in (10).

It can be interesting to investigate how the predictive probability PPm is affected by the ratio between the amount of current information and the weight of future data, with the aim of better understand the behavior of the stopping boundaries of the LLm design as n increases. Let us refer again to the trial settings considered in the previous section: $N = 40$, $N_{min} = 10$, $\delta = 0.1$, $\pi(p_S) = \text{beta}(p_S; 63, 94)$ and $\pi(p_E) = \text{beta}(p_E; 1.4, 1.6)$. In practice, the experimental treatment is considered sufficiently promising if p_E exceeds $p_S + 0.1$, under the prior assumption that p_S is centred on 0.4 and varies in the interval $[0.3, 0.5]$ with high probability. Moreover, we assume that the study is monitored continuously end set the probability threshold θ_T equal to 0.8. We consider fixed values for the observed response rate obtained at the interim stage and, for each value of n between N_{min} and $N-1$, we compute the corresponding predictive probability of interest. In the left panel of Figure 2, we show the behavior of PPm as a function of n for low values of the fixed response rate observed ad interim, while in the right panel higher values of the current response rate are considered. First of all, let us notice that the saw-toothed behavior of PPm in both the graphs is a consequence of the discrete nature of the predictive distribution of future data [28]. Moreover, as expected, the larger the response rate supposed to be observed out of n patients, the higher the predictive probability of a positive conclusion at the planned end of the trial. More importantly, we can note that in the left panel of Figure 2, even if there are some small fluctuations, the shape of PPm is basically decreasing. The fixed observed response rate can be obtained for different couples of the observed number of successes x_{obs} and the current sample size n. For instance, when it is equal to 0.4, we have that PPm is equal to 0.0763, 0.0069, and 0.0000 for x_{obs}/n equal to 4/10, 8/20 and 12/30, respectively. In practice, if n is small, there is still a high number of patients to be enrolled and, even if the observed response rate is low with respect to the design expectations, there is a non-negligible predictive probability that the study will conclude in favor of the experimental therapy. Instead, when n increases and the same response rate is obtained, the number of potential future patients decreases and it becomes very unlikely that the experimental treatment will be claimed sufficiently promising at the conclusion of the trial. The current information, in fact, has a stronger impact on the value of PPm as the future sample size decreases. The basically increasing behavior of PPm shown in the right panel of Figure 2 can be explained with an analogous reasoning. If the fixed response rate registered at the interim stage is high, as the number of future patients decreases, we have a stronger confidence that the superiority of the experimental treatment will be claimed at the scheduled end of the trial. This explain the behavior of PPm.

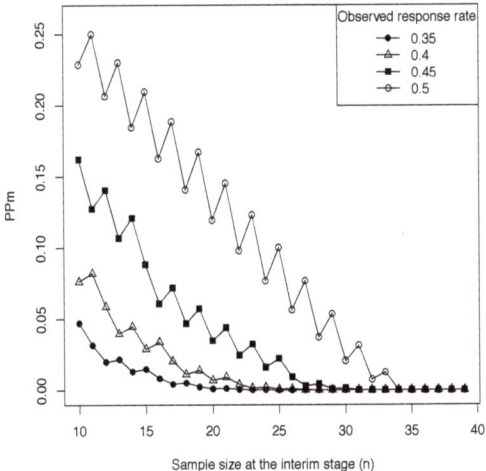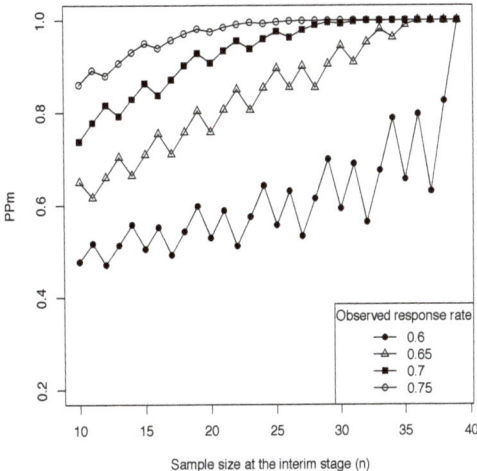

Figure 2. Behavior of PPm as a function of n for different values of the response rate assumed to be observed at the interim stage, when $N = 40$, $N_{min} = 10$, $\delta = 0.1$, $\pi(p_S) = \text{beta}(p_S; 63, 94)$, $\pi(p_E) = \text{beta}(p_E; 1.4, 1.6)$ and $\theta_T = 0.8$.

Furthermore, since PPm is a monotonic function of the number of current responses, it is possible to obtain the stopping boundaries of the LLm design before the beginning of the study. The smaller n, the lower the number of responses needed to let PPm reach the desired level θ_L to go on with the trial. Therefore, similarly to the BOP2m design, the predictive design typically makes it harder to stop the trial when the accumulated information at the interim stage is limited because based on a few patients. In order to have a fair comparison between the designs, under the trial settings previously considered, we use simulations to adjust the probability thresholds θ_L and θ_T, so that the statistical power is maximized when p_E is equal to 0.6 and the type I error rate is controlled at the level 0.1 when the true p_E is 0.4. The resulting calibrated values are $\theta_L = 0.011$ and $\theta_T = 0.59$, and we provide the corresponding stopping boundaries in Table 3.

Table 3. Stopping boundaries of the modified version of the design by Lee and Liu [11], when $N = 40$, $N_{min} = 10$, $\delta = 0.1$, $\pi(p_S) = \text{beta}(p_S; 63, 94)$, $\pi(p_E) = \text{beta}(p_E; 1.4, 1.6)$ and the nominal level for the type I error rate is 0.1.

n	10	11	13	15	17	19	21	23	25	27	28	30	32	33	35	36	37	38	39	40
r_n	1	2	3	4	5	6	7	8	9	10	11	12	13	14	15	16	17	18	19	20

In Figure 3, these stopping boundaries are compared with those of the TS and BOP2m designs provided in the previous sections and based on probability thresholds similarly calibrated. With respect to both the Bayesian designs based on posterior probabilities, the futility rules of the predictive design are less stringent at the initial stages of the trial. For small values of n, the LLm design requires lower values for the minimum number of responses necessary to let the trial proceed. On the contrary, when n is close to the maximum planned sample size, more responses are needed to avoid the termination of the study under the LLm design.

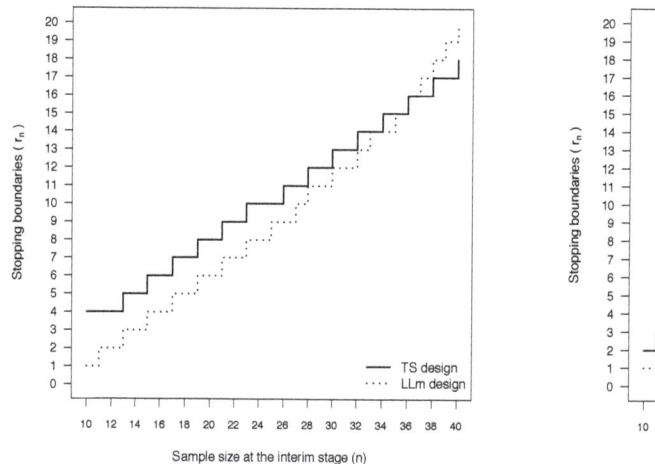
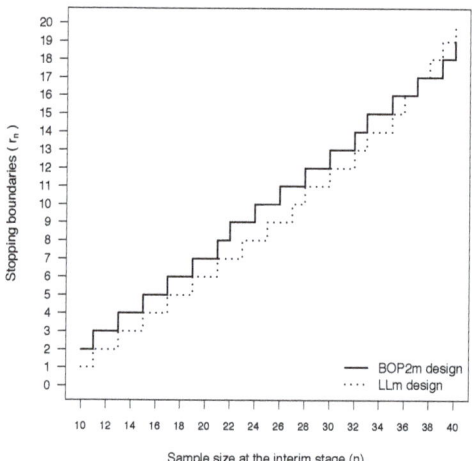

Figure 3. Comparison of stopping boundaries (TS vs. LLm (**left panel**) and BOP2m vs LLm (**right panel**)), when $N = 40$, $N_{min} = 10$, $\delta = 0.1$, $\pi(p_S) = \text{beta}(p_S; 63, 94)$, $\pi(p_E) = \text{beta}(p_E; 1.4, 1.6)$ and the nominal level for the type I error rate is 0.1.

To compare the performance of the three Bayesian designs, we consider a dense set of values for p_E in the interval [0.3, 0.8] and, for each value, we simulate 100,000 clinical trials to empirically evaluate the probability of rejecting H_0. Its behavior as a function of the true p_E is shown in Figure 4 for each design. As expected, when p_E is equal to 0.4, the probability of rejecting H_0 is below the level 0.1 for all the Bayesian designs. This is in fact a consequence of the calibration procedure of the probability cut-offs that ensures a type I error rate controlled at 0.1 under the null scenario where the response rate of the experimental drug is 0.4. When p_E is higher than 0.4, the probability of rejecting H_0 corresponds to the statistical power, i.e., the probability of correctly concluding in favor of the experimental treatment. As p_E varies, the BOP2m design and LLm design yield very similar power levels, which are substantially higher compared with those of the TS design. Thus, more power is gained by using futility rules that gradually become stringent as more patients are enrolled.

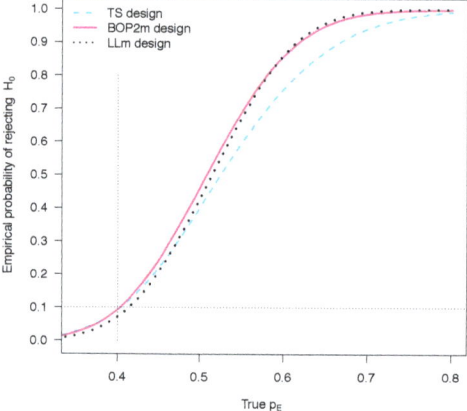

Figure 4. Behavior of the empirical probability of rejecting H_0 for different values of the true p_E, when $N = 40$, $N_{min} = 10$, $\delta = 0.1$, $\pi(p_S) = \text{beta}(p_S; 63, 94)$, and $\pi(p_E) = \text{beta}(p_E; 1.4, 1.6)$. The stopping boundaries used are provided in Sections 3.1, 3.2.1 and 4.1.1 for the TS, the BOP2m and the LLm designs, respectively.

5. Comparison of the Operating Characteristics

In this section, we present the results of simulation studies aimed at evaluating and comparing the performance of the Bayesian futility rules previously described. More specifically, we consider the TS design and the modified versions of the BOP2 design and the predictive design due to Lee and Liu [11], presented in Sections 3.2.1 and 4.1.1.

We assume that the first interim analysis is conducted after observing $N_{min} = 10$ patients and, subsequently, data are monitored using cohorts of size m (with m equal to 1 or 5) until the maximum sample size N is reached (with N equal to 40 or 80). To calibrate the probability thresholds of the Bayesian designs, we specify different scenarios by identifying two values for p_E: one under the null hypothesis ($p_E^{H_0}$) and the other one under the alternative ($p_E^{H_1}$). In particular, we consider four possible values for $p_E^{H_0}$ and fix the corresponding $p_E^{H_1}$ equal to $p_E^{H_0} + 0.2$. For each scenario, we elicit specific prior distributions for p_E and p_S obtained by expressing the hyperparameters in terms of the desired prior mode and a suitable prior sample size, as described in Section 2. The modes of both the beta prior densities are set equal to $p_E^{H_0}$, but their variability is quite different. In fact, the prior sample size of $\pi(p_S)$ is selected to ensure that a large prior probability is assigned to a short interval centred at the prior mode. Specifically, we assign a prior probability about equal to 0.99 to the interval ($p_E^{H_0} - 0.1, p_E^{H_0} - 0.1$). Instead, the prior sample size of $\pi(p_E)$ is set equal to 1, in order of to obtain a flat density based on very weak information. We show the resulting prior distributions in Figure 5 for each of the four scenarios taken into account.

Let us recall that, when we simulate a high number of clinical trials under the assumption that the true p_E is $p_E^{H_0}$, the proportion of trials that conclude in favor of the experimental treatment (i.e., that lead to the rejection of the null hypothesis) represents an empirical evaluation of the type I error rate, while it represents an evaluation of the statistical power if the true value of p_E used to simulate is $p_E^{H_1}$. Given N, m and a specified scenario ($p_E^{H_0}, p_E^{H_1}$), we calibrate the probability cut-off of the TS design by considering a dense set of possible values of C. For each value in the set, we simulate 100,000 trials assuming that the true p_E is $p_E^{H_0}$, compute the empirical type I error probability and select the smallest value of C that controls the type I error rate at the nominal level 0.1. For the BOP2m design, a grid search is used to calibrate the tuning parameters λ and γ. For both of them, we consider a dense set of values in the interval $(0, 1]$ and exhaustively enumerate all possible combinations. For each combination, we simulate 100,000 trials assuming that the true p_E is $p_E^{H_0}$ and find the set of values of (λ, γ) that jointly yield a type I error rate lower than or equal to 0.1. Among the elements of this set of couples, we identify the one that maximizes the empirical statistical power obtained by simulating 100,000 trials under the assumption that the true p_E is $p_E^{H_1}$. An analogous procedure is used to calibrate the probability thresholds of the LLm design. In this latter case, the grid search is performed by considering a dense set of values for θ_T and θ_L in the intervals $(0.3, 0.99)$ and $(0.01, 0.5)$, respectively.

Once the probability boundaries of the Bayesian design have been calibrated to have good frequentist operating characteristics, for each scenario we simulate 100,000 trials using different true values of p_E, that are $p_E^{H_0}$, $p_E^{H_0}+0.1$, $p_E^{H_0}+0.2$, and $p_E^{H_0}+0.3$. The performance of the Bayesian designs are evaluated by computing (i) the proportion of simulated trials where the null hypothesis is rejected (PRH$_0$), (ii) the probability of early termination (PET), empirically obtained through the proportion of simulated trials that terminate before reaching the maximum sample size, and (iii) the average of the actually achieved sample size (ASS). The obtained results are provided in Tables 4 and 5 for different values of N and m, when $\delta = 0.1$. For each scenario used to calibrate the probability thresholds, we have highlighted in gray the operating characteristics under the null hypothesis. Thus, the values of PRH$_0$ in gray represent the empirical type I error rate, that in all cases is no higher of 0.1 for construction. Generally, the BOP2m and the LLm designs show similar operating characteristics. When the true p_E is larger than $p_E^{H_0}$, these two designs yield higher power levels and smaller risks of incorrectly terminating the trial early than the TS design. For instance, let us consider the scenario where $p_E^{H_0} = 0.3$ and $p_E^{H_1} = 0.5$. When $N = 40$ and $m = 5$, if the true response rate of E is 0.5, the empirical power is equal to 0.783, 0.886, and 0.875 for the TS, the BOP2m and the LLm designs, respectively. Moreover, the percentage of trials incorrectly terminated early is 21.2%, 8.8%, and 9.5% under the three designs, respectively. On the other hand, the TS design shows a higher probability of early termination under the null hypothesis. Furthermore, the TS design has a higher tendency to terminate the trial at the early stages and, as a consequence, it is characterized by lower expected values of the actually achieved sample size, which are especially desired under the null hypothesis. We can note that the LLm design generally yields the highest value of average sample size when p_E is equal to $p_E^{H_0}$. This is because, when n is close to the maximum sample size, the predictive design typically requires higher observed response rates to let the trial proceed with respect to the other designs.

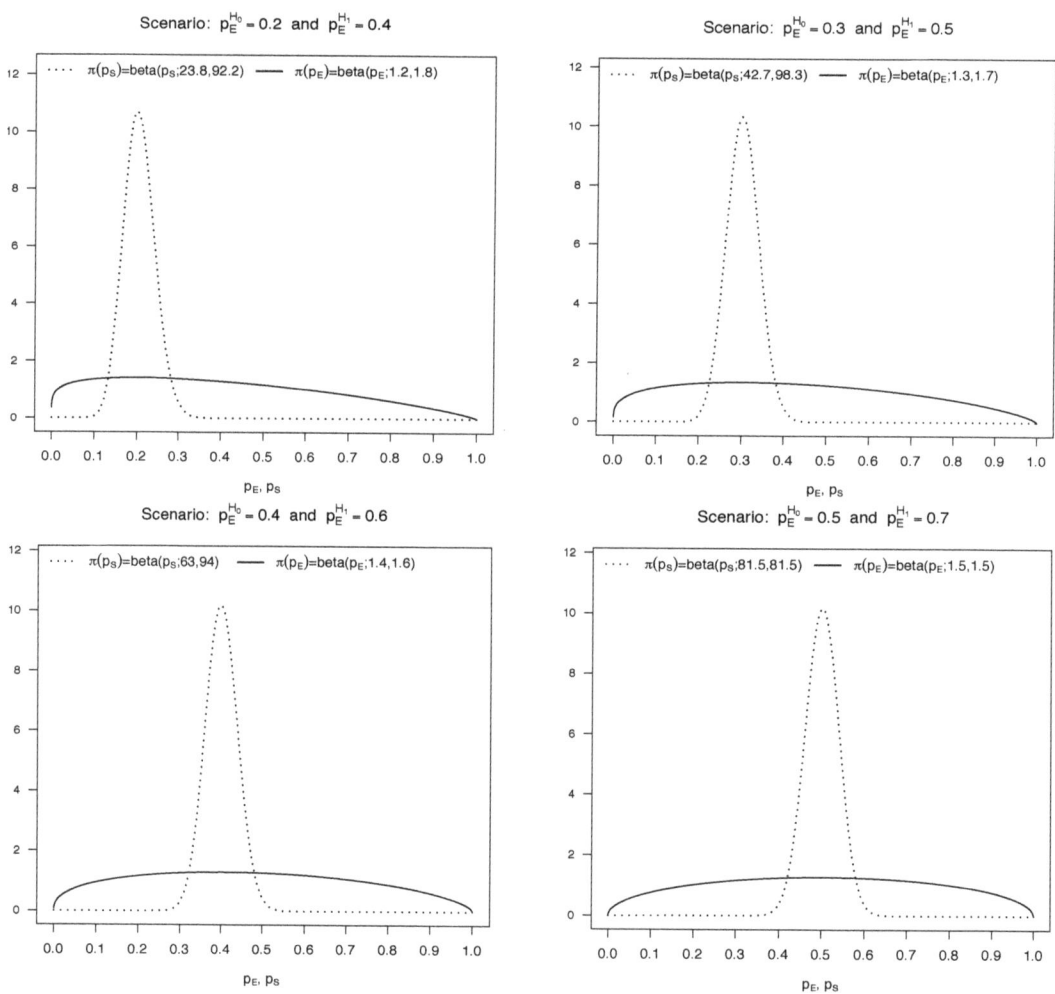

Figure 5. Beta prior distributions of p_E and p_S for each of the scenarios used in the simulation studies.

Table 4. Operating characteristics of the TS, BOP2m and LLm designs, when $N_{min} = 10$, $\delta = 0.1$, $N = 40$ and the type I error rate is controlled at the level 0.1. The lines in gray represent the operating characteristics under the null hypothesis.

Scenarios Used to Calibrate			Operating Characteristics When $N = 40$ and $m = 1$								
			TS			BOP2m			LLm		
$p_E^{H_0}$	$p_E^{H_1}$	True p_E	PRH_0	PET	ASS	PRH_0	PET	ASS	PRH_0	PET	ASS
0.2	0.4	0.2	0.098	0.902	16.56	0.099	0.901	20.88	0.084	0.868	28.11
		0.3	0.475	0.525	27.04	0.540	0.460	31.79	0.548	0.364	36.68
		0.4	0.819	0.181	35.33	0.894	0.106	38.01	0.923	0.053	39.55
		0.5	0.957	0.043	38.81	0.987	0.013	39.7	0.996	0.003	39.97
0.3	0.5	0.3	0.091	0.898	16.52	0.099	0.901	20.44	0.097	0.872	22.43
		0.4	0.428	0.561	26.04	0.483	0.517	30.53	0.502	0.447	32.48
		0.5	0.786	0.212	34.54	0.860	0.140	37.42	0.882	0.103	38.16
		0.6	0.952	0.048	38.70	0.984	0.016	39.64	0.988	0.011	39.73
0.4	0.6	0.4	0.093	0.900	15.97	0.094	0.888	20.57	0.072	0.903	25.56
		0.5	0.401	0.591	24.76	0.462	0.512	30.35	0.428	0.514	34.38
		0.6	0.762	0.236	33.64	0.860	0.132	37.51	0.864	0.110	39.01
		0.7	0.943	0.057	38.37	0.987	0.013	39.72	0.992	0.006	39.94
0.5	0.7	0.5	0.093	0.899	15.80	0.094	0.893	20.14	0.074	0.904	24.90
		0.6	0.405	0.587	24.69	0.463	0.516	30.09	0.433	0.519	34.06
		0.7	0.777	0.222	33.95	0.872	0.123	37.62	0.879	0.102	39.07
		0.8	0.958	0.042	38.80	0.992	0.008	39.80	0.996	0.003	39.97

Scenarios Used to Calibrate			Operating Characteristics When $N = 40$ and $m = 5$								
			TS			BOP2m			LLm		
$p_E^{H_0}$	$p_E^{H_1}$	True p_E	PRH_0	PET	ASS	PRH_0	PET	ASS	PRH_0	PET	ASS
0.2	0.4	0.2	0.093	0.869	18.41	0.070	0.881	22.28	0.086	0.626	30.99
		0.3	0.499	0.467	29.10	0.487	0.436	32.53	0.553	0.157	37.99
		0.4	0.852	0.142	36.60	0.883	0.098	38.31	0.926	0.016	39.77
		0.5	0.973	0.027	39.31	0.989	0.010	39.80	0.996	0.001	39.99
0.3	0.5	0.3	0.098	0.878	16.92	0.096	0.826	23.89	0.097	0.815	22.70
		0.4	0.442	0.534	26.28	0.501	0.397	33.23	0.497	0.388	32.42
		0.5	0.783	0.212	34.19	0.886	0.088	38.51	0.875	0.095	37.90
		0.6	0.941	0.058	38.30	0.991	0.008	39.85	0.984	0.015	39.60
0.4	0.6	0.4	0.097	0.890	16.69	0.097	0.856	21.93	0.073	0.727	28.22
		0.5	0.415	0.572	25.58	0.469	0.470	31.22	0.432	0.286	36.04
		0.6	0.776	0.222	34.09	0.865	0.119	37.80	0.868	0.041	39.42
		0.7	0.947	0.053	38.46	0.989	0.011	39.78	0.993	0.002	39.97
0.5	0.7	0.5	0.097	0.885	16.10	0.096	0.873	21.59	0.075	0.766	28.10
		0.6	0.408	0.575	24.85	0.469	0.489	31.06	0.439	0.319	35.98
		0.7	0.775	0.222	33.96	0.877	0.114	37.93	0.883	0.042	39.51
		0.8	0.958	0.042	38.80	0.993	0.007	39.84	0.997	0.001	39.99

Table 5. Operating characteristics of the TS, BOP2m and LLm designs, when $N_{min} = 10$, $\delta = 0.1$, $N = 80$ and the type I error rate is controlled at the level 0.1. The lines in gray represent the operating characteristics under the null hypothesis.

Scenarios Used to Calibrate			Operating Characteristics When $N = 80$ and $m = 1$								
$p_E^{H_0}$	$p_E^{H_1}$	True p_E	TS			BOP2m			LLm		
			PRH$_0$	PET	ASS	PRH$_0$	PET	ASS	PRH$_0$	PET	ASS
0.2	0.4	0.2	0.099	0.901	29.02	0.095	0.905	38.91	0.065	0.910	50.73
		0.3	0.643	0.357	59.85	0.723	0.277	69.21	0.709	0.241	75.26
		0.4	0.926	0.074	75.22	0.979	0.021	78.93	0.989	0.008	79.75
		0.5	0.987	0.013	79.09	0.999	0.001	79.92	1.000	0.000	79.99
0.3	0.5	0.3	0.100	0.900	27.64	0.099	0.901	37.47	0.087	0.888	51.87
		0.4	0.579	0.421	55.80	0.664	0.336	66.29	0.696	0.262	74.73
		0.5	0.900	0.100	73.52	0.967	0.033	78.35	0.987	0.011	79.68
		0.6	0.983	0.017	78.81	0.998	0.002	79.89	1.000	0.000	79.98
0.4	0.6	0.4	0.099	0.901	26.68	0.096	0.898	37.57	0.100	0.878	51.55
		0.5	0.548	0.452	53.46	0.639	0.355	65.59	0.693	0.273	74.20
		0.6	0.887	0.113	72.66	0.967	0.033	78.33	0.987	0.011	79.64
		0.7	0.982	0.018	78.81	0.999	0.001	79.91	1.000	0.000	79.98
0.5	0.7	0.5	0.098	0.902	26.26	0.100	0.893	36.87	0.098	0.884	46.84
		0.6	0.547	0.453	53.23	0.649	0.344	65.51	0.688	0.286	72.22
		0.7	0.896	0.104	73.17	0.973	0.027	78.58	0.987	0.012	79.48
		0.8	0.988	0.012	79.20	0.999	0.001	79.95	1.000	0.000	79.98

Scenarios Used to Calibrate			Operating Characteristics When $N = 80$ and $m = 5$								
$p_E^{H_0}$	$p_E^{H_1}$	True p_E	TS			BOP2m			LLm		
			PRH$_0$	PET	ASS	PRH$_0$	PET	ASS	PRH$_0$	PET	ASS
0.2	0.4	0.2	0.098	0.895	29.59	0.082	0.887	40.49	0.066	0.794	55.39
		0.3	0.645	0.352	60.38	0.713	0.255	70.04	0.717	0.129	76.89
		0.4	0.929	0.071	75.44	0.979	0.020	78.96	0.991	0.003	79.89
		0.5	0.987	0.013	79.11	0.999	0.001	79.91	1.000	0.000	80.00
0.3	0.5	0.3	0.093	0.894	28.38	0.098	0.882	42.09	0.088	0.796	55.70
		0.4	0.577	0.415	56.26	0.687	0.293	69.43	0.703	0.168	76.08
		0.5	0.900	0.100	73.54	0.977	0.022	78.99	0.988	0.006	79.80
		0.6	0.982	0.018	78.78	0.999	0.001	79.95	1.000	0.000	79.99
0.4	0.6	0.4	0.099	0.885	29.00	0.097	0.893	39.49	0.099	0.815	51.69
		0.5	0.571	0.420	56.22	0.644	0.346	66.67	0.690	0.212	74.20
		0.6	0.907	0.093	74.10	0.970	0.029	78.60	0.986	0.009	79.62
		0.7	0.987	0.013	79.12	0.999	0.001	79.94	1.000	0.000	79.98
0.5	0.7	0.5	0.093	0.896	27.21	0.082	0.880	39.39	0.099	0.800	48.58
		0.6	0.549	0.444	54.19	0.631	0.326	67.09	0.691	0.205	72.98
		0.7	0.904	0.096	73.82	0.977	0.022	78.98	0.988	0.009	79.54
		0.8	0.990	0.010	79.33	1.000	0.000	79.98	1.000	0.000	79.99

6. Discussion

The aim of this paper is to describe and compare Bayesian procedures used for futility monitoring of single-arm trials based on binary data. In this context, the Bayesian TS design [2] is very popular and has inspired several extensions and variations. We compare this design with the BOP2 design proposed by Zhou et al. [7] and the predictive design of Lee and Liu [11]. To have a fair comparison and to add flexibility to the decision rules, in line with Thall and Simon [2] we introduce a little change in these two latter designs to take into account the uncertainty in the response rate of the standard therapy.

The stopping boundaries of the Bayesian designs reflect the intent expressed by their futility rules. For instance, compared with the design of Thall and Simon, the BOP2 aims at introducing more relaxed rules at the early stages of the trial and, as a consequence, the minimum observed response rate required at the interim stage to avoid the termination of the trial increases as a function of the current sample size. Analogous considerations applies for the predictive design. The simulation results show that the statistical power is higher for the designs that define early stopping boundaries that take into account the ratio between the number of patients enrolled and the amount of future data. These designs also ensure lower probabilities of incorrectly terminating the trial early. However, they yield higher expected values of the actually achieved sample size under the assumption that the null hypothesis is true. We summarize below the main features of the three designs along with their advantageous characteristics shown in the simulation studies.

TS	• Simpler and easier to implement • Lower values of the ASS under H_0
BOP2m	• Takes into account the ratio between n and N • Higher power and lower PET under H_1 if compared with TS
LLm	• Takes into account the number of remaining patients • Resembles more closely the clinical decision-making process • Higher power and lower PET under H_1 if compared with TS

Clearly, the decision rules compared are affected by the procedures used to calibrate the probability cut-offs of the designs. These adjustments are usually required by regulatory authorities to control the false positive rate of Bayesian procedures in a frequentist sense. Different calibration methods could be used, in order for instance to minimize the expected sample size under the null hypothesis, while controlling the type I error rate at a desired level.

Finally, let us notice that Thall and Simon [2] and Lee and Liu [11] also consider stopping rules for superiority of the experimental treatment. The same criteria could be implemented in the BOP2 design. However, in phase II single-arm trials investigators generally prefer to allow early stopping due to futility but not due to efficacy, because it is not considered unethical to continue the trial if the new treatment shows to be extremely effective [29]. This way of proceeding is consistent with the "ethical imperative for early termination" that characterizes the well-known two-stage scheme for single-arm phase II studies proposed by Simon [30] and that occurs when the treatment has unacceptably low efficacy. Instead, if the drug has substantial activity, there is interest in studying additional patients to better assess its safety and response. Many Bayesian two-stage designs exploit the Simon's scheme to conduct a phase II study (see [19,26,31], among others).

Funding: This research received no external funding.

Institutional Review Board Statement: Not applicable.

Informed Consent Statement: Not applicable.

Data Availability Statement: Not applicable.

Acknowledgments: The author wishes to thank the guest editors of this Special Issue and three anonymous reviewers.

Conflicts of Interest: The authors declare no conflict of interest.

Abbreviations

List of Abbreviations
TS   Design due to Thall and Simon [2]
BOP2m   Modified version of the BOP2 design due to Zhou et al. [7] to account for uncertainty
LLm   Modified version of the design of Lee and Liu [11] to account for uncertainty in p_s
PRH_0 Proportion of simulated trials where the null hypothesis is rejected
PET   Probability of early termination
ASS   Average of the actually achieved sample size

References

1. Zohar, S.; Teramukai, S.; Zhou, Y. Bayesian design and conduct of phase II single-arm clinical trials with binary outcomes: A tutorial. *Contemp. Clin. Trials* **2008**, *29*, 608–616. [CrossRef] [PubMed]
2. Thall, P.F.; Simon, R. Practical guidelines for phase IIB clinical trials. *Biometrics* **1994**, *50*, 337–349. [CrossRef] [PubMed]
3. Matano, F.; Sambucini, V. Accounting for uncertainty in the historical response rate of the standard treatment in single-arm two-stage designs based on Bayesian power functions. *Pharm. Stat.* **2016**, *15*, 517–530. [CrossRef]
4. Thall, P.F.; Simon, R.; Estey, E.H. Bayesian sequential monitoring designs for single-arm clinical trials with multiple outcomes. *Stat. Med.* **1995**, *14*, 357–379. [CrossRef] [PubMed]
5. Thall, P.F.; Simon, R.; Estey, E.H. New statistical strategy for monitoring safety and efficacy in single-arm clinical trials. *J. Clin. Oncol.* **1996**, *14*, 296–303. [CrossRef] [PubMed]
6. Thall, P.F.; Sung, H.G. Some extensions and applications of a Bayesian strategy for monitoring multiple outcomes in clinical trials. *Stat. Med.* **1998**, *17*, 1563–1580. [CrossRef]
7. Zhou, H.; Lee, J.J.; Yuan, Y. BOP2: Bayesian optimal design for phase II clinical trials with simple and complex endpoints. *Stat. Med.* **2017**, *36*, 3302–3314. [CrossRef]
8. Jiang, L.; Yan, F.; Thall, P.F.; Huang, X. Comparing Bayesian early stopping boundaries for phase II clinical trials. *Pharm. Stat.* **2020**, *19*, 928–939. [CrossRef]
9. Berry, S.M.; Carlin, B.P.; Lee, J.J.; Muller, P. *Bayesian Adaptive Methods for Clinical Trials*; Chapman and Hall/CRC: Boca Raton, FL, USA, 2011.
10. Dmitrienko, A.; Wang, M.D. Bayesian predictive approach to interim monitoring in clinical trials. *Stat. Med.* **2006**, *25*, 2178–2195. [CrossRef]
11. Lee, J.J.; Liu, D.D. A predictive probability design for phase II cancer clinical trials. *Clin. Trials* **2008**, *5*, 93–106. [CrossRef]
12. Saville, B.R.; Connor, J.T.; Ayers, G.D.; Alvarez, J. The utility of Bayesian predictive probabilities for interim monitoring of clinical trials. *Clin. Trials* **2014**, *11*, 485–493. [CrossRef]
13. Lin, R.; Lee, J.J. Novel bayesian adaptive designs and their applications in cancer clinical trials. In *Computational and Methodological Statistics and Biostatistics*; Bekker, A., Chen, D.G., Ferreira, J.T., Eds.; Springer: Cham, Switzerland, 2020; pp. 395–426.
14. Yin, G.; Chen, N.; Lee, J.J. Phase II trial design with Bayesian adaptive randomization and predictive probability. *J. R. Stat. Soc. Ser. C* **2012**, *61*, 219–235. [CrossRef]
15. Hobbs, B.P.; Chen, N.; Lee, J.J. Controlled multi-arm platform design using predictive probability. *Stat. Methods Med. Res.* **2018**, *27*, 65–78. [CrossRef] [PubMed]
16. Sambucini, V. Bayesian predictive monitoring with bivariate binary outcomes in phase II clinical trials. *Comput. Stat. Data Anal.* **2019**, *132*, 18–30. [CrossRef]
17. Yin, G.; Chen, N.; Lee, J.J. Bayesian Adaptive Randomization and Trial Monitoring with Predictive Probability for Time-to-event Endpoint *Stat. Biosci.* **2018**, *10*, 420–438.
18. Zhou, M.; Tang, Q.; Lang, L.; Xing, J.; Tatsuoka, K. Predictive probability methods for interim monitoring in clinical trials with longitudinal outcomes. *Stat. Med.* **2018**, *37*, 2187–2207. [CrossRef] [PubMed]
19. Sambucini, V. A Bayesian predictive two-stage design for phase II clinical trials. *Stat. Med.* **2008**, *27*, 1199–1224. [CrossRef]
20. Ibrahim, J.G.; Chen, M.H. Power prior distributions for regression models. *Stat. Sci.* **2000**, *15*, 46–60.
21. De Santis, F. Using historical data for Bayesian sample size determination. *J. R. Stat. Soc. Ser. A* **2007**, *170*, 95–113. [CrossRef]
22. Chen C.; Chaloner, K. A Bayesian stopping rule for a single arm study: With a case study of stem cell transplantation. *Stat. Med.* **2006**, *25*, 2956–2966. [CrossRef]
23. Mayo, M.S.; Gajewski, B.J. Bayesian sample size calculations in phase II clinical trials using informative conjugate priors. *Control Clin Trials* **2004**, *25*, 157–167. [CrossRef]
24. Gajewski, B.J.; Mayo, M.S. Bayesian sample size calculations in phase II clinical trials using a mixture of informative priors. *Stat. Med.* **2006**, *25*, 2554–2566. [CrossRef] [PubMed]
25. Heitjan, D.F. Bayesian interim analysis of phase II cancer clinical trials. *Stat. Med.* **1997**, *16*, 1791–1802. [CrossRef]

26. Tan, S.B.; Machin, D. Bayesian two-stage designs for phase II clinical trials. *Stat. Med.* **2002**, *21*, 1991–2012. [CrossRef]
27. Ventz S.; Trippa L. Bayesian designs and the control of frequentist characteristics: A practical solution. *Biometrics* **2015**, *71*, 218–226. [CrossRef] [PubMed]
28. Sambucini, V. Bayesian vs. Frequentist Power Functions to Determine the Optimal Sample Size: Testing One Sample Binomial Proportion Using Exact Methods. In *Bayesian Inference*; Tejedor, J.P., Ed.; IntechOpen: Rijeka, Croatia, 2017; pp. 77–95.
29. Yin, G. *Clinical Trial Design: Bayesian and Frequentist Adaptive Methods*; Wiley: Hoboken, NJ, USA, 2012.
30. Simon, R. Optimal two-stage designs for phase II clinical trials. *Control. Clin. Trials* **1989**, *10*, 1–10. [CrossRef]
31. Dong, G.; Shih, W.J.; Moore, D.; Quan, H.; Marcella, S. A Bayesian-frequentist two-stage single-arm phase II clinical trial design. *Stat. Med.* **2012**, *31*, 2055–2067. [CrossRef]

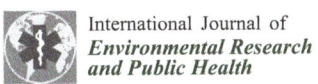

Article

Bayesian Design for Identifying Cohort-Specific Optimal Dose Combinations Based on Multiple Endpoints: Application to a Phase I Trial in Non-Small Cell Lung Cancer

Bethany Jablonski Horton [1,*], Nolan A. Wages [1] and Ryan D. Gentzler [2]

[1] Division of Translational Research and Applied Statistics, Department of Public Health Sciences, University of Virginia, Charlottesville, VA 22904, USA; naw7n@virginia.edu
[2] Division of Hematology/Oncology, University of Virginia Cancer Center, Charlottesville, VA 22904, USA.; rg2uc@virginia.edu
* Correspondence: bjh8f@virginia.edu

Citation: Horton, B.J.; Wages, N.A.; Gentzler, R.D. Bayesian Design for Identifying Cohort-Specific Optimal Dose Combinations Based on Multiple Endpoints: Application to a Phase I Trial in Non-Small Cell Lung Cancer. *Int. J. Environ. Res. Public Health* **2021**, *18*, 11452. https://doi.org/10.3390/ijerph182111452

Academic Editors: Paola Berchialla and Ileana Baldi

Received: 29 September 2021
Accepted: 27 October 2021
Published: 30 October 2021

Publisher's Note: MDPI stays neutral with regard to jurisdictional clai-ms in published maps and institutio-nal affiliations.

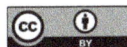

Copyright: © 2021 by the authors. Licensee MDPI, Basel, Switzerland. This article is an open access article distributed under the terms and conditions of the Creative Commons Attribution (CC BY) license (https://creativecommons.org/licenses/by/4.0/).

Abstract: Immunotherapy and chemotherapy combinations have proven to be a safe and efficacious treatment approach in multiple settings. However, it is not clear whether approved doses of chemotherapy developed to achieve a maximum tolerated dose are the ideal dose when combining cytotoxic chemotherapy with immunotherapy to induce immune responses. This trial of a modulated dose chemotherapy and Pembrolizumab, with or without a second immunomodulatory agent, uses a Bayesian design to select the optimal treatment combination by balancing both safety and efficacy of the chemotherapy and immunotherapy agents within each of two cohorts. The simulation study provides evidence that the proposed Bayesian design successfully addresses the primary study aim to identify the optimal dose combination for each of the two independent patient cohorts. This conclusion is supported by the high percentage of simulated trials which select a treatment combination that is both safe and highly efficacious. The proposed trial was funded and was being finalized when the sponsoring company decided not to proceed due to negative findings in another patient population. The proposed trial design will continue to be relevant as multiple chemotherapy and immunotherapy combinations become the standard of care and future research will require evaluating the appropriate doses of various components of multiple drug regimens.

Keywords: Bayesian trial design; early phase dose finding; treatment combinations; optimal dose combination; oncology

1. Introduction

The global incidence of lung cancer was 2.2 million in 2020, resulting in an estimated 1.7 million deaths [1]. In the United States, the 2021 estimated incidence of new diagnoses is 235,760 and the estimated number of deaths was 131,880. Lung cancer represents 12.4% of all new cancer cases in the US and remains the leading cause of cancer death for both men and women. Only 18% of patients are diagnosed with localized disease and an additional 22% are diagnosed with regional disease with the remaining having distant spread at the time of diagnosis. The 5-year survival for patients with localized and regional disease is 59.8% and 32.9% respectively [2].

Immune checkpoint inhibitors (ICI), such as those that inhibit programmed death ligand 1 (PD-1) or its ligand (PD-L1), have been approved as first and second-line treatments for non-small cell lung cancer (NSCLC) and are currently being evaluated in the neo-adjuvant and adjuvant setting. Pembrolizumab, a PD-1 inhibitor, is commonly used to treat patients with advanced NSCLC, either alone or in combination with chemotherapy. These agents have improved overall survival and can result in durable disease control and meaningful increases in long-term survival. Although treatment with anti-PD-1 or anti-PD-L1 antibodies can induce clinical responses in the setting of many advanced cancers, these ICIs fail to induce durable responses in a large proportion of patients. Thus, there remains a critical need to identify combinatorial approaches to augment anti-PD-1 responses and overcome immune resistance mechanisms. The efficacy of checkpoint inhibitors may be further enhanced by overcoming immune resistance mechanisms within the tumor microenvironment. Various agents have demonstrated potential to synergize with ICIs to enhance an immune response, including agents that target indoleamine 2,3-dioxygenase (IDO), vascular endothelial growth factor (VEGF), histone deacetylase (HDAC), or poly-ADP-ribose polymerase (PARP), among others. In addition, combinations of other checkpoint inhibitors (CPIs), such as those that target CTLA4, TIGIT, and LAG-3 have shown promise. In advanced NSCLC, a combination of PD-1 and CTLA4 has been shown to improve overall survival compared to chemotherapy alone and this strategy is now FDA approved [3,4].

Immunotherapy and chemotherapy combinations have proven to be a safe and efficacious treatment approach in multiple settings and there is potential to further elucidate a synergistic relationship between these modalities [5–7]. It is not clear whether approved doses of chemotherapy, which were developed to achieve a maximum tolerated dose (MTD), are the ideal dose when combining cytotoxic chemotherapy with immunotherapy to induce immune responses. Lower doses of chemotherapy may maximize this synergistic effect and allow for a combination with less toxicity. Further exploring the role of immunotherapy combinations with chemotherapy offers even more potential to improve response rates and survival in a disease with significant morbidity and mortality. The Checkmate 9LA study evaluated a combination of ipilimumab, a CTLA4 inhibitor, with nivolumab, a PD-1 inhibitor, with only two cycles of chemotherapy rather than the standard four cycles. This trial showed superior overall survival with this combination compared to four cycles of chemotherapy alone. However, the doses of chemotherapy given for those two cycles were at the standard dose [3].

The clinical question of interest for this study of patients with NSCLC is to explore potential benefits of lower doses of chemotherapy as well as adding a second immunotherapy agent to the commonly used standard of care regimen of platinum-doublet chemotherapy and pembrolizumab. To address this clinical question, the trial was proposed with a Bayesian design to select the optimal treatment combination by balancing both safety and efficacy of the chemotherapy and immunotherapy agents within each of two cohorts. For an overview of Bayesian design of adaptive clinical trials, we refer the reader to Giovagnoli [8] and the references therein. There are no existing dose-finding methods available to address the multitude of challenges presented by research objectives of this study. Our team adapted relevant components of existing methods to develop an appropriate and flexible design strategy. There is an increased demand to tailor early-phase clinical trial designs to the trial's research objectives in order to treat study participants as efficiently as possible rather than reorienting the objectives to apply an "off-the-shelf" method, potentially missing the opportunity to answer promising and relevant research questions. Details of the design are provided in Section 2, followed by simulation results in Section 3. Discussion and conclusion follow in Sections 4 and 5, respectively.

2. Methods

This trial is an early phase study evaluating the safety and efficacy of the combination of modulated dose chemotherapy and Pembrolizumab, with or without second immunomodulatory agent as neoadjuvant therapy for stage IB-IIIA surgically resectable NSCLC patients in two cohorts. The patient cohorts are defined by patients with adenocarcinoma (Cohort A) and squamous cell carcinoma (Cohort B). Standard histology-based chemotherapy regimens vary for the two patient cohorts, and it is not known whether one cohort is expected to have systematically greater or lesser toxicity than the other cohort. Thus, the cohorts are considered independently. Patients will receive 4 cycles of neoadjuvant combination therapy followed by surgical resection with a primary objective of determining the optimal dose combination (ODC). The ODC will incorporate both safety and efficacy and will be defined as the combination with the highest response rate among combinations with an acceptable level of toxicity. The primary outcomes guiding accrual decisions include the frequency of treatment-related dose-limiting toxicities (DLTs) and the frequency of pathologic response, assessed between 12 and 28 weeks from the start of treatment.

2.1. Treatment Combinations by Patient Cohort

It is anticipated that 65% of the participant population will be from Cohort A and 35% from Cohort B based on prevalence of squamous and non-squamous histology. Treatment details are provided in Table 1, where treatment combinations are labeled as Arms A1 through A6 for Cohort A and Arms B1 through B6 for Cohort B. The ODC in each cohort is the combination that is estimated to have an acceptable toxicity profile, as measured by DLTs, and a good response profile as measured by pathologic response. Adverse events are assessed and graded using the National Cancer Institute's Common Terminology Criteria (CTCAE).

Table 1. Treatment combinations by cohort.

	Cohort A: Adenocarcinoma Patients			
	Pembrolizumab 200 mg IV Q3W			
		Chemotherapy (mg/m^2)		
	Cisplatin	25	50	75
	Pemetrexed	150	375	500
Immune agent 2	Dose level 1	A4	A5	A6
	0	A1	A2	A3
	Cohort B: Squamous Cell Carcinoma Patients			
	Pembrolizumab 200 mg IV Q3W			
		Chemotherapy (mg/m^2)		
	Cisplatin	25	50	75
	Gemcitabine	400	800	1200
Immune agent 2	Dose level 1	B4	B5	B6
	0	B1	B2	B3

As data accumulate, each evaluable participant is classified as experiencing a DLT (yes/no) and experiencing a response (yes/no). Based on the expectedness of adverse events, the maximum allowable DLT rate is 30%. Any combination with an estimated DLT probability $\leq 30\%$ is considered "acceptable" in terms of safety.

2.2. Bayesian Dose-Finding Design

The intention of this design is to determine cohort-specific ODC where treatment combination allocation is based on a Bayesian continual reassessment method accounting for both toxicity and efficacy [9]. The study is designed to accrue eligible participants using cohorts of size one. Allocation to treatment combinations is implemented for each patient cohort independently, and the process is the same in both cohorts. With regard to safety, it is assumed that increasing the dose level while holding the other agent fixed will result in an increased probability of DLT. Using this assumption, modeling incorporates a set of four possible orderings for DLT probabilities among the treatment combinations in Table 2 and a working model for DLT probabilities corresponding to the four possible orders in Table 3. This process is considered separately for each of the two patient cohorts.

Table 2. Possible orders of DLT probabilities.

Order (m)	Combination
1	1–2–4–3–5–6
2	1–2–4–5–3–6
3	1–4–2–5–3–6
4	1–4–2–3–5–6

Table 3. Working model of DLT probabilities under each ordering.

Order (m)	Combination					
	1	2	3	4	5	6
1	0.03	0.10	0.15	0.10	0.22	0.30
2	0.03	0.05	0.22	0.10	0.15	0.30
3	0.03	0.10	0.22	0.05	0.15	0.30
4	0.03	0.10	0.15	0.05	0.22	0.30

The continual reassessment method (CRM) is fit for toxicity within each ordering using the working model and the accumulated data. For each working model in each cohort, $m = 1, \ldots, 4$ in Table 3, the DLT probabilities are modeled using a class of one-parameter power models $\Pr(\text{DLT at combination } i) \approx p_{mci}^{\exp(\theta_{mc})}$, where the p_{mci} are the working model values for order m given in Table 3, i indexes the dose combination and c indexes the cohort.

DLT probability estimation embodies characteristics of the continual reassessment method (CRM) [10], so we use its features to specify design parameters. The skeleton values for toxicity were selected using to the algorithm of Lee and Cheung [11], using recommended specifications that yield good operating characteristics. CRM designs have been shown to be robust and efficient with the use of "reasonable" skeletons, where adjacent values have adequate spacing. The algorithm is available as a function, getprior, within the R [12] package dfcrm [13] and requires a spacing measure ρ to generate reasonable spacing between adjacent combinations in the skeleton. Simulation results in Lee and Cheung [11] indicate that the optimal range of ρ is [0.04, 0.10] for common target toxicity rates (i.e., 0.20–0.33). The value $\rho = 0.04$ lies in the optimal range and provides a set of reasonably spaced skeleton values. The skeletons should represent the various possible orderings of regimen–toxicity curves, according to the toxicity assumptions displayed in Table 2. The class of skeletons in Table 3 was generated using the algorithm and the locations of these values were adjusted to correspond to the six orderings in Table 2 using the getwm function in R package pocrm [14].

The prior distribution on the parameter θ for all working models is given by $g(\theta) = N(0, 0.48)$, a normal distribution with mean 0 and standard deviation 0.48. The standard deviation for the prior distribution was chosen according to Algorithm 9.1 in Cheung [15] using values of $\sigma_\theta^{LI} = 0.75$, $\lambda_1 = 0.6, \lambda_2 = 1.4$ and a grid width of 0.03. According to Cheung [15], there are two practical advantages for choosing a normal distribution in this setting. First, posterior computations using Gauss–Hermite quadrature [16] under the above parametrization are accurate, and the second, Bayesian CRM utilizing a class of one-parameter models that includes the power model is invariant to the mean of a prior that forms a location-scale family. This property allows for the prior mean to be zero and the prior to be completely specified by its standard deviation, simplifying the process of calibration. A uniform prior distribution, $\tau(m) = 1/m$, is placed on each working model for each cohort so that all working models are considered equally likely a priori. Based on the observed toxicity data $D_c = \{(y_{ci}, n_{ci}); i = 1, \ldots, 6\}$, where y_{ci} is the number of DLTs, n_{ci} is the number of subjects treated on combination i, and c specifies the cohort. The likelihood for ordering m is given by

$$L_m(D_c|\theta) \propto \prod_{i=1}^{6} \left(p_{mci}^{\exp(\theta_m)}\right)^{y_{ci}} \left(1 - p_{mci}^{\exp(\theta_m)}\right)^{n_{ci}-y_{ci}} \quad (1)$$

Using Bayes theorem, the posterior probability for each working model given the data can then be calculated as

$$P(m|D_c) = \frac{\tau(m) \int L_m(D_c|\theta)g(\theta)d\theta}{\sum_{m=1}^{5} \tau(m) \int L_m(D_c|\theta)g(\theta)d\theta} \quad (2)$$

After accrual of each participant into the trial the model associated with the largest posterior probability is selected and the DLT probability estimates, $\hat{\pi}_{ci}$, are updated using the chosen working model using the Bayesian form of the CRM [9] so that

$$\hat{\pi}_{ci} = \frac{\int p_{mci}^{\exp(\theta_m)} L_m(D_c|\theta)g(\theta)d\theta}{\int L_m(D_c|\theta)g(\theta)d\theta} \quad (3)$$

If a tie occurs between the posterior model probabilities of two or more models, then the selected model would be randomly chosen from among the tied models. The estimated DLT probabilities are used to define a set of "acceptable" combinations with regard to safety. The maximum tolerated dose combination (MTDC) is defined as the combination with estimated DLT probability closest to the maximum allowable DLT rate of 30%. Any combination with estimated DLT rate less than or equal to that of the MTDC would be considered acceptable in terms of safety.

The probability of response δ_{ci} at combination i in cohort c is modeled using a beta-binomial model

$$z_{ci}|\delta_{ci} \sim \text{Binomial}(\delta_{ci}); \quad \delta_{ci} \sim \text{Beta}(\tau_{ci}, \nu_{ci}) \quad (4)$$

where $\text{Beta}(\tau_{ci}, \nu_{ci})$ is a beta distribution with parameters τ_{ci} and ν_{ci}. Based on the number of responses z_{ci} and the number of treated participants n_{ci} on combination i in cohort c, the posterior distribution of δ_{ci} follows a beta distribution so that

$$\delta_{ci}|(z_{ci}, n_{ci}) \sim \text{Beta}(\tau_{ci} + z_{ci}, \nu_{ci} + n_{ci} - z_{ci}) \quad (5)$$

Using a non-informative $\text{Beta}(0.5, 0.5)$ prior distribution in each cohort, the probabilities of pathologic response for each combination are estimated based on the posterior mean $\hat{\delta}_{ci} = (z_{ci} + 0.5)/(n_{ci} + 1)$, separately for each cohort. Once the set of acceptable combinations is determined in each cohort, the recommended combination varies depending on how many participants have entered the study to that point. For the first third of the trial (1/3 the maximum sample size), the combination recommendation in each cohort is based on randomization using a weighted allocation scheme. The recommended combination for the next entered participant is chosen at random from the set of acceptable combinations, with each acceptable combination weighted by its estimated response probability. Based on the estimates $\hat{\delta}_{ci}$, we calculate the randomization probability

$$R_{ci} = \frac{\hat{\delta}_{ci}}{\sum \hat{\delta}_{ci}} \quad (6)$$

and randomize the next participant in cohort c to an acceptable combination i with probability R_{ci}. This approach allows for acceptable combinations with higher estimated response probabilities to have a higher chance of being randomly chosen as the next recommended combination. For the latter two-thirds of the trial (final 2/3 of maximum sample size), the recommended combination for the next entered participant is defined as the acceptable combination with the highest estimated response probability so that the next participant is assigned the combination i satisfying argmax$\hat{\delta}_{ci}$. As each participant enters the study, a new recommended combination is obtained, and the next entered participant would be allocated to the updated recommended combination. The trial is designed to stop once sufficient information about the optimal combination in each cohort is obtained, according to the stopping rules defined in the following section.

2.3. Sample Size and Stopping Rules

The maximum target sample size is 60 based on obtaining sufficient information to determine the optimal dose combination in each cohort, which is defined by the combination with the highest response rate among combinations with acceptable toxicity. Stopping rules are incorporated for both safety considerations and efficient use of participants by stopping accrual to a cohort once a sufficient number of patients are treated at the ODC. If the set of acceptable combinations is empty at any point, accrual to the study will be halted. This stopping guideline will trigger a review by the study investigators and DSMC to determine if the study should be modified or permanently closed to further accrual. Accrual to the study for a cohort will end if the recommended treatment combination for the next participant is to a combination that already has 12 patients treated at that combination. If occurring, this treatment combination is determined to be the optimal dose combination for the cohort. Otherwise, accrual will continue until 60 patients are accrued to the study.

Twelve patients receiving the optimal combination will allow for adequate data to assess the pathologic response rate. Based on a Beta(0.5, 0.5) prior, if 5 out of 12 patients receiving the ODC experience pathologic response, then the posterior distribution of δ_{ci} is Beta(5.5, 7.5) according to Equation (5). The probability that the response rate for the optimal combination exceeds the standard of care is given by,

$$\Pr(\delta_{ci} > 0.28 | z_{ci} = 5, n_{ci} = 12) \tag{7}$$

$$= \int_{0.28}^{1} \frac{\Gamma(13)}{\Gamma(5.5)\Gamma(7.5)} \delta_{ci}^{4.5} (1 - \delta_{ci})^{6.5} \tag{8}$$

$$\approx 0.853, \tag{9}$$

where i and c indicate the combination and cohort, respectively.

3. Simulation Results

A simulation study provides operating characteristics that convey the design's ability to address the aims of the study. In dose-finding clinical trials, operating characteristics provide the scientific justification for the selected design and sample size, similar to that of a power analysis in a phase III clinical trial [17].

3.1. Design of Simulation Study

Simulations were run in R to display the performance of the design described in Section 2, with results presented in Tables 4 and 5. Six scenarios are considered, allowing for a broad range of possible relationships between treatment dosage, DLT, and efficacy rates. In each scenario, 1000 simulated trials were run. For each treatment combination, Table 4 presents the true DLT and efficacy rates (row 1), percentage of selection as the ODC (row 2), and the average number of participants treated (row 3). In Table 4, optimal combinations are indicated in bold type, and unsafe combinations are indicated in red type. Table 5 displays the average sample size overall and by cohort. While the overall maximum sample size is 60 participants, it is assumed that 65% of participants are diagnosed with adenocarcinoma, and the remaining 35% are diagnosed with squamous cell carcinoma. This provides maximum sample sizes of 39 and 21 for Cohorts A and B, respectively. The following six scenarios were chosen to display the operating characteristics for this design, providing a wide variety of dose-toxicity-efficacy relationships.

1. All doses are safe. Intermediate chemo dose maximizes efficacy.
2. All doses are safe. More chemo yields better efficacy.
3. Highest chemo dose with immune agent 2 is unsafe. More chemo yields better efficacy.
4. Highest chemo dose with immune agent 2 is unsafe. Intermediate chemo dose maximizes efficacy.

5. Highest chemo dose with and without immune agent 2 are unsafe. Intermediate chemo dose maximizes efficacy.
6. Two cohorts have different safety and efficacy profiles.

Table 4. Operating characteristics for Cohorts A and B.

Row 1: (True % DLT, True % Efficacy); Row 2: % Selection as OTC; Row 3: Average Participants Treated.	Immune Agent 2	Cohort A			Cohort B		
		Cisplatin, Pemetrexed (mg/m^2)			Cisplatin, Gemcitabine (mg/m^2)		
		25, 150	50, 375	75, 500	25, 400	50, 800	75, 1200
Scenario 1: All doses are safe. Intermediate chemo dose maximizes efficacy.	Dose 1	(0.03, 0.35) 11.4 3.9	(0.08, 0.50) 33.4 5.8	(0.20, 0.45) 18.7 4.2	(0.03, 0.35) 13.0 3.2	(0.08, 0.50) 30.3 4.4	(0.20, 0.45) 18.1 2.7
	0	(0.01, 0.25) 4.7 3.1	(0.05, 0.40) 21.5 5.3	(0.15, 0.35) 10.2 3.7	(0.01, 0.25) 6.7 2.6	(0.05, 0.40) 20.8 4.3	(0.15, 0.35) 11.1 2.6
Scenario 2: All doses are safe. More chemo yields better efficacy.	Dose 1	(0.03, 0.55) 9.5 3.5	(0.08, 0.67) 19.9 4.4	(0.20, 0.78) 30.9 5.0	(0.03, 0.55) 14.1 3.1	(0.08, 0.67) 21.0 3.3	(0.20, 0.78) 24.6 3.3
	0	(0.01, 0.45) 4.3 2.9	(0.05, 0.57) 13.2 4.7	(0.15, 0.68) 22.2 4.5	(0.01, 0.45) 5.7 2.3	(0.05, 0.57) 16.5 4.2	(0.15, 0.68) 18.1 3.1
Scenario 3: Highest chemo dose with immune agent 2 is unsafe. More chemo yields better efficacy.	Dose 1	(0.22, 0.55) 22.2 5.2	(0.27, 0.67) 16 3.9	(0.32, 0.78) 5.9 1.5	(0.22, 0.55) 20 3.8	(0.27, 0.67) 17.8 3.2	(0.32, 0.78) 6.7 1.3
	0	(0.20, 0.45) 12.7 4.2	(0.25, 0.57) 28 6.5	(0.30, 0.68) 15.2 3.8	(0.20, 0.45) 12.2 3.1	(0.25, 0.57) 28.3 5.6	(0.30, 0.68) 14.7 2.7
Scenario 4: Highest chemo dose with immune agent 2 is unsafe. Intermediate chemo dose maximizes efficacy.	Dose 1	(0.22, 0.60) 9 3.7	(0.27, 0.85) 19.3 4.2	(0.32, 0.70) 1.7 1	(0.22, 0.60) 8.6 2.5	(0.27, 0.85) 15.8 2.7	(0.32, 0.70) 1.7 0.7
	0	(0.20, 0.55) 6.7 3.3	(0.25, 0.83) 57.5 9.2	(0.30, 0.68) 5.8 2.5	(0.20, 0.55) 10.3 2.7	(0.25, 0.83) 58.9 8.6	(0.30, 0.68) 4.5 1.6
Scenario 5: Highest chemo dose with/out immune agent 2 is unsafe. Intermediate chemo dose maximizes efficacy.	Dose 1	(0.10, 0.70) 12.6 5.2	(0.22, 0.85) 26.8 4.2	(0.42, 0.70) 1.6 1.2	(0.10, 0.70) 10.9 2.7	(0.22, 0.85) 23.2 3.5	(0.42, 0.70) 1.7 0.8
	0	(0.08, 0.65) 7.5 3.5	(0.20, 0.83) 47.5 8.3	(0.40, 0.68) 4 2.5	(0.08, 0.65) 9.7 2.7	(0.20, 0.83) 50.7 7.8	(0.40, 0.68) 3.8 1.5
Scenario 6: Two cohorts have different safety and efficacy profiles.	Dose 1	(0.03, 0.55) 7.4 2.6	(0.08, 0.67) 20.5 4.6	(0.20, 0.78) 33.7 4.6	(0.10, 0.70) 13.5 2.8	(0.22, 0.85) 19.6 3.1	(0.42, 0.70) 2 0.8
	0	(0.01, 0.45) 3 3.2	(0.05, 0.57) 13.6 4.6	(0.15, 0.68) 21.8 5.5	(0.08, 0.65) 11 2.7	(0.20, 0.83) 49.3 7.2	(0.40, 0.68) 4.6 1.6

Table 5. Average sample size across simulations.

Scenario	Cohort A	Cohort B	Overall
1	25.4	19.8	45.2
2	24.8	19.2	44
3	25.1	19.7	44.8
4	23.9	18.8	42.7
5	24.9	19	43.9
6	25.1	18.2	43.3

3.2. Sample Size and Accrual

Accrual to the study for a cohort was designed to end once the next recommendation is to assign the next participant to a combination that already has 12 patients treated at that combination. Accrual is estimated to be 2–3 patients per month, allowing for accrual to be complete within two years. If the minimum follow-up period for participants already on study is not satisfied at the time a new participant is ready to be put on study, then the participant may be accrued to any combination by random allocation, which has accrued at least one participant and is in the acceptable safety set. At the time of combination allocation for the next participant, model-based estimates are calculated for both DLT and response probabilities using the available observed data from all participants accrued to the study at that time. It is important to note that in this design approach, some model-based decisions may be made using slightly less efficacy data than DLT data due to the longer minimum observation window for efficacy. Adjusting for 10% dropout and ineligibility, the maximum sample size should not exceed 67 patients.

3.3. Summary of Operating Characteristics

The selected design performs well by providing a high rate of ODC selection in the optimal combinations and a low rate of ODC selection in less desirable treatment combinations, either because of safety concerns or insufficient efficacy. Consider Scenario 1 in Cohorts A and B, where the optimal combination is the treatment combination of immune agent 2 and the intermediate dosage of chemotherapy (indicated in bold type). While all treatment combinations are considered safe, three treatment combinations with low DLT rates and high rates efficacy are highlighted in gray. For Cohort A, these three treatment combinations comprise more than 70% of the recommended ODCs while treating, on average, 58.7% of the trial participants. In Cohort B, these three treatment combinations comprise 69.9% of the recommended ODCs while treating, on average, 59.6% of the trial participants. In contrast, consider Scenario 4, where the treatment combination with immune agent 2 and the highest level of chemotherapy is unsafe. Treatment combinations with the intermediate dosage of chemotherapy, both with and without immune agent 2, have the highest level of efficacy as well as acceptable toxicity. Very few simulated trials resulted in an ODC recommendation of the unsafe treatment combination (1.7% for both Cohorts A and B). The two optimal treatment combinations comprise 76.8% and 74.7% of the ODC recommendations for Cohorts A and B, respectively. Additionally, more than half of simulated trial participants are treated on the two optimal combinations (56.1% and 60.1% for Cohorts A and B, respectively).

The maximum sample size is 60 eligible participants; however, the simulation results in Table 5 indicate that across all scenarios considered, the maximum average trial size is 46 participants. The design used for the trial both performs well and uses resources efficiently by stopping the study once the design recommends a treatment combination in which 12 participants have been treated in the cohort.

4. Discussion

The design for this study was chosen by balancing the primary study aims and adaptation of existing methods in developing a flexible design strategy. Careful selection of the dose-finding method allows the study design to address the primary study aim without reorienting the study goals to fit a simpler design. In this case, the primary aim of the study is to identify the ODC for each of the two independent patient cohorts. Simulation studies are provided to evaluate the operating characteristics of this design and highlight the ability of the design to identify the ODC and other desirable treatment combinations in a high percentage of trials. Additionally, simulations guide the anticipated final sample size needed to draw meaningful conclusions about the efficacy of the selected ODC.

Treatment regimens varied for the two patient cohorts, and it was not anticipated that either cohort would have systematically greater or lesser toxicity than the other cohort. Because of this, the cohorts were considered independently. If prior information indicated that one cohort was expected to have greater or lesser toxicity, appropriate changes in the design would have been made to use this order information in identifying the ODC for each cohort. Study design options for treatment combinations are limited, especially when considering the additional complexity of clinical aims. While several methods are available to account for two or more groups of participants, these designs consider dose-finding for a single agent [18–21]. The approach outlined in this paper to tailor the study design to the complex research objectives provides the framework that demonstrates how adaptive designs can be modified within a single trial to address the objectives specific to the study while advancing early development of novel treatment regimens. This manuscript aims to provide an example for designing complex early-phase trials with multiple objectives in various cohorts.

5. Conclusions

This phase I study design aims to identify the optimal dose combination for each of two cohorts of patients with non-small cell lung cancer, based on multiple endpoints. Simulation studies indicate that the design is well suited to address the study aims while conserving study resources.

During the finalization of this trial protocol, the company sponsoring the study decided not to move forward with this trial due to recent negative findings in another patient group [22]. While this trial was not initiated, plans were near completion and this example highlights the benefits of using a Bayesian design for early phase clinical trials.

As multiple chemotherapy and immunotherapy combinations become the standard of care, future research will likely require evaluating the appropriate doses of the various components of the multiple drug regimen. The Bayesian phase I design described here allows for evaluation of both safe and efficacious doses for various drug combinations commonly used in NSCLC and incorporates standard histology-based chemotherapy regimens in the same trial.

Author Contributions: Conceptualization, B.J.H., N.A.W. and R.D.G.; methodology, B.J.H. and N.A.W.; validation, B.J.H. and N.A.W.; writing—original draft preparation, B.J.H.; writing—review and editing, B.J.H., N.A.W. and R.D.G.; All authors have read and agreed to the published version of the manuscript.

Funding: This research was funded by National Cancer Institute, grant number R01CA247932; the Biostatistics Shared Resource, Cancer Center Support Grant, University of Virginia Cancer Center, University of Virginia (P30 CA044579); and the APC was funded by Elizabeth Cronly and the Patients & Friends Research Fund of University of Virginia Cancer Center.

Institutional Review Board Statement: Not applicable.

Informed Consent Statement: Not applicable.

Data Availability Statement: Not applicable.

Conflicts of Interest: The authors declare no conflict of interest.

Abbreviations

Abbreviations
CPI	Checkpoint inhibitor
DLT	Dose-limiting toxicity
HDAC	Histone deacetylase
ICI	Immune checkpoint inhibitor
IDO	Indoleamine 2,3-dioxygenase
MTD	Maximum tolerated dose
NSCLC	Non-small cell lung cancer
ODC	Optimal dose combination
PARP	Poly-ADP-ribose polymerase
PD-1	Programmed death-1
PD-L1	Programmed death ligand-1
VEGF	Vascular endothelial growth factor

References

1. Cancer Today. Available online: http://gco.iarc.fr/today/home (accessed on 14 September 2021).
2. Cancer of the Lung and Bronchus—Cancer Stat Facts. SEER. Available online: https://seer.cancer.gov/statfacts/html/lungb.html (accessed on 14 September 2021).
3. Paz-Ares, L.; Ciuleanu, T.E.; Cobo, M.; Schenker, M.; Zurawski, B.; Menezes, J.; Richardet, E.; Bennouna, J.; Felip, E.; Juan-Vidal, O.; et al. First-line nivolumab plus ipilimumab combined with two cycles of chemotherapy in patients with non-small-cell lung cancer (CheckMate 9LA): An international, randomised, open-label, phase 3 trial. *Lancet Oncol.* **2021**, *22*, 198–211. [CrossRef]
4. Hellmann, M.D.; Paz-Ares, L.; Caro, R.B.; Zurawski, B.; Kim, S.W.; Costa, E.C.; Park, K.; Alexandru, A.; Lupinacci, L.; De La Mora Jimenez, E.; et al. Nivolumab plus Ipilimumab in Advanced Non-Small-Cell Lung Cancer. *N. Engl. J. Med.* **2019**, *381*, 2020–2031. [CrossRef]
5. Socinski, M.A.; Jotte, R.M.; Cappuzzo, F.; Orlandi, F. Atezolizumab for First-Line Treatment of Metastatic Nonsquamous NSCLC. *N. Engl. J. Med.* **2018**, *378*, 2288–2301. [CrossRef] [PubMed]
6. Gandhi, L.; Rodríguez-Abreu, D.; Gadgeel, S.; Esteban, E.; Felip, E.; De Angelis, F.; Domine, M.; Clingan, P.; Hochmair, M.J.; Powell, S.F.; et al. Pembrolizumab plus Chemotherapy in Metastatic Non-Small-Cell Lung Cancer. *N. Engl. J. Med.* **2018**, *378*, 2078–2092. [CrossRef] [PubMed]
7. Paz-Ares, L.; Luft, A.; Vicente, D.; Tafreshi, A.; Gümüş, M.; Mazières, J.; Hermes, B.; Şenler, F.Ç.; Csőszi, T.; Fülöp, A.; et al. Pembrolizumab plus Chemotherapy for Squamous Non-Small-Cell Lung Cancer. *N. Engl. J. Med.* **2018**, *379*, 2040–2051. [CrossRef] [PubMed]
8. Giovagnoli, A. The Bayesian Design of Adaptive Clinical Trials. *Int. J. Environ. Res. Public Health* **2021**, *18*, 530. [CrossRef] [PubMed]
9. Wages, N.A.; Conaway, M.R.; O'Quigley, J. Continual Reassessment Method for Partial Ordering. *Biometrics* **2011**, *67*, 1555–1563. [CrossRef] [PubMed]
10. O'Quigley, J.; Pepe, M.; Fisher, L. Continual Reassessment Method: A Practical Design for Phase 1 Clinical Trials in Cancer. *Biometrics* **1990**, *46*, 33–48. [CrossRef]
11. Lee, S.M.; Cheung, Y.K. Model calibration in the continual reassessment method. *Clin. Trials* **2009**, *6*, 227–238. [CrossRef]
12. R Core Team. *R: A Language and Environment for Statistical Computing*; R Foundation for Statistical Computing: Vienna, Austria, 2021. Available online: https://www.R-project.org (accessed on 16 September 2021).
13. Cheung, K. dfcrm: Dose-Finding by the Continual Reassessment Method. 2019. Available online: https://CRAN.R-project.org/package=dfcrm (accessed on 21 September 2021).
14. Wages, N.A. pocrm: Dose Finding in Drug Combination Phase I Trials Using PO-CRM. 2021. Available online: https://CRAN.R-project.org/package=pocrm (accessed on 21 September 2021).
15. Cheung, Y.K. *Dose Finding by the Continual Reassessment Method*; Chapman and Hall/CRC: Boca Raton, FL, USA, 2011.
16. Naylor, J.C.; Smith, A.F.M. Applications of a Method for the Efficient Computation of Posterior Distributions. *J. R. Stat. Soc. Ser. C (Appl. Stat.)* **1982**, *31*, 214–225. [CrossRef]
17. Wages, N.A.; Horton, B.J.; Conaway, M.R.; Petroni, G.R. Operating characteristics are needed to properly evaluate the scientific validity of phase I protocols. *Contemp. Clin. Trials* **2021**, *108*, 106517. [CrossRef] [PubMed]
18. O'Quigley, J.; Iasonos, A. Bridging solutions in dose-finding problems. *Stat. Biopharm. Res.* **2014**, *6*, 185–197. [CrossRef] [PubMed]
19. Horton, B.J.; Wages, N.A.; Conaway, M.R. Shift models for dose-finding in partially ordered groups. *Clin. Trials* **2018**, *16*, 32–40. [CrossRef] [PubMed]
20. Conaway, M. Isotonic designs for phase I trials in partially ordered groups. *Clin. Trials* **2017**, *14*, 491–498. [CrossRef] [PubMed]
21. Conaway, M.R. A design for phase I trials in completely or partially ordered groups. *Stat. Med.* **2017**, *36*, 2323–2332. [CrossRef] [PubMed]
22. Long, G.V.; Dummer, R.; Hamid, O.; Gajewski, T.F.; Caglevic, C.; Dalle, S.; Arance, A.; Carlino, M.S.; Grob, J.J.; Kim, T.M.; et al. Epacadostat plus pembrolizumab versus placebo plus pembrolizumab in patients with unresectable or metastatic melanoma (ECHO-301/KEYNOTE-252): A phase 3, randomised, double-blind study. *Lancet Oncol.* **2019**, *20*, 1083–1097. [CrossRef]

MDPI
St. Alban-Anlage 66
4052 Basel
Switzerland
Tel. +41 61 683 77 34
Fax +41 61 302 89 18
www.mdpi.com

International Journal of Environmental Research and Public Health Editorial Office
E-mail: ijerph@mdpi.com
www.mdpi.com/journal/ijerph

www.ingramcontent.com/pod-product-compliance
Lightning Source LLC
LaVergne TN
LVHW070706100526
838202LV00013B/1042